ANNUAL REVIEW OF GERONTOLOGY AND GERIATRICS

VOLUME 34, 2014

Editors

Annual Review of Gerontology and Geriatrics

Genetics

VOLUME 34, 2014

Volume Editor

RICHARD L. SPROTT, PhD

Series Editor

TONI C. ANTONUCCI, PhD

SPRINGER PUBLISHING COMPANY
NEW YORK

Springer Publishing Company, LLC
11 West 42nd Street
New York, NY 10036
www.springerpub.com

Acquisitions Editor: Sheri W. Sussman
Composition: Absolute Service, Inc.

ISBN: 978-0-8261-9965-2
E-book ISBN: 978-0-8261-9966-9
ISSN: 0198-8794
Online ISSN: 1944-4036

14 15 16/ 5 4 3 2 1

Printed in the United States of America by Gasch Printing

Contents

About the Volume Editor

Richard L. Sprott, PhD, began his undergraduate studies at Franklin and Marshall College in Lancaster, Pennsylvania. He completed them at the University of North Carolina (UNC) at Chapel Hill, earning a BA with honors in Psychology. After receiving his PhD in Experimental Psychology (Behavior Genetics) at UNC, he went on to a post-doctoral fellowship in Behavior Genetics at the Jackson Laboratory in Bar Harbor, Maine. Following two years of teaching at Oakland University, Dr. Sprott returned to The Jackson Laboratory, where he conducted a research program on single-gene influences on behavior and the interaction of aging variables with those genes.

After a decade in Maine, Dr. Sprott moved to the National Institute on Aging where he directed the Institute's programs on the biology of aging. A major focus of his career has been the development of animal models for aging research. He developed a nationwide research program of research on biomarkers of aging and the effects of dietary restriction on longevity. He is the author of many books and articles. He is an internationally recognized expert on animal model development and plays an active role in model development in countries around the world. He is the past president of the International Biogerontological Resource Institute (IBRI) in Friuli, Italy, and current president of the International Healthspan Institute with headquarters at Pennsylvania State University. Dr. Sprott left the National Institute on Aging in 1998 to become the first executive director of the Ellison Medical Foundation, created to support basic biological and biomedical research on aging. He retired from The Ellison Medical Foundation in 2012.

Contributors

Steve Austad, PhD, Department of Biology, University of Alabama Birmingham, Birmingham, AL

Gil Atzmon, PhD, Institute for Aging Research, Departments for Medicine and Genetics, Albert Einstein College of Medicine, Bronx, NY

Nir Barzilai, MD, Institute for Aging Research, Departments for Medicine and Genetics, Albert Einstein College of Medicine, Bronx, NY

Anne Brunet, BSc, PhD, Department of Genetics, Stanford University, Stanford, CA, and Glenn Laboratories for the Biology of Aging at Stanford, Stanford, CA

Sean P. Curran, BSc, PhD, Davis School of Gerontology, University of Southern California, Los Angeles, and Center for Academic Research and Training in Anthropogeny (CARTA), La Jolla, CA

Anna K. Dahl, PhD, Department of Medical Epidemiology and Biostatistics, Karolinska Institutet, Stockholm, Sweden

Caleb Finch, BS, PhD, Davis School of Gerontology and Dornsife College, University of Southern California, Los Angeles, CA

Deborah Finkel, BS, PhD, Indiana University Southeast, New Albany, IN

Lotte Gerritsen, Bsc, Msc, PhD, Department of Medical Epidemiology and Biostatistics, Karolinska Institutet, Stockholm, Sweden

Matt Kaeberlein, PhD, Department of Pathology, University of Washington, Seattle, WA

Scott F. Leiser, BSc, PhD, Department of Pathology, University of Washington, Seattle, WA

David B. Lombard, BA, MD, PhD, Geriatrics Center, University of Michigan, Ann Arbor, MI

Salah Mahmoudi, BSc, PhD, Department of Genetics, Stanford University, Stanford, CA

Elena Mancini, BSc, PhD, Department of Genetics, Stanford University, Stanford, CA

George M. Martin, BS, MD, Departments of Pathology and Genome Sciences, University of Washington, Seattle, WA, and Visiting Scholar, University of California, Los Angeles, Los Angeles, CA

Roger J. McCarter, MsC, PhD, Department of Biobehavioral Health, The Pennsylvania State University, State College, PA

Mark A. McCormick, BS, PhD, Buck Institute for Research on Aging, Novato, CA

Gerald E. McClearn, BS, MA, PhD, Department of Biobehavioral Health, The Pennsylvania State University, State College, PA

Richard A. Miller, MD, PhD, Geriatrics Center, University of Michigan, Ann Arbor, MI

Nancy L. Pedersen, BA, MA, PhD, Karolinska Institutet, Stockholm, Sweden, and University of Southern California, Los Angeles, CA

Jason N. Pitt, BSc, PhD, Department of Pathology, University of Washington, Seattle, WA

Daniel E. L. Promislow, PhD, Department of Pathology, University of Washington, Seattle, WA

Victoria A. Rafalski, BSc, PhD, Gladstone Institute, University of California, San Francisco, CA

Chandra A. Reynolds, BA, MA, PhD, Department of Psychology, University of California, Riverside, CA

J. Tobias Stout, MA, PhD, Department of Biobehavioral Health, The Pennsylvania State University, State College, PA, Retired

David J. Vandenberg, BS, PhD, Department of Biobehavioral Health, The Pennsylvania State University, State College, PA

Ashley E. Webb, BSc, PhD, Department of Genetics, Stanford University, Stanford, CA

Previous Volumes in the Series

Vol. 33, 2013: Healthy Longevity: A Global Approach
Editors: Jean-Marie Robine, DEA, DED, Carol Jagger, PhD, and Eileen M. Crimmins, PhD

Vol. 32, 2012: Emerging Perspectives on Resilience in Adulthood and Later Life
Editors: Bert Hayslip Jr., PhD, and Gregory C. Smith, PhD

Vol. 31, 2011: Pathways Through the Transitions of Care for Older Adults
Editors: Peggye Dilworth-Anderson, PhD, and Mary H. Palmer, PhD

Vol. 30, 2010: Biobehavioral Perspectives on Health in Later Life
Editor: Keith E. Whitfield, PhD

Vol. 29: Life-Course Perspectives on Late Life Health Inequalities
Editors: Toni C. Antonucci, PhD, and James S. Jackson, PhD

Vol. 28: Gerontological and Geriatric Education
Editors: Harvey L. Sterns, PhD, and Marie A. Bernard, MD

Vol. 27: Biopsychosocial Approaches to Longevity
Editors: Leonard W. Poon, PhD, DPhil, and Thomas T. Perls, MD, MPH

Vol. 26: The Crown of Life Dynamics of the Early Postretirement Period
Editors: Jacquelyn Boone James, PhD, and Paul Wink, PhD

Vol. 25: Aging Health Care Workforce Issues
Editors: Toni Miles, MD, PhD, and Antonio Furino, PhD, JD

Vol. 24: Focus on Intergenerational Relations Across Time and Place
Editors: Merril Silverstein, PhD, and K. Warner Schaie, PhD

Vol. 23: Focus on Aging in Context: Socio-Physical Environments
Editors: Hans Werner Wahl, PhD, Rick J. Scheidt, PhD, and Paul G. Windley, PhD

Vol. 22: Focus on Economic Outcomes in Later Life
Editors: Stephen Crystal, PhD, and Dennis Shea, PhD

Vol. 21: Focus on Modern Topics in the Biology of Aging
Editors: Vincent C. Cristofalo, PhD, and Richard Adelman, PhD

Forthcoming Volume in the Series

Volume 35, 2015

Research on Subjective Aging: New Developments and Future Directions

Volume Editors: Manfred Diehl and Hans-Werner Wahl

Preface

The last volume in this series to address the biology of aging, Modern Topics in the Biology of Aging, *Annual Review of Gerontology and Geriatrics, Volume 21*, 2001, came 11 years after the publication of Biology of Aging, *Annual Review of Gerontology and Geriatrics, Volume 10*, 1990. This review follows after a 12-year wait for an update on the state of biological research on aging. Much has happened in that dozen-year span.

The 1990 volume focused sharply on mechanisms of aging and on the then-current themes and theories of aging. As a field of research, aging had only been a National Institutes of Health (NIH) institute for 15 years and the field was still working to define its subject matter and research approach. Quoting from Vincent Cristofalo's preface to that volume,

> There are some themes about which most scientists would agree; the general scenario of aging is similar in all the metazoa studied. Regulation of the process is probably multifactorial and contains both genetic and environmental components. Maximum life-span potential is genetically regulated. Finally, most investigators believe that aging is regulated by a highly conserved clock-like mechanism that runs at different and species-specific rates.

Contributors to that volume were asked to address the questions: "What is aging, why do we age, and how does the process work?"

In the 2001 volume, editors Vincent Cristofalo and Richard Adelman asked contributors to update mechanisms research, and they brought three approaches to the effort: demography, evolutionary studies, and biology, including "perspectives of the social and behavioral sciences." This expansion of the research agenda recognized the growing importance of a broader field of aging research, as society became more aware of the "aging demographic" and the promise and problems that would arrive with increased longevity. The volume recognized both the increased specialization in the biology of aging research and the simultaneous broadening of the interest in and concern about the approaching baby boom age cohort.

So, where are we now? This volume is focused on the genetics of aging, from the level of very basic organisms like worms (*Caenorhabditis elegans*) to humans. Biological research on aging has evolved to the point that we are now focused on the actions of single genes and their products on the course of the lives of organisms across the animal spectrum (plants have fallen out of favor as aging research subjects). This genetic focus is a reflection of the dramatic increase in our understanding of basic aging processes that has resulted from the discovery of single genes and gene products that can profoundly affect aging processes, lengthening or shortening lifespans and health spans. As will be obvious from the chapters that follow, there is no longer agreement that ". . . aging is regulated by a highly conserved clock-like mechanism that runs at different and species-specific rates." Rather, it is now generally accepted that aging processes (not the process of aging) are the result of the interactions of many genetic factors and are sensitive to environmental manipulation. The volume is also organized from the "simplest" organisms to the most complex (humans). This results in increasing attention to complexity as an issue in itself.

In Chapter 1, Brunet, Mahmoudi, Mancini, Rafalski, and Webb describe aging at the stem cell level. The key questions are why adult stem cells functionally decline while embryonic stem cells do not. Many of the basic themes of current aging research are raised in their discussion of stem cell function including tissue repair and regeneration, cellular reprogramming, and longevity pathways such as insulin-FOXO, target of rapamycin (TOR), AMP-activated protein kinase (AMPK), and the Sirtuins. These themes appear time and again in subsequent chapters, suggesting that the field is rapidly coming to agreement on fruitful approaches if not on specific mechanisms.

In Chapter 2, Curran introduces essential genes as longevity regulators that have essential roles in development. These are genes essential in earlier development that then have anti-longevity effects in later life. This difference in early versus late-life gene effect is an example of antagonistic pleiotropy, one of the emerging themes in current biology. His work in the worm, *C. elegans*, describes well-conserved loci (e.g., daf, FOXO, TOR) in the worms that are found in higher organisms and that are likely to be of interest in mammalian studies as well. He also introduces the hormesis hypothesis that basically postulates that a small amount of stress can be beneficial and protect against larger subsequent stressors. The relevance of hormesis to aging is somewhat controversial, but the hypothesis has led to much interesting research.

In Chapter 3, Pitt, Leiser, and Kaeberlein examine the role of oxygen in the aging of organisms from worms to humans. Of the various "rate of aging" theories, the most durable are those that invoke reactive oxygen species (ROS) as causative agents in DNA damage, mutation, and cell senescence. This chapter provides an extensive review of the many ways oxygen levels affect aging processes. The calorie restriction manipulations that affect longevity in many species have been sometimes assumed to have their effects by reducing oxygen consumption and subsequent oxidative damage from ROS. This literature is fraught with contradictions and failed experimental confirmations of basic assumptions. Pitt et al. have sorted the evidence in a new and useful way leading to a novel focus on the hypoxia inducible transcription factor (HIF) and its effects on aging gene actions and aging pathways (FOXO, mechanistic target of rapamycin [mTOR], daf, and Sirtuins).

In Chapter 4, Lombard and Miller describe the various interventions (mutations, diets, or drugs) that can affect lifespan and examine the mechanisms for those effects. Whether interventions change longevity by altering rates of aging or by manipulating disease states is a central question at the core of lifespan extension research. This chapter reviews an informative selection of the existing literature and provides an assessment of the research. Perhaps more importantly, it provides an exhaustive discussion of the critical steps that should be undertaken to sort out the mechanisms and relevance of the results of interventions to the biology of aging as distinct from the biology of disease. This is a chapter that should be on the shelf of every investigator engaged in aging intervention research.

In Chapter 5, Finch and Austad introduce the species comparison approach to investigate genetic influences on aging. By examining age-related neurodegeneration in closely related primate species, they are able to suggest innovative approaches to the investigation of major effects of minor genetic differences. Although the great apes, including Homo sapiens, are largely genetically identical, there are major differences in neurological age-related disease progression and longevity consequences. A major contribution of this chapter is the discussion of the use of various potential primate models for longevity research. This topic is particularly timely given the recent NIH decision to retire most chimpanzees from research.

In Chapter 6, Barzilai and Atzmon argue for the use of research in families with exceptional longevity to understand the genetic and environmental underpinnings of successful long life. Among the issues to be sorted out are the relative contributions of genes that directly affect aging processes from those that exert their effects through resistance to disease. The basic process/disease dichotomy is first discussed in Chapter 4, the first mammalian chapter. Disease must play a role in lower organisms as well, but we simply do not know enough about possible diseases of worms and flies to ask the right questions. This chapter advocates the utilization of a three-pronged approach to finding genes relevant to longevity: look for well-conserved genes, for genes that are associated with age-related disease, and for protective genes in centenarians.

In Chapter 7, Finkel, Gerritsen, Reynolds, Dahl, and Pedersen present an exhaustive inventory of individual differences in human age-related behaviors and health. These differences are examined using varied genetic approaches including the Swedish Twin studies, candidate gene studies, and genome-wide association studies. The authors highlight the complexity of human health and behavior and provide an exhaustive review of the studies of subjective and objective health, stress, frailty, and longevity. Complexity is a major issue in this chapter and the authors discuss various approaches for dealing with complexity.

In Chapter 8, McClearn, Vandenberg, Stout, and McCarter take on the subject of complexity by presenting an experimental example of the degrees of complexity within a set of controlled studies. Using end of life as a simple outcome measure and quantitative trait loci to nominate potential genes for analysis, the authors set out to confirm the effects and study the actions of lifespan increasing and lifespan decreasing genotypes. Using the unexpected results of these studies, the authors describe the problems of complexity even at the level of simple experiments and provide a discussion of methods for dealing with complexity.

In Chapter 9, McCormick and Promislow approach complexity in another dimension. They argue that a molecular network approach has the potential to clarify the relationships among a vast array of pathways that affect aging and disease. The chapter first introduces the range of age-relevant questions that are subjects of investigation and then offers specific advice on how the use of network analysis could improve research in these areas. This too is a chapter that should be on every investigator's shelf.

In Chapter 10, Martin reminds us that to fully understand the biology of aging, it is not sufficient only to investigate the influence of the constitutional genome, the environment, and their many interactions. Stochastic events also play important roles. Although there is general recognition of the fact that there can be different phenotypic outcomes as a result of random somatic mutations, stochastic variations in gene expression, epigenetic or otherwise, are likely to also be of importance. In particular, he argues that age-related epigenetic drifts in gene expression may be responsible for a range of important geriatric pathologies.

CHAPTER 1

Longevity Pathways in Mammalian Stem Cells

Anne Brunet, Salah Mahmoudi, Elena Mancini, Victoria A. Rafalski, and Ashley E. Webb

ABSTRACT

Aging is accompanied by a general decline in tissue function and a striking increase in diseases. With their ability to self-renew and differentiate, adult stem cells represent a regenerative reserve for the aging tissue. Understanding the mechanisms underlying the age-dependent decline in adult stem cell function should help identify ways to preserve tissue homeostasis during aging. Tapping into the potential of adult stem cells should also allow tissue repair and regeneration in the case of degenerative diseases linked with age. In contrast to adult stem cells, embryonic stem cells have unlimited self-renewal and pluripotency, and the mechanisms underlying their "immortality" may give clues into fundamental principles governing cellular youth or rejuvenation. The advent of cellular reprogramming, which allows the generation of patient-specific pluripotent stem cells, has opened new avenues for therapeutic treatments of age-related diseases. This chapter reviews how longevity pathways influence stem cell function in mammalian adult stem cells, embryonic stem cells, and induced pluripotent stem cells. We specifically discuss genetic pathways that play a conserved role in lifespan, such as the insulin-FOXO pathway and the mechanistic target of rapamycin (mTOR) pathway, as well as metabolic enzymes that are involved in health span, such as AMP-activated protein kinase (AMPK) and Sirtuins.

http://dx.doi.org/10.1891/0198-8794.34.1

INTRODUCTION

Age is the prime risk factor for a wide range of diseases—including Alzheimer's and Parkinson's diseases, heart disease, diabetes, as well as many cancers—posing a formidable societal challenge. Even in the absence of diseases, aging is associated with functional decline—for example, cognitive abilities deteriorate with age. As the age of the population is increasing worldwide, so are these debilitating age-dependent disorders and decline. Stem cells, with their ability to self-renew and produce differentiated cells, have an amazing potential for tissue regeneration during aging. They also represent an attractive source of cells for regenerative medicine for aging-related diseases.

There exist different categories of stem cells, each of which could inform the aging process in different ways. Adult mammals possess tissue-specific stem cells that reside in specialized niches, and these cells are thought to be important for maintenance and repair of tissue. During aging, however, tissue-specific stem cells exhibit an age-related decline in functionality, which may contribute to tissue deterioration with age. For adult stem cells, an important question is how to maintain them the longest time possible or how to "reactivate" them if they become too dormant during the aging process.

Another type of stem cells with relevance to aging research in a related yet different way are embryonic stem cells (ESCs). ESCs have the potential to give rise to cell types of all three germ layers (endoderm, mesoderm, and ectoderm) and seemingly have unlimited self-renewal properties. These cells have been proposed as a source of various cell types for regenerative medicine. The advent of technologies to reprogram differentiated cells into induced pluripotent stem cells (iPSCs) with ESC properties allows the generation of patient-specific embryonic-like stem cells, a key step toward "personalized stem cell therapies" that would alleviate ethical and immunological concerns of ESCs as well as some safety concerns. Understanding how stem cells deal with damages that occur during aging in a manner that differs from their differentiated counterparts could provide keys to understanding basic principle of youthfulness or immortality.

LONGEVITY PATHWAYS

Insulin/IGF1-FOXO Pathway

The insulin/insulin-like growth factor 1 (IGF1)-FOXO signaling pathway has been shown to regulate longevity in a conserved manner from worms to humans (Kenyon, 2010). Insulin/IGF1 binding to its receptor triggers the activation of the phosphoinositide 3 kinase (PI3K), which in turn activates the protein kinases AKT and serum- and glucocorticoid-induced protein kinase (SGK; see Figure 1.1). Both protein kinases have been shown to phosphorylate FOXO transcription

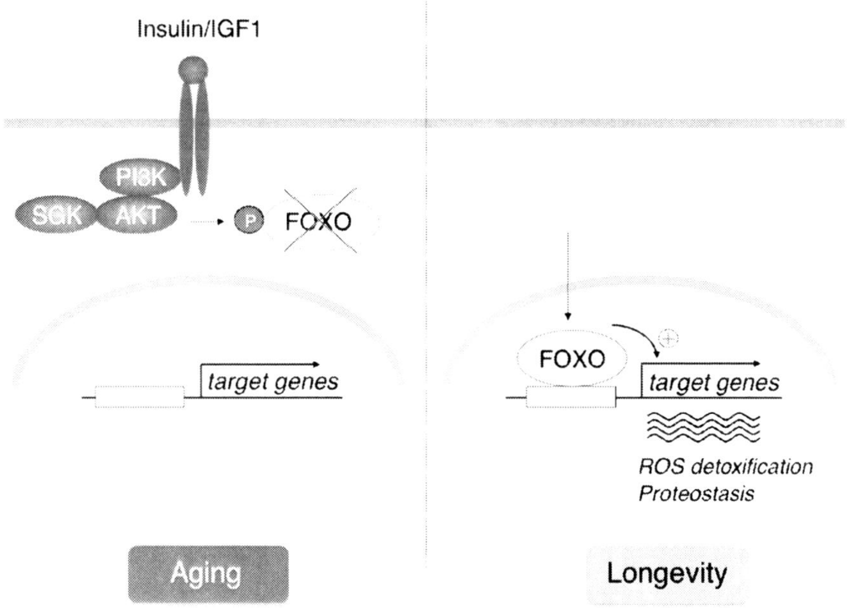

FIGURE 1.1 The insulin/IGF1-FOXO pathway in the regulation of organismal longevity. Selected members of the insulin/IGF1-FOXO pathway are presented. P = phosphorylation; ROS = reactive oxygen species.

factors at three conserved sites, thereby preventing them from regulating their programs of gene expression (Biggs, Meisenhelder, Hunter, Cavenee, & Arden, 1999; Brunet et al., 1999; Brunet et al., 2001; Kops et al., 1999). In *Caenorhabditis elegans*, lowering the expression or activity of the insulin receptor—or that of PI3K, AKT, or SGK—extends lifespan and delays signs of aging (Friedman & Johnson, 1988; Hertweck, Gobel, & Baumeister, 2004; Kenyon, Chang, Gensch, Rudner, & Tabtiang, 1993; Kimura, Tissenbaum, Liu, & Ruvkun, 1997; Paradis, Ailion, Toker, Thomas, & Ruvkun, 1999; Paradis & Ruvkun, 1998), although the role of SGK in lifespan significantly differs from that of AKT (A. T. Chen, Guo, Dumas, Ashrafi, & Hu, 2013; Soukas, Kane, Carr, Melo, & Ruvkun, 2009). The Kenyon and Ruvkun labs showed that longevity resulting from low insulin signaling requires an intact FOXO (termed DAF-16 in *C. elegans*; Kenyon et al., 1993; K. Lin, Dorman, Rodan, & Kenyon, 1997; Ogg et al., 1997). Consistently, overexpression of FOXO/DAF-16 in worms can be sufficient to extend lifespan (Henderson & Johnson, 2001). FOXO/DAF-16 encompasses several isoforms that can mediate different phenotypes, with the DAF-16d/f isoform being particularly important for longevity (Kwon, Narasimhan, Yen, & Tissenbaum, 2010.). The program of genes regulated by FOXO/DAF-16 includes genes involved in cellular resistance to stress (e.g., *sod-3*), protein homeostasis (e.g., *rpn-6*), and changes in energy metabolism (e.g., *mdt-15*; S. S. Lee, Kennedy, Tolonen, & Ruvkun, 2003; Murphy et al., 2003; Oh et al., 2006; Vilchez, Morantte, et al., 2012; P. Zhang, Judy, Lee, & Kenyon, 2013) and requires the interaction between FOXO and the SWItch/Sucrose NonFermentable (SWI/SNF) chromatin remodeler (Riedel et al., 2013). The insulin-FOXO pathway functions primarily in the intestine and the nervous system to regulate the lifespan of the whole organism (Libina, Berman, & Kenyon, 2003; Murphy, Lee, & Kenyon, 2007; Wolkow, Kimura, Lee, & Ruvkun, 2000). Accordingly, FOXO target genes can act in a cell-autonomous or cell-nonautonomous manner (Murphy et al., 2003; P. Zhang et al., 2013). Other transcription factors are also involved in the longevity triggered by low insulin signaling, for example, the heat shock transcription factor 1 (HSF1; Chiang, Ching, Lee, Mousigian, & Hsu, 2012; Hsu, Murphy, & Kenyon, 2003) and the SKN-1/NRF2 (Tullet et al., 2008). Thus, the insulin pathway coordinates various cellular and systemic responses that contribute to longevity in worms.

The ability of the insulin signaling pathway to impact organismal lifespan is conserved in other species. In *Drosophila*, decreased insulin signaling also extends lifespan in a manner that requires the FOXO isoform (termed *dFOXO*) in this organism (Clancy et al., 2001; Tatar et al., 2001). Expression of dFOXO is sufficient to cause lifespan extension in flies (Giannakou et al., 2004; Hwangbo, Gershman, Tu, Palmer, & Tatar, 2004), particularly when dFOXO is expressed in the fat bodies (Giannakou et al., 2004). dFOXO regulates a program of genes involved in neuroendocrine signaling, metabolism, and stress resistance (Alic et al., 2011; Gershman et al., 2007; Puig, Marr, Ruhf, & Tjian, 2003). In mice, conditional knock out of the insulin receptor in fat tissue or knock out of one allele of the IGF1 receptor (IGF1R), results in lifespan extension, particularly in females (Blüher, Kahn, & Kahn, 2003; Holzenberger et al., 2003). Consistently, knock out of the insulin receptor substrate 1 (IRS1) also leads to lifespan extension in mice (Selman et al., 2008). Overexpression of the phosphatase and tensin homolog (PTEN), which prevents activation of the PI3K-AKT pathway, extends the lifespan of mice (Ortega-Molina et al., 2012). FOXO1 has been shown to function downstream of IRS1 in nutrient homeostasis in mice (Dong et al., 2008). Whether FOXO overexpression extends lifespan in mice and whether FOXO acts downstream of the insulin pathway for the regulation of longevity in this organism have not yet been addressed. Remarkably, in humans, single nucleotide polymorphisms (SNPs) in genes that encode IGF1R, AKT, and FOXO3 are associated with exceptional human longevity (Anselmi et al., 2009; Flachsbart et al., 2009; Pawlikowska et al., 2009; Suh et al., 2008; Willcox et al., 2008). The link between these FOXO3 genetic variants and exceptional longevity has been replicated in independent cohorts of centenarians of different ethnicity (Anselmi et al., 2009; Li et al., 2009; Soerensen et al., 2010), highlighting the conserved role of this pathway in human longevity.

Whether the insulin pathway mediates the beneficial effects of dietary restriction (DR) on lifespan and health has been subject to debate. A priori, it would seem that a pathway that senses insulin levels (and therefore replete conditions) or lack of insulin (and therefore nutrient poor conditions) could play a role in mediating longevity by DR. In *C. elegans*, however, the insulin pathway appears to function independently of several methods of dietary restriction used in this organism: the genetic mimic called *eat-2*, dietary deprivation (DD), and DR regimens in liquid medium (BDR or lDR; Bishop & Guarente, 2007; Greer, Dowlatshahi, et al., 2007; Mair & Dillin, 2008; Panowski, Wolff, Aguilaniu, Durieux, & Dillin, 2007). On the other hand, FOXO is necessary for longevity induced by two dietary restriction regimens: a method where feeding bacteria are restricted (sDR; Greer, Dowlatshahi, et al., 2007) and intermittent fasting (IF; Honjoh, Yamamoto, Uno, & Nishida, 2009). In flies, dFOXO is not absolutely necessary for longevity induced by DR, but overexpression of dFOXO mimics, at least in part, a dietary restriction phenotype (Giannakou, Goss, & Partridge, 2008). In mammals, the jury is still out on whether the longevity benefits imparted by DR are influenced by the insulin-FOXO pathway, but the PI3K-FOXO pathway has been involved in the beneficial impact of dietary restriction on cancer in mice (Kalaany & Sabatini, 2009). Together, these findings suggest that there is a link between the insulin-FOXO pathway and the integration of low nutrient benefits on lifespan and health span. The extent of the role played by the insulin-FOXO pathway in longevity by DR may be linked to the type of diet that is fed to each organism—and therefore the way in which dietary restriction is established. The insulin pathway may be crucial for the benefits of DR on lifespan only when the diet is rich in carbohydrates (which lead to the production of insulin by the organism) but may not be involved when the diet is rich in proteins or lipids.

Mechanistic Target of Rapamycin (mTOR) Pathway

The protein kinase termed mechanistic target of rapamycin (mTOR) affects lifespan in a conserved manner from yeast to mammals. mTOR is part of two distinct multiprotein complexes, mTORC1 and mTORC2, that are known to be involved in cellular and organismal growth (D. H. Kim et al., 2002; Laplante & Sabatini, 2012; Sarbassov et al., 2004). The mTORC1 protein complex receives inputs both from nutrient-sensing pathways (e.g., PI3K-AKT) and from amino acids (Laplante & Sabatini, 2012; see Figure 1.2). The regulation of mTORC1 by nutrient pathways involves the phosphorylation of tuberous sclerosis 2 (TSC2), a GTPase-activating protein (GAP) for the GTPase Ras homolog enriched in brain (RHEB). TSC2 can be phosphorylated by AKT (Inoki, Li, Zhu, Wu, & Guan, 2002; Manning, Tee, Logsdon, Blenis, & Cantley, 2002; Potter, Pedraza, & Xu, 2002), which leads to TSC2 degradation and the subsequent activation of RHEB (Inoki, Li, Xu, & Guan, 2003). In turn, activated RHEB binds to the mTORC1 complex and activate

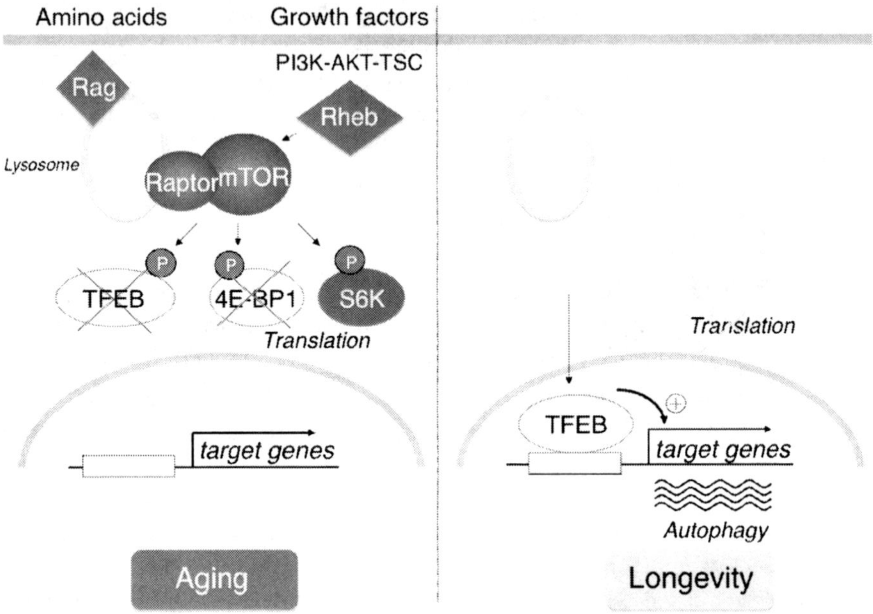

FIGURE 1.2 The mTOR pathway in the regulation of organismal longevity. Selected members of the mTOR pathway are presented. P = phosphorylation.

the mTOR protein kinase within this complex. The activation of mTORC1 by amino acids involves lysosomes. In the presence of amino acids, mTORC1 translocates from the cytoplasm to lysosomes, where mTORC1 is activated by Rag GTPases present in a complex called Ragulator (Sancak et al., 2010; Sancak et al., 2008). Upon activation, mTORC1 is responsible for phosphorylating substrates involved in the regulation of protein translation (e.g., Ribosomal protein S6 kinase 70 KD [S6K1], Eukaryotic translation initiation factor 4E-binding protein 1 [4E-BP1]; reviewed in Ma & Blenis, 2009), autophagy (e.g., UNC51-like kinase 1 [ULK1], T cell transcription factor EB [TFEB]; J. Kim, Kundu, Viollet, & Guan, 2011; Peña-Llopis et al., 2011; Roczniak-Ferguson et al., 2012; Settembre et al., 2012), as well as lipid metabolism (e.g., lipin; Peterson et al., 2011). Importantly, the macrolide rapamycin can specifically inhibit the activity of the mTORC1 complex (D. H. Kim et al., 2002; Sabatini, Erdjument-Bromage, Lui, Tempst, & Snyder, 1994), thereby providing a powerful handle to dissect mTORC1 action in vitro and in vivo. In contrast to the mTORC1 complex, which has been well characterized, comparatively little is known on the regulation and mode of action of the mTORC2 complex. Rapamycin does not efficiently inhibit the mTORC2 complex. mTORC2 substrates include the protein kinases AKT and SGK (Sarbassov, Guertin, Ali, & Sabatini, 2005), which connects the mTOR and the PI3K-AKT pathways.

Knock down of mTOR or a component of the mTORC1 complex (Raptor) was initially found to extend lifespan in *C. elegans* (Vellai et al., 2003). Subsequent studies in yeast and flies demonstrated the importance of reducing the activity of the mTORC1 complex for lifespan extension (Kaeberlein et al., 2005; Kapahi et al., 2004; Medvedik, Lamming, Kim, & Sinclair, 2007). The effect of mTORC1 complexes on longevity is mediated by various substrates, including the translation factors 4E-BP in flies (Zid et al., 2009) and eIF4H in worms (Ching, Paal, Mehta, Zhong, & Hsu, 2010), as well as the transcription factors FOXO/DAF-16, SKN-1, and TFEB/HLH-30 in *C. elegans* (Lapierre et al., 2013; Robida-Stubbs et al., 2012). Interestingly, rapamycin extends lifespan in mice, particularly in females, when initiated at midlife (Harrison et al., 2009), consistent with the observation that mTORC1 activity increases with age (Sengupta, Peterson, Laplante, Oh, & Sabatini, 2010). Females heterozygous for mTOR also exhibit lifespan extension (Lamming et al., 2012). Finally, knock out of a key mTORC1 substrate, S6K1, can also extend mouse lifespan, specifically in females (Selman et al., 2009). Together, these studies show that excess mTORC1 activity is detrimental for longevity from yeast to mammals. In contrast, lowering mTORC2 activity appears to decrease lifespan in *C. elegans* (Soukas et al., 2009), raising the possibility that specific mTOR-containing complexes may have opposing roles on lifespan. Whether the opposing roles of mTORC1 and mTORC2 in aging are caused by different substrates of these complexes or by the degrees in which the activity of the mTOR kinase is changed is not known yet.

The mTOR pathway is critical in the response to dietary restriction-induced longevity in yeast, worms, and flies. In yeast, the lifespan extension caused by mTOR inhibition is not further extended by DR (Kaeberlein et al., 2005), suggesting a genetic interaction between both pathways. In the worm *C. elegans*, RHEB, the GTPase that activates mTORC1, is necessary for lifespan extension by the IF method of DR (Honjoh et al., 2009). Furthermore, mTOR deficiency extends lifespan in ad lib fed animals but not in the DR genetic mimetic *eat-2* mutant worms (Hansen et al., 2008). Together, these findings indicate that mTORC1 mediates part of longevity by DR. However, deficiency in one substrate of mTORC1, S6K, can further extend the lifespan of DR mimetic mutants in *C. elegans* (Hansen et al., 2007), indicating that there is also an mTORC1-independent component of DR. This is supported by the observation that rapamycin still further extends the lifespan of DR-treated flies (Bjedov et al., 2010). The importance of the mTOR pathway in mammalian DR has not been fully tested yet, but it is interesting to note that the transcriptional profile of S6K1 deficient mice resembles that of dietary-restricted mice (Selman et al., 2009). However, rapamycin-treated animals and dietary-restricted animals differ in terms of insulin sensitivity, adiposity, and gene expression, suggesting that inhibiting mTORC1 and restricting food intake are not entirely equivalent (Fok et al., 2012). The mTOR pathway may be particularly critical to mediate dietary restriction regimens that involve changes in amino acids but may not be universally involved in all methods of DR.

AMP-Activated Protein Kinase

AMP-activated protein kinase (AMPK) is a central energy-sensor in cells (see Figure 1.3). Contrary to TOR and the PI3K-AKT pathway, which sense energy-replete states (or excess of energy), AMPK senses low energy levels. In response to decrease in energy levels, AMPK switches on ATP-generating pathways and switches off ATP-consuming pathways (Hardie, Ross, & Hawley, 2012). A heterotrimeric protein kinase, AMPK, is activated when the AMP:ATP ratio increases, and its activation requires the presence of one of several upstream kinases, including the tumor suppressor liver kinase B1 (LKB1) and Ca^{2+}/Calmodulin-dependent protein kinase kinase β (CAMKKβ; reviewed in Kahn, Alquier, Carling, & Hardie, 2005; Mihaylova & Shaw, 2011). In mammalian cells, AMPK directly phosphorylates many substrates that are involved in glucose and lipid metabolism (e.g., acetyl-CoA carboxylase alpha [ACC1]; Kahn, Alquier, Carling, & Hardie, 2005), autophagy (e.g., ULK1; Egan et al., 2011; J. Kim et al.,

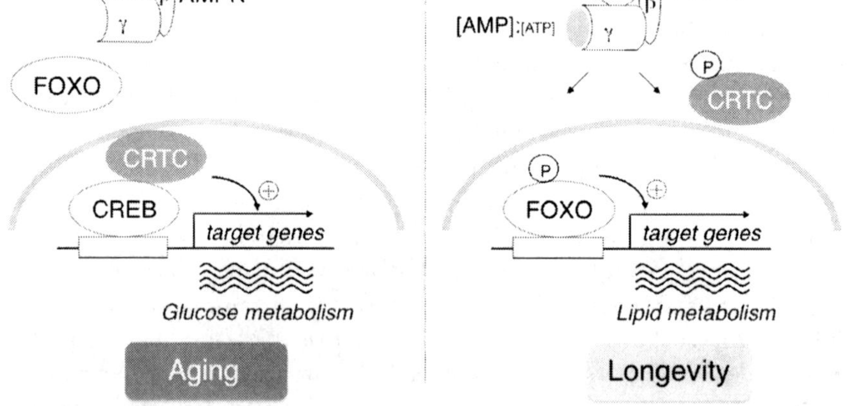

FIGURE 1.3 The AMPK pathway in the regulation of organismal longevity. Selected members of the AMPK pathway are presented. P = phosphorylation.

2011), transcriptional regulation (e.g., histone deacetylases [HDACs], FOXO3, CREB-regulated transcription coactivator 2 [CRTC2]; Greer, Oskoui, et al., 2007; Koo et al., 2005; Mihaylova et al., 2011; Shaw et al., 2005), as well as cell cycle and cytoskeletal regulation (e.g., protein phosphatase 1 regulatory subunit 12C (PPP1R12C), cell division cycle 27 [CDC27]; Banko et al., 2011).

AMPK was shown to be critical for longevity in invertebrates. Expressing wild type or constitutively active AMPK leads to lifespan extension in *C. elegans* (Apfeld, O'connor, McDonagh, DiStefano, & Curtis, 2004; Greer, Dowlatshahi, et al., 2007; Mair et al., 2011). AMPK exerts its beneficial effects on lifespan via FOXO and CRTC1, the worm ortholog of CRTC2 (Greer, Dowlatshahi, et al., 2007; Mair et al., 2011). The importance of AMPK in longevity was corroborated in yeast (Lu et al., 2011) and flies (Stenesen et al., 2013). In flies, AMPK expression in the fat body is sufficient to extend lifespan (Stenesen et al., 2013). Several compounds that activate AMPK (among several other pathways), such as the antidiabetic drug metformin and resveratrol, have been tested for their impacts on health span and lifespan. Metformin extends lifespan in worms (Cabreiro et al., 2013; Onken & Driscoll, 2010) but not in flies (Slack, Foley, & Partridge, 2012). In mice, metformin has been shown to activate AMPK in vivo and to slightly, but significantly, extend the lifespan of middle-aged mice (Martin-Montalvo et al., 2013). The compound resveratrol, which can activate AMPK in vivo (as well as Sirtuins, see below), provides metabolic benefits in mice and extends the lifespan in mice on a high-fat diet (Baur et al., 2006), although it does not extend lifespan of mice on a regular diet (Pearson et al., 2008).

Interestingly, AMPK was found to be necessary for lifespan extension by some DR methods in worms (e.g., sDR; Greer & Brunet, 2009; Greer, Dowlatshahi, et al., 2007), although not all (e.g., *eat-2*; Curtis, O'Connor, & DiStefano, 2006; Greer & Brunet, 2009; Mair, Panowski, Shaw, & Dillin, 2009). A recent study indicates that AMPK is also important for lifespan extension by DR in flies (Stenesen et al., 2013). The importance of AMPK on the longevity induced by DR in mammals has not yet been assessed, but AMPK is necessary for some of the health benefits induced by DR in mice. Overall, AMPK likely mediates the benefits on health of DR regimens that trigger a sharp increase in the AMP:ATP ratio, for example, by rationing glucose.

Sirtuins

The Sirtuin family of protein deacetylases was initially shown to be implicated in lifespan in the yeast *Saccharomyces cerevisiae* by the Guarente lab (Kaeberlein, McVey, & Guarente, 1999). Since this initial discovery, Sirtuins have been extensively studied (Imai & Guarente, 2010; see Figure 1.4). Mammalian Sirtuins encompass seven family members (SIRT1 to SIRT7) that are localized

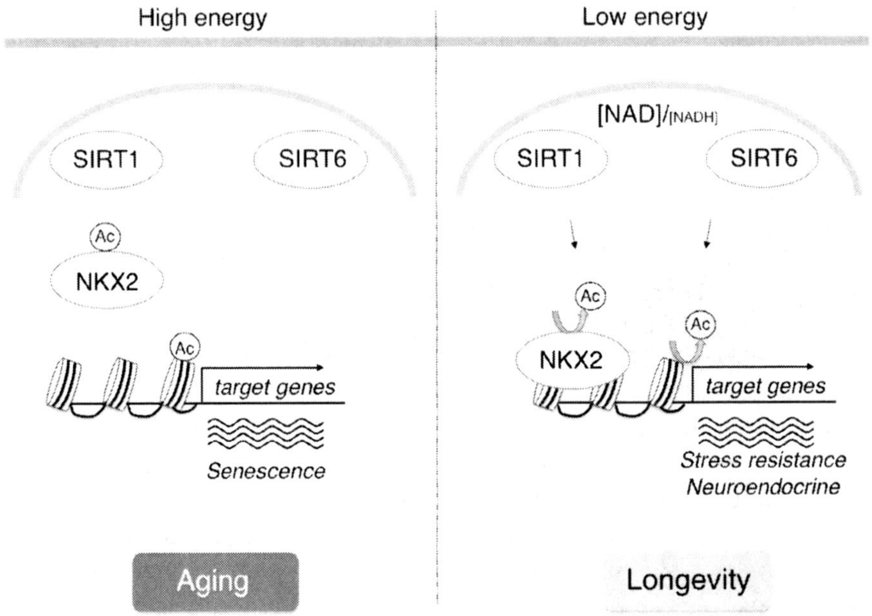

FIGURE 1.4 Sirtuin pathways in the regulation of organismal longevity. Selected members of the Sirtuin pathway are presented. Ac = acetylation.

in different subcellular compartments: nucleus (SIRT1, SIRT6, and SIRT7), cytoplasm (SIRT2), and mitochondria (SIRT3, SIRT4, and SIRT5; Nakagawa & Guarente, 2011). Yeast SIR2, as well as some of its orthologs in mammals (SIRT1, SIRT3, SIRT6, and SIRT7), function as protein deacetylases (Imai, Armstrong, Kaeberlein, & Guarente, 2000), although Sirtuins also have other enzymatic activity including ADP-ribosyltransferase enzymatic activity (all Sirtuins; Tanner, Landry, Sternglanz, & Denu, 2000) and lysine demalonylase and desuccinylase activity (SIRT5; Du et al., 2011). Sirtuin enzymatic activity is enhanced when the ratio between NAD+ and NADH is high, a state associated with low energy and oxidative stress (Imai & Guarente, 2010). Sirtuins can deacetylate a wide range of substrates, including histones and nonhistone proteins. For example, SIRT1 can deacetylate specific histone residues (e.g., lysine 16 on histone H4 [H4K16] and lysine 9 on histone H3 [H3K9]; Imai et al., 2000; Vaquero et al., 2004), transcription factors (e.g., FOXO and p53; Brunet et al., 2004; Luo et al., 2001; Motta et al., 2004; Vaziri et al., 2001), and transcriptional coactivators (e.g., Peroxisime proliferator-activated receptor-gamma coactivator 1 [PGC1] and CRTC2; Y. Liu et al., 2008; Rodgers, Lerin, Gerhart-Hines, & Puigserver, 2008).

Although the importance of Sirtuins in lifespan is still subject to debate, it is clear that this family of proteins has beneficial effects on energy metabolism and several aspects of longevity. SIR2 overexpression is sufficient to extend the replicative lifespan of *S. cerevisiae* (Kaeberlein et al., 1999). In worms and flies, a first set of reports had shown that the lifespan extension by SIR2 overexpression was also observed in these organisms (Rogina & Helfand, 2004; Tissenbaum & Guarente, 2001), although these data were challenged in 2011 (Burnett et al., 2011). In 2013, two studies indicated that SIR2 expression can extend the lifespan of worms (Mouchiroud et al., 2013) and flies (Hoffmann, Romey, Fink, Yong, & Roeder, 2013). Collectively, this work indicates that Sirtuins can play a role in aspects of longevity in invertebrates, but that the extent by which they affect lifespan may depend on other factors, possibly nutrient status. The mechanisms by which SIR2 acts to extend lifespan in invertebrates involve both epigenetic chromatin changes and specific pathways. In yeast, deacetylation of H4K16 by SIR2 appears to be crucial for replicative lifespan: H4K16 acetylation accumulates in old mothers at subtelomeric regions and SIR2 prevents this accumulation (Dang et al., 2009). In worms, longevity induced by SIR2 overexpression requires FOXO transcription factors to extend lifespan in worms (Mouchiroud et al., 2013; Tissenbaum & Guarente, 2001) as well as the mitochondrial unfolded protein response (UPR; Mouchiroud et al., 2013). In mice, SIRT1 expression in the whole organism is not sufficient to extend maximal lifespan, although SIRT1 improves various markers of metabolic health, for example, reduction in circulating cholesterol levels (Bordone et al., 2007; Herranz et al., 2010). SIRT1 also improves both the peripheric and central circadian clocks (Chang & Guarente, 2013; Nakahata et al., 2008), particularly in aged mice (Chang & Guarente, 2013). Interestingly, Imai and colleagues recently found that SIRT1 expression in the brain is sufficient to extend lifespan via neuroendocrine mechanisms (Satoh et al., 2013). SIRT1 can interact with the homeobox protein Nkx2-1 and regulate the expression of the receptor for orexin, a peptide involved in several aspect of wakefulness and appetite, in specific nuclei of the hypothalamus (Satoh et al., 2013). Thus, SIRT1 expression in the brain may be beneficial for preventing the effects of age on the dysregulation of the circadian clock and metabolic regulation. SIRT1 expression in the brain also provides protection against neurodegenerative diseases, particularly Alzheimer's disease (Donmez, Wang, Cohen, & Guarente, 2010; D. Kim et al., 2007), although it would be interesting to determine if this is a cell autonomous phenomenon or is caused by the neuroendocrine systemic action of SIRT1. Resveratrol and other small molecule activators of SIRT1 (termed STACS) can extend lifespan in yeast, worms, and flies (Howitz et al., 2003; Wood et al., 2004). These compounds can also extend mean lifespan and promote health in mice, particularly when mice are obese (Baur et al., 2006; Milne et al., 2007; Minor et al., 2012; Pearson et al., 2008). Whether STACS act via SIRT1 or via other pathways (e.g., AMPK) has been the subject of another controversy, but STACS have recently been shown to act at least in large part by directly activating SIRT1 (Hubbard et al., 2013). Together, these studies highlight a crucial role of SIRT1 in health span and suggest that SIRT1 may have more effects on maximal lifespan when expressed in the nervous system than in peripheral tissues.

The field is also starting to assess the role of other Sirtuin family members in the regulation of lifespan. Mice lacking SIRT6, a member of the Sirtuin family that is localized in the nucleus, display signs of progeria (Kawahara et al., 2009). SIRT6 acts by deacetylating H3K9 at genes regulated by NF-κB transcription factor and by directly interacting with NF-κB (Kawahara et al., 2009). Conversely, mice overexpressing SIRT6 exhibit lifespan extension, at least in males (Kanfi et al., 2012). It will be interesting to test the importance of mitochondrial Sirtuins (e.g., SIRT3) on lifespan and health span.

Sirtuins mediate some aspects of longevity by dietary restriction. In yeast, SIR2 is necessary for DR-induced longevity (S. J. Lin, Defossez, & Guarente, 2000). In worms, and flies, activation of SIR2 extends lifespan in a manner that is no longer further extended by DR (Wood et al., 2004), and SIR2 is important to mediate longevity by some DR regimens in worms (e.g., *eat-2*; Wang & Tissenbaum, 2006). However, for other pathways, some aspects of DR-induced longevity do not require Sirtuins. For example, in yeast, longevity by DR can occur independently of SIR2 (Kaeberlein, Kirkland, Fields, & Kennedy, 2004); and in worms, other methods of DR do not require SIR2 for lifespan extension (e.g., sDR; Greer & Brunet, 2009). In mammals, it is interesting to note that expression of the SIRT1 gene is induced by nutrient restriction (Cohen et al., 2004), and the phenotypes seen with SIRT1 overexpression resemble that of caloric-restricted mice (Bordone et al., 2007). Consistently, resveratrol induces gene expression patterns and metabolic phenotypes that mimic that of DR (Pearson et al., 2008; Timmers et al., 2011). Finally, SIRT1 is essential for the regulation of energy metabolism in mice in response to caloric restriction (Boily et al., 2008), although whether Sirtuins are required for the longevity extension by DR in mammals is not known. Taken together, these observations indicate that Sirtuins are pivotal hubs in the network of pathways that mediate health span in response to dietary restriction.

LONGEVITY PATHWAYS IN ADULT STEM CELLS IN MAMMALS

Role of FOXO Transcription Factors in Mammalian Adult Stem Cells

Several members of the insulin-FOXO pathway have been implicated in the regulation of adult stem cell homeostasis. Here we will focus on the role of FOXO transcription factors in mammalian adult stem cells (see Figure 1.5), drawing

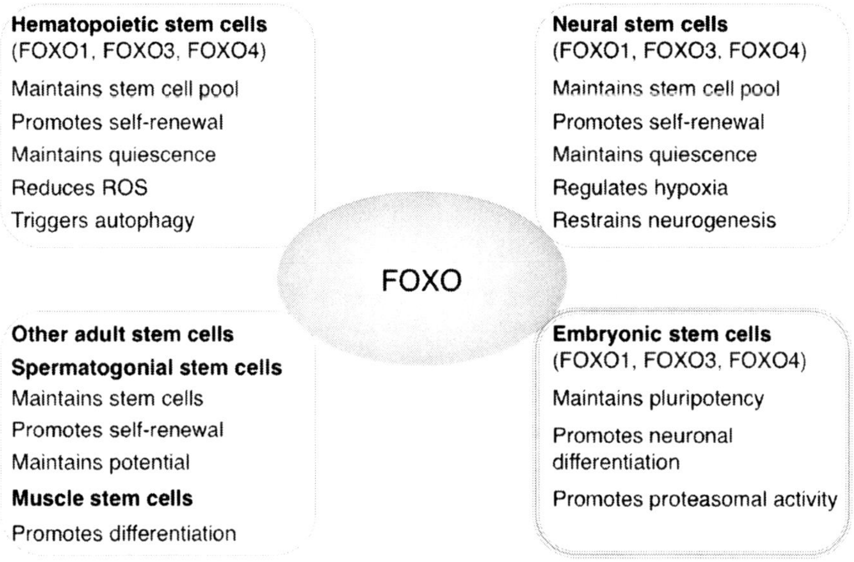

FIGURE 1.5 Role of FOXO transcription factors in mammalian adult and embryonic stem cells. ROS = reactive oxygen species.

from examples in adult hematopoietic stem cells (HSCs), adult neural stem cells (NSCs), and postnatal spermatogonial stem cells (SSCs). FOXO factors are critical for adult HSC function. Triple knockout (TKO) of *Foxo1*, FOXO3, and FOXO4 in the mouse hematopoietic lineage or complete knockout of FOXO3 alone results in decreased long-term hematopoietic reconstitution, indicating disruptions in HSC self-renewal (Miyamoto et al., 2007; Tothova et al., 2007). TKO and FOXO3$^{-/-}$ HSCs have elevated reactive oxygen species (ROS), fail to maintain quiescence, and exhibit myeloid expansion (Miyamoto et al., 2007; Tothova et al., 2007). Treatment with N-acetylcysteine (NAC), an antioxidant, reverses most defects in FOXO-deficient HSCs (Tothova et al., 2007). Interestingly, FOXO3 is crucial for the induction of an autophagy gene expression program in response to starvation in HSCs, and accordingly FOXO3$^{-/-}$ HSCs are deficient in their ability to induce autophagy (Warr et al., 2013). The induction of autophagy by FOXO3 protects HSCs under conditions of metabolic stress, and appears to be essential for the maintenance of HSCs during aging (Warr et al., 2013). Thus, FOXO transcription factors are important regulators of HSC homeostasis in basal states as well as in response to metabolic stress and aging.

Similar to HSCs, adult NSCs require FOXO transcription factors to maintain self-renewal capacity over time. Complete loss of FOXO3, or adult NSC (and astrocyte)-specific TKO (GFAP-TKO), results in decreased NSC self-renewal in vitro, and depletion of NSCs with age in vivo (Paik et al., 2009; Renault et al., 2009). NSCs lacking FOXO transcription factors lose their quiescent state and display premature differentiation (Paik et al., 2009; Renault et al., 2009), thereby leading to the progressive exhaustion of the pool of these cells over time. Conversely, expression of FOXO3 can limit neuronal differentiation of NSCs (Webb et al., 2013), which may participate in preserving the NSC pool throughout life. The molecular mechanisms underlying FOXO function in NSCs have yet to be fully elucidated. Like FOXO-deficient HSCs, FOXO-deficient NSCs have elevated ROS, although treatment with the reducing agent NAC only partially rescues the self-renewal defect (Paik et al., 2009), indicating that other mechanisms are likely involved. Characterization of the program of genes regulated by FOXO3 in NSCs uncovered genes involved in cellular quiescence (*p27*^{Kip1}*/Cdkn1b*, *Ccng2*), glucose metabolism (*Pdk1*, *Slc2a3*), hypoxia regulation (*Selenbp1*; Renault et al., 2009), and glial differentiation (*Mbp*, *Plp1*; Paik et al., 2009). The maintenance of quiescence, prevention of premature differentiation, and switch in metabolism could all cooperate to preserve the homeostasis of NSCs (Paik et al., 2009; Renault et al., 2009). Chromatin immunoprecipitation followed by ultra-high throughput sequencing (ChIP-Seq) has revealed the ensemble of FOXO3 direct targets in adult NSC cultures (Webb et al., 2013). These targets comprise genes involved in telomere protection (e.g., *Pot1a*) as well as components of the Notch and Wnt pathways that are involved in the balance between NSC maintenance and neuronal differentiation (Webb et al., 2013). Furthermore, this study also revealed that FOXO3 co-occurred genome-wide with the proneuronal transcription factor Achaete-scute complex homolog 1 (ASCL1; Webb et al., 2013), and that FOXO3 could inhibit ASCL1's proneuronal function. Thus, FOXO3 may also contribute to the maintenance of the NSC reservoir by fine-tuning the balance between NSCs and neurons. Precisely how various FOXO targets contribute to stem cell functionality is unknown, but FOXO3 appears to have multiple mechanisms of action, each contributing to stem cell maintenance. Identifying which FOXO targets in the transcriptional network participate in these different mechanisms of stem cell maintenance and if some targets are more important than others will be a key step in delaying the age-dependent loss of NSCs.

FOXO factors also play a role in the homeostasis of other types of stem cells. FOXO3 regulates adult muscle stem cells (called satellite cells; Hu, Geles, Paik, DePinho, & Tjian, 2008). FOXO3 can directly bind to the *MyoD* promoter in satellite cells, and *MyoD* transcription is deficient in *Foxo3*$^{-/-}$ satellite cells (Hu et al., 2008). Although FOXO3-deficient muscles appear normal overall, satellite cells isolated from *Foxo3*$^{-/-}$ mice display defects in differentiation, as assessed by myosin staining (Hu et al., 2008). Interestingly, FOXO3-deficient mice also display defects in muscle regeneration upon injury (Hu et al., 2008). These studies were conducted in juvenile animals, and it would be interesting to determine the importance of FOXO3 in the defects in muscle regeneration that occur as a consequence of aging. FOXO1 regulates postnatal SSCs. Germline-specific knock out of FOXO1 or germline-specific TKO (Vasa-FOXO1$^{lox/lox}$ or Vasa-TKO) disrupts both self-renewal and differentiation of SSCs (Goertz, Wu, Gallardo, Hamra, & Castrillon, 2011). Analysis of FOXO targets in these cells identified the *Ret* gene, a receptor for the glial cell line-derived neurotrophic factor (GDNF) ligand and key regulator of germ cell maintenance, as a downstream effector of FOXO function in these cells, although whether *Ret* is a direct FOXO target remains to be determined.

Together, these studies reveal the importance of FOXO transcription factors in the maintenance of several adult stem cell pools in the blood, brain, muscle, and germline. It will be interesting to determine whether FOXO transcription factors also play significant roles in other populations of adult stem cells (e.g., in the intestine or skin), and if so, which transcriptional program they regulate in each stem cell type. Given the importance of the non-cell-autonomous action of FOXO in invertebrates, it will be important to dissect the cell-autonomous and non-cell-autonomous action of FOXO factors in adult stem cells.

mTOR Pathway in Mammalian Adult Stem Cells

The activation of the "pro-aging" pathway mTOR is deleterious for the maintenance of adult stem cells (see Figure 1.6). Maintaining lower mTOR activity, which is known to extend lifespan in many organisms, also prevents exhaustion of the adult HSC pool. For example, deletion of tuberous sclerosis protein 1 (TSC1), a negative regulator of mTORC1, leads to defects in the ability of HSCs

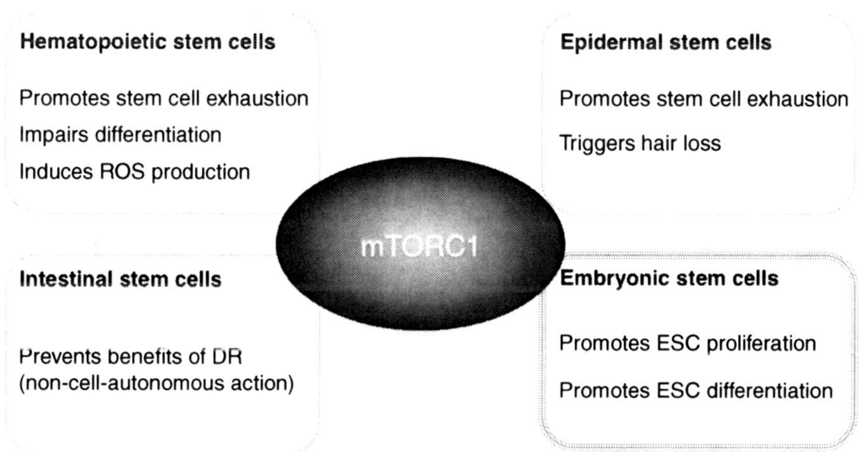

FIGURE 1.6 Role of mTORC1 in mammalian adult and embryonic stem cells. DR = dietary restriction; ESC = embryonic stem cell; ROS = reactive oxygen species.

to properly differentiate and impairs their capacity for bone marrow reconstitution (C. Chen et al., 2008). Overactive mTORC1 signaling resulting from TSC deletion may impair cellular quiescence, which is required to preserve the pool of adult stem cells (Kippin, Martens, & van der Kooy, 2005; Morshead et al., 1994). mTORC1 hyperactivation is associated with increased numbers of mitochondria and higher ROS levels in adult HSCs (C. Chen et al., 2008). Lowering ROS levels by treatment with the antioxidant NAC partially rescues these HSC defects (C. Chen et al., 2008), similar to what was seen for FOXO-deficient HSCs (Tothova et al., 2007). The increase in mTOR signaling with age in HSCs (C. Chen et al., 2008) might underlie the defects of age-dependent deterioration of these cells. Indeed, treatment of old mice with the mTORC1 inhibitor rapamycin confers "youthful" phenotypes to old HSCs and improves the function of the mouse immune system (C. Chen et al., 2008). Although reducing mTOR activity is beneficial for HSCs, the complete deficiency of mTOR activity can actually prove detrimental for HSCs. For example, complete deficiency in Raptor results in an impairment of HSC function following transplantation (Kalaitzidis et al., 2012). Deficiency in Raptor is associated with changes in lipid and cholesterol metabolism in HSCs (Kalaitzidis et al., 2012). In epidermal stem cells, mTOR activation following chronic Wnt signaling triggers the premature exhaustion of these cells and untimely hair loss (Castilho, Squarize, Chodosh, Williams, & Gutkind, 2009). Although the action of the mTOR pathway in stem cells appears to be in part cell-autonomous (Kalaitzidis et al., 2012; Magri et al., 2011), mTORC1 can also prevent the beneficial impact of dietary restriction on adult intestinal stem cells by acting in a non-cell-autonomous manner in Paneth cells, which constitute the intestinal stem cell niche (Yilmaz et al., 2012).

AMPK in Mammalian Adult Stem Cells

The role of AMPK in mammalian adult stem cells has not yet been clearly established (see Figure 1.7). HSCs that lack both catalytic α subunits of AMPK have decreased levels of ATP and mitochondrial DNA (Nakada, Saunders, & Morrison, 2010). Deficiency in AMPK activity leads to significant decrease in the numbers of HSCs in the bone marrow (Nakada et al., 2010), suggesting that the regulation of mitochondrial homeostasis by AMPK contribute to the control of HSC number. However, AMPK activity is not necessary for HSCs to reconstitute the blood in bone marrow transplantation assays (Nakada et al., 2010). The impact of AMPK deficiency on HSCs is much less drastic than that of the upstream regulator LKB1, raising the possibility that AMPK-related kinases may be important for the function of LKB1 in this context (Gan et al., 2010; Gurumurthy et al., 2010; Nakada et al., 2010). Because AMPK is activated by low energy levels, it is possible that the effects of AMPK abrogation may be accentuated in starved animals.

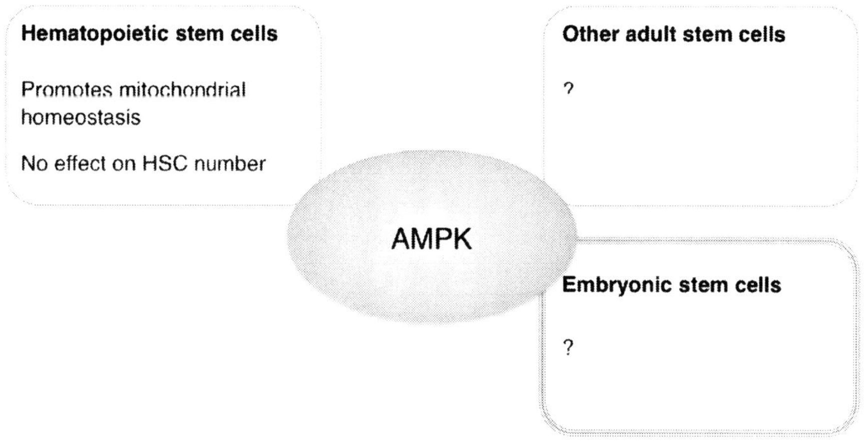

FIGURE 1.7 Role of AMPK in mammalian adult and embryonic stem cells. HSC = hematopoietic stem cell.

Although the role of AMPK in adult NSCs has not been characterized yet, deficiency in AMPK activity leads to defective mitosis of neural progenitor cells during mouse brain development (Dasgupta & Milbrandt, 2009). Under low-energy conditions, AMPK activity may ensure the completion of mitosis in stem/progenitor cells that are actively cycling because cell cycle arrest at this stage could have disastrous consequences for the genomic stability of a cell. However, the exact importance and mode of action of AMPK in adult stem cells, as well as the substrates that mediate AMPK actions in these cells, remain to be more thoroughly examined.

Sirtuins in Mammalian Adult Stem Cells

Although chronic SIRT1 deficiency in mice does not affect HSC function and normal hematopoiesis (Leko et al., 2012; Narala et al., 2008), recent evidence indicates that inducible SIRT1 deficiency in adult mice leads to the expansion of hematopoietic progenitors (Singh et al., 2013; see Figure 1.8). This expansion is dependent on stress signals and ultimately leads to the depletion of the pool of HSCs (Singh et al., 2013). The effect of SIRT1 in hematopoietic progenitors is cell-autonomous, and SIRT1 loss leads to genomic instability in HSCs (Singh et al., 2013). SIRT3, a mitochondrial Sirtuin, has recently been found to be important to HSC self renewal. In the absence of SIRT3, HSCs are prematurely depleted and this is particularly evident in older animals (Brown et al., 2013). SIRT3 levels in HSCs decrease with age (Brown et al., 2013), which may underlie the progressive deficit of normal HSCs during aging. Strikingly, lentiviral-based overexpression of SIRT3 in old HSCs can restore survival and proliferative

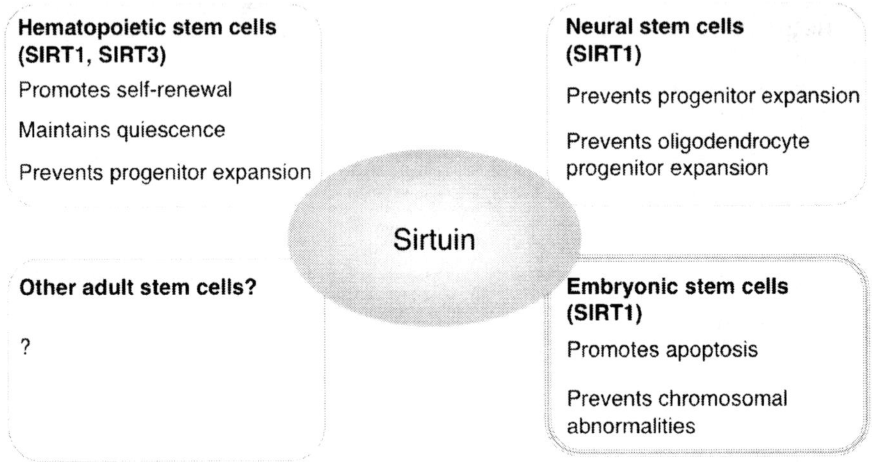

FIGURE 1.8 Role of Sirtuins in mammalian adult and embryonic stem cells.

function of aged HSCs (Brown et al., 2013). The mechanism by which SIRT3 protects HSCs may involve, at least in part, the regulation of the mitochondrial superoxide dismutase 2 (SOD2; Brown et al., 2013).

SIRT1 has recently been found to play an important role in adult NSCs (Rafalski et al., 2013). The specific deletion of the *Sirt1* gene in adult NSCs with a tamoxifen-inducible Cre system results in the expansion of neural progenitors (Rafalski et al., 2013). SIRT1 deficiency results in a particularly striking increase in oligodendrocyte progenitors in a manner that depends on platelet-derived growth factor (PDGF) signaling (Rafalski et al., 2013). The oligodendrocytes produced upon SIRT1 deficiency are functional. Interestingly, SIRT1-deficient mice have improved remyelination upon demyelinating injury and show less paralysis in a mouse model for multiple sclerosis (Rafalski et al., 2013). Whether the expansion in oligodendrocyte production upon SIRT1 deletion ultimately leads to the depletion of the NSC pool has not been tested yet. Deleting a pro-longevity gene might transiently favor the production of differentiated cells, at the expense of ultimately depleting the reservoir of stem cells. As shown in embryonic neural progenitors, SIRT1 may play a particularly important role under oxidative conditions (Prozorovski et al., 2008).

The role of SIRT1 in other pools of stem cells has not been thoroughly tested yet, although SIRT1 deficient muscle progenitor cells display defects in proliferation and differentiation (Fulco et al., 2008; Rathbone, Booth, & Lees, 2009). Furthermore, resveratrol, an SIRT1 activator, has been shown to rescue the decline in several adult stem cell types, such as mesenchymal stem cells and HSCs, in progeroid mouse models (B. Liu et al., 2012), raising the possibility for a more general role of SIRT1 (or AMPK) in various adult stem cells during aging.

LONGEVITY PATHWAYS IN MAMMALIAN EMBRYONIC STEM CELLS

FOXO Transcription Factors in Embryonic Stem Cells

FOXO transcription factors have recently emerged as important regulators of ESC pluripotency (see Figure 1.5). FOXO1 was found to be highly expressed in H1 human ESCs (hESCs) and was reportedly more abundantly expressed than all three other FOXO family members (FOXO3, FOXO4, or FOXO6; X. Zhang et al., 2011). FOXO1 expression is downregulated during differentiation of ESCs, suggesting a more prominent role for FOXO1 in ESCs than in differentiated progeny (X. Zhang et al., 2011). FOXO1 knockdown in H1 ESCs results in a decrease in pluripotency markers and in the ability of ESCs to differentiate into the different germ layers (X. Zhang et al., 2011). Knock down of either FOXO1 or FOXO3 also leads to defect in pluripotency in mouse ESCs (X. Zhang et al., 2011). FOXO1 appears to act by directly affecting the pluripotency network via binding of octamer-binding transcription factor 4 (OCT4) and SOX2 regulatory regions rather than by regulating ESC proliferation or ROS content. The Dillin lab investigated the role of FOXO transcription factors in human ESC pluripotency and differentiation into the neuronal fate, revealing an important role for FOXO4 in this context. In H9 ESCs, FOXO4 knock down results in a defect in ESC pluripotency, whereas knock down of FOXO1 or FOXO3 has no effects on ESC function (Vilchez, Boyer, et al., 2012). The implication of FOXO4, but not FOXO1, in ESCs contrasts with the study by the Ghaffari lab (X. Zhang et al., 2011). The differences between both studies might be explained by the extent of the FOXO knock down or by differences in the ESC cultures and clones. Interestingly, FOXO4 upregulates proteasome activity in ESCs, in particular Proteasome 26S subunit non-ATPas 11 (PSMD11), a regulatory subunit of the proteasome (Vilchez, Boyer, et al., 2012). ESCs are characterized by high levels of proteasome activity compared to differentiated cells, and this increased proteostasis is critical for stem cell potential (Vilchez, Boyer, et al., 2012). FOXO4 is also necessary for neuronal differentiation of human ESCs into neurons (Vilchez et al., 2013). Thus, FOXO1, FOXO3, and FOXO4 are important for the pluripotency of ESCs, although these transcription factors have varying degrees of importance and appear to act via distinct mechanisms (regulation of the pluripotency network for FOXO1 and upregulation of proteasome activity for FOXO4). FOXO4 appears to be particularly important for the ability of ESCs to differentiate into the neuronal lineage. Thus, although FOXO transcription factors play important roles in adult stem cells and ESCs, their function in these cell types seem to be quite different. In adult stem cells, FOXO factors mostly prevent exhaustion of the stem cell reserves by preserving adult stem cell quiescence and preventing premature differentiation (Renault et al., 2009; Webb et al., 2013). In ESCs,

FOXO appears to be important for pluripotency and necessary for differentiation (Vilchez et al., 2013). It would be interesting to perform direct comparative studies of the various mechanisms that have been implicated downstream of FOXO transcription factors to determine whether there are shared pathways as well as specific mechanisms depending on stem cell types.

mTOR Pathway in ESCs

mTOR signaling plays an important role in ESC self-renewal (see Figure 1.6). Inhibition of mTOR by rapamycin or by knockdown in mouse and human ESCs reduces the expression of pluripotency markers and impairs the self-renewal of ESCs in vitro (Schieke et al., 2008; Zhou et al., 2009). Furthermore, deletion of mTOR inhibits proliferation in early mouse embryos (Murakami et al., 2004). Somewhat surprisingly, mTOR also appears to promote ESC differentiation. For example, the transition from ESCs to more differentiated cell types is associated with increased activation of mTORC1 signaling (Easley et al., 2010; Sampath et al., 2008). Furthermore, overexpression of a constitutively active form of S6K1, a substrate of mTORC1, promotes differentiation of ESCs (Easley et al., 2010). It will be important to understand the circumstances under which TOR promotes either ESC self-renewal/pluripotency or differentiation and whether different mTOR substrates are involved in mediating these diverse functions of mTOR.

AMPK and Sirtuins in ESCs

The role of AMPK in ESCs has not been studied yet, but there is evidence for a role of Sirtuins in ESCs (see Figure 1.8). In vitro differentiation of mouse ESCs into the hematopoietic lineage is defective in the absence of SIRT1 (Ou et al., 2010). SIRT1 is highly expressed in human and mouse ESCs, and its expression declines during multilineage differentiation, suggesting that SIRT1 plays a more important role in ESCs than in differentiated progeny (Calvanese et al., 2010; Saunders et al., 2010). Under basal conditions, mouse ESCs that lack SIRT1 show no obvious defects (McBurney et al., 2003), but exposure to mild oxidative stress activates SIRT1 to promote ESC apoptosis (Chae & Broxmeyer, 2011; Han et al., 2008). In response to stress stimuli, SIRT1 also prevents the accumulation of chromosomal abnormalities in mouse ESCs (Oberdoerffer et al., 2008). These findings that SIRT1 triggers ESC apoptosis under stress stimuli contrast with previously reported roles for SIRT1 in preventing apoptosis in response to oxidative stress in mouse embryonic fibroblasts and differentiated neurons (Brunet et al., 2004; Motta et al., 2004). The ability of SIRT1 to induce or prevent apoptosis may depend on stem versus differentiated cells or on the amount and source of oxidative stress.

LONGEVITY PATHWAYS AND REPROGRAMMING TO iPSCs

Insulin/IGF1-FOXO Pathway in Reprogramming

Does manipulating longevity pathways impact the ability of differentiated cells to generate functional iPSCs? The study of longevity pathways in reprogramming is still in its infancy. However, chemical inhibitors of the insulin-IGF1 signaling pathway have been shown to ameliorate reprogramming (see Figure 1.9). For example, the IGF1 receptor inhibitor PQ401 and the PI3K inhibitor LY294002 improved the reprogramming efficiency of mouse embryonic fibroblasts (MEFs; T. Chen et al., 2011). Inhibition of the insulin/IGF-1 pathway was shown to act in the initial phase of reprogramming (T. Chen et al., 2011). These results suggest that "pro-longevity signaling" (i.e., inhibition of the insulin pathway) may improve reprogramming. Whether inhibitors of the insulin pathway also help the reprogramming of adult cells or even old cells is not yet known but would be interesting to test.

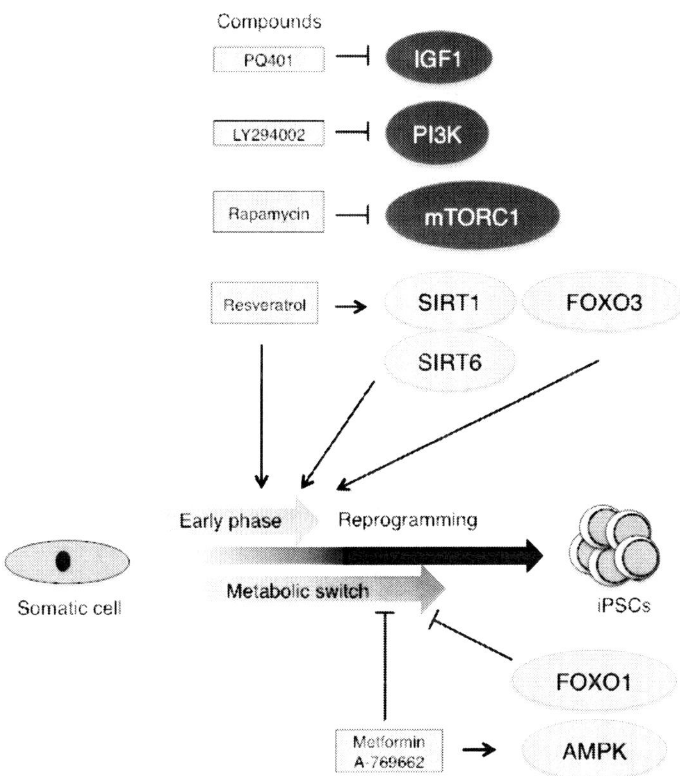

FIGURE 1.9 Longevity pathways in cellular reprogramming.

FOXO transcription factors have recently been implicated in the process of reprogramming and iPSC function. *Foxo3*$^{-/-}$ MEFs can reprogram into iPSCs that are normal in terms of markers and ability to generate the three germ lineages (endoderm, mesoderm, and ectoderm; Wang, Tian, & Zheng, 2013). However, *Foxo3*$^{-/-}$ MEFs do exhibit a delay in the reprogramming process, which can be rescued by expression of FOXO3 (Wang et al., 2013). In contrast, another study reported that FOXO1 acted as a barrier to reprogramming in that overexpression of a dominant negative mutant of FOXO1 ameliorated reprogramming efficiency, whereas overexpression of a constitutively active mutant of FOXO1 inhibited reprogramming (Yu et al., 2013). Consistent with what was observed for FOXO4 in human ESCs (Vilchez et al., 2013), FOXO3 deficiency also impairs the potential of mouse iPSCs to differentiate into cells that are positive for various markers along the neuronal lineage (SOX2, NESTIN, and TUJ1; Wang et al., 2013). It will be interesting to characterize further the role of various FOXO transcription factors in reprogramming and iPSC quality, particularly in cells from older individuals.

mTOR Pathway in Reprogramming

Similar to what was observed for inhibitors of the insulin pathway, the mTORC1 inhibitor rapamycin has been found to significantly improve the reprogramming efficiency of MEFs (T. Chen et al., 2011; see Figure 1.9). The resulting iPSC lines expressed pluripotency markers, were karyotypically normal, and could give rise to chimeras with germline transmission (T. Chen et al., 2011). It will be interesting to further explore the molecular and cellular mechanisms by which modulation of the mTORC1 pathways influences reprogramming and iPSC quality in cells from individuals of different ages.

AMPK in Reprogramming

The role of AMPK in reprogramming has been tested via chemical compounds (see Figure 1.9). Metformin, which activates AMPK, was shown to have no significant effects on iPSC generation in one study (T. Chen et al., 2011), whereas it was reported to decrease the ability of both MEFs and adult human fibroblasts to generate iPSCs in another study (Vazquez-Martin, Vellon, et al., 2012). The more specific AMPK activator A-769662 was also found to decrease reprogramming efficiency (Vazquez-Martin, Vellon, et al., 2012). The mechanisms of action of AMPK activating compound in reprogramming are not yet completely characterized, but these compounds have been proposed to prevent the metabolic switch from oxidative to glycolytic metabolism (Vazquez-Martin, Vellon, et al., 2012), a key step in the transition to iPSCs (Folmes et al., 2011; Panopoulos et al., 2012; Varum et al., 2011). Interestingly, systemic injection of metformin was also shown to limit to the tumorigenicity of iPSCs that were implanted in mice, without decreasing their pluripotency (Vazquez-Martin, Cufi, et al., 2012), raising the possibility that AMPK activation could be used to prevent tumor risks of stem cell therapies.

Sirtuins in Reprogramming

So far, the role of two Sirtuin family members, SIRT1 and SIRT6, has been examined and both Sirtuins appear to ameliorate the reprogramming process (see Figure 1.9). SIRT1 expression is high in human H9 ESCs, but lower when these cells differentiate (Y. L. Lee et al., 2012), raising the possibility that SIRT1 is critical for stemness. Knock down of SIRT1 impairs the reprogramming efficiency of MEFs, particularly in the early phases (Y. L. Lee et al., 2012). Overexpression of SIRT1 improves reprogramming efficiency (Y. L. Lee et al., 2012). Consistently, resveratrol was found to improve reprogramming efficiency in MEFs in two independent studies (T. Chen et al., 2011; Y. L. Lee et al., 2012). It is somewhat surprising that AMPK and SIRT1, which have similar function and have both been found to be activated by resveratrol, have opposing role on reprogramming. It would be interesting to compare more directly AMPK and SIRT1 and test the downstream mechanism of their action.

SIRT6, combined with the four reprogramming factors, improved the reprogramming of old human fibroblasts, but had no influence on young human fibroblast's ability to reprogram (Sharma et al., 2013).

Together, these studies indicate that "longevity genes" tend to ameliorate the efficiency of the reprogramming process, although there may also be some instances where longevity genes (e.g., AMPK, FOXO1) act as a barrier to the reprogramming process, maybe because they change the metabolism of these cells in a way that antagonizes reprogramming. It will be important to delineate the specific roles and mode of action of longevity genes in reprogramming, and importantly in the quality of iPSCs that are generated. This will be particularly important in instances where reprogramming has to be done from older patients, for example for personalized stem cell therapies.

CONCLUSION

Longevity pathways play a critical role in several types of stem cells. In adult stem cells, pro-longevity genes appear to act by preserving the pool of adult stem cells, preventing exit from stem cell quiescence and premature differentiation. In ESCs and in the transition from differentiated cells to iPSCs, the role of pro-longevity pathways is still not completely understood. On the one hand, some pro-longevity genes appear to help promote ESC function and reprogramming to iPSCs, perhaps highlighting common paths toward "youthfulness" and longevity. On the other hand, some pro-longevity genes appear to actually prevent ESC proliferation and reprogramming. In this case, maintenance of the organism and stem cell renewal may represent a classical example of "antagonistic pleiotropy."

More experiments will be needed to determine the specific conditions in which longevity pathways have a positive versus negative role in stem cells. Unraveling the mechanisms that can uncouple the effects of longevity genes on different features of stem cell function will be a key step in harnessing the potential of stem cells for longevity and rejuvenation.

So far, the studies that have tested the importance and mode of action of longevity genes and stem cells have only captured the tip of the iceberg. Indeed, most of the work has focused so far on one longevity pathway, one stem cell type, and one condition (often the basal condition). The full story is likely to be far more complex. It will be important to perform a more systematic study of longevity pathways in stem cells, viewing these pathways as a network rather than simple linear pathways. Significant crosstalk exists between the different longevity pathways, for example, between the PI3K-AKT and TOR pathways as well as between the AMPK and Sirtuin pathways. How perturbating one hub in the longevity network affects the other nodes has yet to be studied in stem cells. It will also be key to perform a more systematic comparison between different stem cell types. Furthermore, it is important to note that longevity pathways may be particularly induced or activated in response to certain circumstances, for example, starvation, or at different times of the circadian cycle. Thus, it will be critical to reexamine the role of these longevity pathways not just under basal conditions but also as a function of the organism's diet, time during the day, and so forth. Finally, another level of complexity arises from the fact that adult stem cells are present within an intricate niche in the tissue and are thus subjected to influences of other cell types and from the blood circulation (Conboy et al., 2005; Ruckh et al., 2012; Villeda et al., 2011). Whether longevity genes influence stem cell function by acting solely in stem cells or by also acting in the niche or even by controlling the systemic environment is a key axis for future research. It will be interesting to dissect the cell-autonomous versus non-cell-autonomous role of longevity pathways in adult stem cells.

Could the study of longevity pathways in stem cells teach us about rejuvenation? As was done for some longevity genes (Brown et al., 2013), it will be exciting to manipulate the longevity pathways in stem cells that are already old and test if this can reverse some aspects of aging in these cells, and if so which ones. The process of reprogramming differentiated cells into iPSCs has a rejuvenating capacity because it converts a somatic cell (even from an old organism) back into a cell with pluripotency (Rando & Chang, 2012). Indeed, some aspects of aged cells, such as telomere lengths and gene expression changes, are reversed to young states by the process of reprogramming followed by redifferentiation (Lapasset et al., 2011). Understanding the rejuvenation properties of the reprogramming process could ultimately help us better grasp the link between youthfulness and stemness. Finally, deciphering the potential rejuvenation properties of longevity genes in stem cells will have important therapeutical applications for diseases of age. Stem cells, and in particular iPSCs, have been proposed as a source of cells for regenerative therapies, which could be particularly helpful for degenerative age-dependent diseases. For these stem cell therapies to be efficient, it will be important to understand how to have good quality patient-specific stem cells (especially if the donor cells are isolated from already aged individuals). It will also be critical to understand the interactions between the stem cells and their niche and the systemic environment of the host, and the potential role of longevity genes in these interactions, so that the transplanted cells are as "young" as possible and remain young even in the face of an older environment in patients with age-dependent diseases.

ACKNOWLEDGMENTS

We thank support from the National Institutes of Health (National Institute on Aging and National Institute of General Medical Sciences), the Ellison Medical Foundation, the California Institute for Regenerative Medicine, and the Glenn Foundation for Medical Research (A.B.). We also thank support from EMBO (S.M.), the American Federation for Aging Research (E.M. and A.E.W), and the National Institute of Neurological Disorders and Stroke (V.A.R.).

REFERENCES

Alic, N., Andrews, T. D., Giannakou, M. E., Papatheodorou, I., Slack, C., Hoddinott, M. P.,. . . Partridge, L. (2011). Genome-wide dFOXO targets and topology of the transcriptomic response to stress and insulin signalling. *Molecular Systems Biology*, 7, 502.

Anselmi, C. V., Malovini, A., Roncarati, R., Novelli, V., Villa, F., Condorelli, G., . . . Puca, A. A. (2009). Association of the FOXO3A locus with extreme longevity in a southern Italian centenarian study. *Rejuvenation Research*, *12*, 95–104.

Apfeld, J., O'Connor, G., McDonagh, T., DiStefano, P. S., & Curtis, R. (2004). The AMP-activated protein kinase AAK-2 links energy levels and insulin-like signals to lifespan in *C. elegans*. *Genes & Development*, *18*, 3004–3009.

Banko, M. R., Allen, J. J., Schaffer, B. E., Wilker, E. W., Tsou, P., White, J. L., . . . Brunet, A. (2011). Chemical genetic screen for AMPKalpha2 substrates uncovers a network of proteins involved in mitosis. *Molecular Cell*, *44*, 878–892.

Baur, J. A., Pearson, K. J., Price, N. L., Jamieson, H. A., Lerin, C., Kalra, A., . . . Sinclair, D. A. (2006). Resveratrol improves health and survival of mice on a high-calorie diet. *Nature*, *444*, 337–342.

Biggs, W. H., III, Meisenhelder, J., Hunter, T., Cavenee, W. K., & Arden, K. C. (1999). Protein kinase B/Akt-mediated phosphorylation promotes nuclear exclusion of the winged helix transcription factor FKHR1. *Proceedings of the National Academy of Sciences of the United States of America*, *96*, 7421–7426.

Bishop, N. A., & Guarente, L. (2007). Two neurons mediate diet-restriction-induced longevity in *C. elegans*. *Nature*, *447*, 545–549.

Bjedov, I., Toivonen, J. M., Kerr, F., Slack, C., Jacobson, J., Foley, A., & Partridge, L. (2010). Mechanisms of life span extension by rapamycin in the fruit fly *Drosophila melanogaster*. *Cell Metabolism*, *11*, 35–46.

Blüher, M., Kahn, B. B., & Kahn, C. R. (2003). Extended longevity in mice lacking the insulin receptor in adipose tissue. *Science*, *299*, 572–574.

Boily, G., Seifert, E. L., Bevilacqua, L., He, X. H., Sabourin, G., Estey, C., . . . McBurney, M. V. (2008). SIRT1 regulates energy metabolism and response to caloric restriction in mice. *PLoS One*, *3*, e1759.

Bordone, L., Cohen, D., Robinson, A., Motta, M. C., van Veen, E., Czopik, A., . . . Guarente, L. (2007). SIRT1 transgenic mice show phenotypes resembling calorie restriction. *Aging Cell*, *6*, 759–767.

Brown, K., Xie, S., Qiu, X., Mohrin, M., Shin, J., Liu, Y., . . . Chen, D. (2013). SIRT3 reverses aging-associated degeneration. *Cell Reports*, *3*, 319–327.

Brunet, A., Bonni, A., Zigmond, M. J., Lin, M. Z., Juo, P., Hu, L. S., . . . Greenberg, M. E. (1999). Akt promotes cell survival by phosphorylating and inhibiting a Forkhead transcription factor. *Cell*, *96*, 857–868.

Brunet, A., Park, J., Tran, H., Hu, L. S., Hemmings, B. A., & Greenberg, M. E. (2001). Protein kinase SGK mediates survival signals by phosphorylating the Forkhead transcription factor FKHRL1 (FOXO3a). *Molecular & Cellular Biology*, *21*, 952–965.

Brunet, A., Sweeney, L. B., Sturgill, J. F., Chua, K. F., Greer, P. L., . . . Greenberg, M. E. (2004). Stress-dependent regulation of FOXO transcription factors by the SIRT1 deacetylase. *Science*, *303*, 2011–2015.

Burnett, C., Valentini, S., Cabreiro, F., Goss, M., Somogyvári, M., Piper, M. D., . . . Gems, D. (2011). Absence of effects of Sir2 overexpression on lifespan in *C. elegans* and *Drosophila*. *Nature*, *477*, 482–485.

Cabreiro, F., Au, C., Leung, K. Y., Vergara-Irigaray, N., Cochemé, H. M., Noori, T., . . . Gems, D. (2013). Metformin retards aging in *C. elegans* by altering microbial folate and methionine metabolism. *Cell*, *153*, 228–239.

Calvanese, V., Lara, E., Suárez-Alvarez, B., Abu Dawud, R., Vázquez-Chantada, M., Martinez-Chantar, M. L., . . . Fraga, M. F. (2010). Sirtuin 1 regulation of developmental genes during differentiation of stem cells. *Proceedings of the National Academy of Sciences of the United States of America*, *107*, 13736–13741.

Castilho, R. M., Squarize, C. H., Chodosh, L. A., Williams, B. O., & Gutkind, J. S. (2009). mTOR mediates Wnt-induced epidermal stem cell exhaustion and aging. *Cell Stem Cell*, *5*, 279–289.

Chae, H. D., & Broxmeyer, H. E. (2011). SIRT1 deficiency downregulates PTEN/JNK/FOXO1 pathway to block reactive oxygen species-induced apoptosis in mouse embryonic stem cells. *Stem Cells and Development*, *20*, 1277–1285.

Chang, H. C., & Guarente, L. (2013). SIRT1 mediates central circadian control in the SCN by a mechanism that decays with aging. *Cell*, *153*, 1448–1460.

Chen, A. T., Guo, C., Dumas, K. J., Ashrafi, K., & Hu, P. J. (2013). Effects of *Caenorhabditis elegans* sgk-1 mutations on lifespan, stress resistance, and DAF-16/FOXO regulation. *Aging Cell*, *12*(5), 932–940.

Chen, C., Liu, Y., Liu, R., Ikenoue, T., Guan, K. L., & Zheng, P. (2008). TSC-mTOR maintains quiescence and function of hematopoietic stem cells by repressing mitochondrial biogenesis and reactive oxygen species. *Journal of Experimental Medicine*, *205*, 2397–2408.

Chen, T., Shen, L., Yu, J., Wan, H., Guo, A., Chen, J., . . . Pei, G. (2011). Rapamycin and other longevity-promoting compounds enhance the generation of mouse induced pluripotent stem cells. *Aging Cell*, *10*, 908–911.

Chiang, W. C., Ching, T. T., Lee, H. C., Mousigian, C., & Hsu, A. L. (2012). HSF-1 regulators DDL-1/2 link insulin-like signaling to heat-shock responses and modulation of longevity. *Cell*, *148*, 322–334.

Ching, T. T., Paal, A. B., Mehta, A., Zhong, L., & Hsu, A. L. (2010). drr-2 encodes an eIF4H that acts downstream of TOR in diet-restriction-induced longevity of C. elegans. *Aging Cell*, *9*, 545–557.

Clancy, D. J., Gems, D., Harshman, L. G., Oldham, S., Stocker, H., Hafen, E., . . . Partridge, L. (2001). Extension of life-span by loss of CHICO, a *Drosophila* insulin receptor substrate protein. *Science*, *292*, 104–106.

Cohen, H. Y., Miller, C., Bitterman, K. J., Wall, N. R., Hekking, B., Kessler, B., . . . Sinclair, D. A. (2004). Calorie restriction promotes mammalian cell survival by inducing the SIRT1 deacetylase. *Science*, *305*, 390–392.

Conboy, I. M., Conboy, M. J., Wagers, A. J., Girma, E. R., Weissman, I. L., & Rando, T. A. (2005). Rejuvenation of aged progenitor cells by exposure to a young systemic environment. *Nature*, *433*, 760–764.

Curtis, R., O'Connor, G., & DiStefano, P. S. (2006). Aging networks in *Caenorhabditis elegans*: AMP-activated protein kinase (aak-2) links multiple aging and metabolism pathways. *Aging Cell*, *5*, 119–126.

Dang, W., Steffen, K. K., Perry, R., Dorsey, J. A., Johnson, F. B., Shilatifard, A., . . . Berger, S. L. (2009). Histone H4 lysine 16 acetylation regulates cellular lifespan. *Nature*, *459*, 802–807.

Dasgupta, B., & Milbrandt, J. (2009). AMP-activated protein kinase phosphorylates retinoblastoma protein to control mammalian brain development. *Development Cell*, *16*, 256–270.

Dong, X. C., Copps, K. D., Guo, S., Li, Y., Kollipara, R., DePinho, R. A., & White, M. F. (2008). Inactivation of hepatic FOXO1 by insulin signaling is required for adaptive nutrient homeostasis and endocrine growth regulation. *Cell Metabolism*, *8*, 65–76.

Donmez, G., Wang, D., Cohen, D. E., & Guarente, L. (2010). SIRT1 suppresses beta-amyloid production by activating the alpha-secretase gene ADAM10. *Cell*, *142*, 320–332.

Du, J., Zhou, Y., Su, X., Yu, J. J., Khan, S., Jiang, H., . . . Lin, H. (2011). SIRT5 is a NAD-dependent protein lysine demalonylase and desuccinylase. *Science*, *334*, 806–809.

Easley, C. A., IV, Ben-Yehudah, A., Redinger, C. J., Oliver, S. L., Varum, S. T., Eisinger, V. M., . . . Schatten, G. P. (2010). mTOR-mediated activation of p70 S6K induces differentiation of pluripotent human embryonic stem cells. *Cellular Reprogramming*, *12*, 263–273.

Egan, D. F., Shackelford, D. B., Mihaylova, M. M., Gelino, S., Kohnz, R. A., Mair, W., . . . Shaw, R. J. (2011). Phosphorylation of ULK1 (hATG1) by AMP-activated protein kinase connects energy sensing to mitophagy. *Science*, *331*, 456–461.

Flachsbart, F., Caliebe, A., Kleindorp, R., Blanché, H., von Eller-Eberstein, H., Nikolaus, S., . . . Nebel, A. (2009). Association of FOXO3A variation with human longevity confirmed in German centenarians. *Proceedings of the National Academy of Sciences of the United States of America*, *106*, 2700–2705.

Fok, W. C., Zhang, Y., Salmon, A. B., Bhattacharya, A., Gunda, R., Jones, D., . . . Pérez, V. I. (2012). Short-term treatment with rapamycin and dietary restriction have overlapping and distinctive effects in young mice. *Journal of Gerontology. Series A, Biological Sciences & Medical Sciences*, *68*, 108–116.

Folmes, C. D., Nelson, T. J., Martinez-Fernandez, A., Arrell, D. K., Lindor, J. Z., Dzeja, P. P., . . . Terzic, A. (2011). Somatic oxidative bioenergetics transitions into pluripotency-dependent glycolysis to facilitate nuclear reprogramming. *Cell Metabolism*, *14*, 264–271.

Friedman, D. B., & Johnson, T. E. (1988). A mutation in the age-1 gene in *Caenorhabditis elegans* lengthens life and reduces hermaphrodite fertility. *Genetics*, *118*, 75–86.

Fulco, M., Cen, Y., Zhao, P., Hoffman, E. P., McBurney, M. W., Sauve, A. A., & Sartorelli, V. (2008). Glucose restriction inhibits skeletal myoblast differentiation by activating SIRT1 through AMPK-mediated regulation of Nampt. *Development Cell*, *14*, 661–673.

Gan, B., Hu, J., Jiang, S., Liu, Y., Sahin, E., Zhuang, L., . . . Depinho, R. A. (2010). Lkb1 regulates quiescence and metabolic homeostasis of haematopoietic stem cells. *Nature*, *468*, 701–704.

Gershman, B., Puig, O., Hang, L., Peitzsch, R. M., Tatar, M., & Garofalo, R. S. (2007). High-resolution dynamics of the transcriptional response to nutrition in *Drosophila*: A key role for dFOXO. *Physiological Genomics*, *29*, 24–34.

Giannakou, M. E., Goss, M., Jünger, M. A., Hafen, E., Leevers, S. J., & Partridge, L. (2004). Long-lived *Drosophila* with overexpressed dFOXO in adult fat body. *Science*, *305*, 361.

Giannakou, M. E., Goss, M., & Partridge, L. (2008). Role of dFOXO in lifespan extension by dietary restriction in *Drosophila melanogaster*: Not required, but its activity modulates the response. *Aging Cell*, *7*, 187–198.

Goertz, M. J., Wu, Z., Gallardo, T. D., Hamra, F. K., & Castrillon, D. H. (2011). FOXO1 is required in mouse spermatogonial stem cells for their maintenance and the initiation of spermatogenesis. *Journal of Clinical Investigation*, *121*, 3456–3466.

Greer, E. L., & Brunet, A. (2009). Different dietary restriction regimens extend lifespan by both independent and overlapping genetic pathways in *C. elegans*. *Aging Cell*, *8*, 113–127.

Greer, E. L., Dowlatshahi, D., Banko, M. R., Villen, J., Hoang, K., Blanchard, D., . . . Brunet, A. (2007). An AMPK-FOXO pathway mediates longevity induced by a novel method of dietary restriction in *C. elegans*. *Current Biology*, *17*, 1646–1656.

Greer, E. L., Oskoui, P. R., Banko, M. R., Maniar, J. M., Gygi, M. P., Gygi, S. P., & Brunet, A. (2007). The energy sensor AMP-activated protein kinase directly regulates the mammalian FOXO3 transcription factor. *Journal of Biological Chemistry*, *282*, 30107–30119.

Gurumurthy, S., Xie, S. Z., Alagesan, B., Kim, J., Yusuf, R. Z., Saez, B., . . . Bardeesy, N. (2010). The Lkb1 metabolic sensor maintains haematopoietic stem cell survival. *Nature*, *468*, 659–663.

Han, M. K., Song, E. K., Guo, Y., Ou, X., Mantel, C., & Broxmeyer, H. E. (2008). SIRT1 regulates apoptosis and Nanog expression in mouse embryonic stem cells by controlling p53 subcellular localization. *Cell Stem Cell*, *2*, 241–251.

Hansen, M., Chandra, A., Mitic, L. L., Onken, B., Driscoll, M., & Kenyon, C. (2008). A role for autophagy in the extension of lifespan by dietary restriction in *C. elegans*. *PLoS Genetics*, *4*, e24.

Hansen, M., Taubert, S., Crawford, D., Libina, N., Lee, S. J., & Kenyon, C. (2007). Lifespan extension by conditions that inhibit translation in *Caenorhabditis elegans*. *Aging Cell*, *6*, 95–110.

Hardie, D. G., Ross, F. A., & Hawley, S. A. (2012). AMPK: A nutrient and energy sensor that maintains energy homeostasis. *Nature Reviews & Molecular Cell Biology*, *13*, 251–262.

Harrison, D. E., Strong, R., Sharp, Z. D., Nelson, J. F., Astle, C. M., Flurkey, K., . . . Miller, R. A. (2009). Rapamycin fed late in life extends lifespan in genetically heterogeneous mice. *Nature*, *460*, 392–395.

Henderson, S. T., & Johnson, T. E. (2001). Daf-16 integrates developmental and environmental inputs to mediate aging in the nematode *Caenorhabditis elegans*. *Current Biology*, *11*, 1975–1980.

Herranz, D., Muñoz-Martin, M., Cañamero, M., Mulero, F., Martinez-Pastor, B., Fernandez-Capetillo, O., & Serrano, M. (2010). *Sirt1* improves healthy ageing and protects from metabolic syndrome-associated cancer. *Nature Commununicatons*, *1*, 3.

Hertweck, M., Gobel, C., & Baumeister, R. (2004). *C. elegans* SGK-1 is the critical component in the Akt/PKB kinase complex to control stress response and life span. *Developmental Cell*, *6*, 577–588.

Hoffmann, J., Romey, R., Fink, C., Yong, L., & Roeder, T. (2013). Overexpression of Sir2 in the adult fat body is sufficient to extend lifespan of male and female *Drosophila*. *Aging (Albany NY)*, *5*, 315–327.

Holzenberger, M., Dupont, J., Ducos, B., Leneuve, P., Géloën, A., Even, P. C., . . . Le Bouc, Y. (2003). IGF-1 receptor regulates lifespan and resistance to oxidative stress in mice. *Nature*, *421*, 182–187.

Honjoh, S., Yamamoto, T., Uno, M., & Nishida, E. (2009). Signalling through RHEB-1 mediates intermittent fasting-induced longevity in *C. elegans*. *Nature*, *457*, 726–730.

Howitz, K. T., Bitterman, K. J., Cohen, H. Y., Lamming, D. W., Lavu, S., Wood, J. G., . . . Sinclair, D. A. (2003). Small molecule activators of sirtuins extend *Saccharomyces cerevisiae* lifespan. *Nature*, *425*, 191–196.

Hsu, A. L., Murphy, C. T., & Kenyon, C. (2003). Regulation of aging and age-related disease by DAF-16 and heat-shock factor. *Science*, *300*, 1142–1145.

Hu, P., Geles, K. G., Paik, J. H., DePinho, R. A., & Tjian, R. (2008). Codependent activators direct myoblast-specific MyoD transcription. *Developmental Cell*, *15*, 534–546.

Hubbard, B. P., Gomes, A. P., Dai, H., Li, J., Case, A. W., Considine, T., . . . Sinclair, D. A. (2013). Evidence for a common mechanism of SIRT1 regulation by allosteric activators. *Science*, *339*, 1216–1219.

Hwangbo, D. S., Gershman, B., Tu, M. P., Palmer, M., & Tatar, M. (2004). *Drosophila* dFOXO controls lifespan and regulates insulin signalling in brain and fat body. *Nature*, *429*, 562–566.

Imai, S., Armstrong, C. M., Kaeberlein, M., & Guarente, L. (2000). Transcriptional silencing and longevity protein Sir2 is an NAD-dependent histone deacetylase. *Nature*, *403*, 795–800.

Imai, S., & Guarente, L. (2010). Ten years of NAD-dependent SIR2 family deacetylases: Implications for metabolic diseases. *Trends in Pharmacological Sciences*, *31*, 212–220.

Inoki, K., Li, Y., Xu, T., & Guan, K. L. (2003). Rheb GTPase is a direct target of TSC2 GAP activity and regulates mTOR signaling. *Genes & Development*, *17*, 1829–1834.

Inoki, K., Li, Y., Zhu, T., Wu, J., & Guan, K. L. (2002). TSC2 is phosphorylated and inhibited by Akt and suppresses mTOR signalling. *Nature Cell Biology*, *4*, 648–657.

Kaeberlein, M., Kirkland, K. T., Fields, S., & Kennedy, B. K. (2004). Sir2-independent life span extension by calorie restriction in yeast. *PLoS Biology*, *2*, E296.

Kaeberlein, M., McVey, M., & Guarente, L. (1999). The SIR2/3/4 complex and SIR2 alone promote longevity in *Saccharomyces cerevisiae* by two different mechanisms. *Genes & Development*, *13*, 2570–2580.

Kaeberlein, M., Powers, R. W., III, Steffen, K. K., Westman, E. A., Hu, D., Dang, N., . . . Kennedy, B. K. (2005). Regulation of yeast replicative life span by TOR and Sch9 in response to nutrients. *Science*, *310*, 1193–1196.

Kahn, B. B., Alquier, T., Carling, D., & Hardie, D. G. (2005). AMP-activated protein kinase: Ancient energy gauge provides clues to modern understanding of metabolism. *Cell Metabolism*, *1*, 15–25.

Kalaany, N. Y., & Sabatini, D. M. (2009). Tumours with PI3K activation are resistant to dietary restriction. *Nature*, *458*, 725–731.

Kalaitzidis, D., Sykes, S. M., Wang, Z., Punt, N., Tang, Y., Ragu, C., . . . Armstrong, S. A. (2012). mTOR complex 1 plays critical roles in hematopoiesis and Pten-loss-evoked leukemogenesis. *Cell Stem Cell*, *11*, 429–439.

Kanfi, Y., Naiman, S., Amir, G., Peshti, V., Zinman, G., Nahum, L., . . . Cohen, H. Y. (2012). The sirtuin SIRT6 regulates lifespan in male mice. *Nature*, *483*, 218–221.

Kapahi, P., Zid, B. M., Harper, T., Koslover, D., Sapin, V., & Benzer, S. (2004). Regulation of lifespan in *Drosophila* by modulation of genes in the TOR signaling pathway. *Current Biology*, *14*, 885–890.

Kawahara, T. L., Michishita, E., Adler, A. S., Damian, M., Berber, E., Lin, M., . . . Chua, K. F. (2009). SIRT6 links histone H3 lysine 9 deacetylation to NF-kappaB-dependent gene expression and organismal life span. *Cell*, *136*, 62–74.

Kenyon, C. J. (2010). The genetics of ageing. *Nature*, *464*, 504–512.

Kenyon, C., Chang, J., Gensch, E., Rudner, A., & Tabtiang, R. (1993). A *C. elegans* mutant that lives twice as long as wild type. *Nature*, *366*, 461–464.

Kim, D., Nguyen, M. D., Dobbin, M. M., Fischer, A., Sananbenesi, F., Rodgers, J. T., . . . Tsai, L. H. (2007). SIRT1 deacetylase protects against neurodegeneration in models for Alzheimer's disease and amyotrophic lateral sclerosis. *The EMBO Journal, 26*, 3169–3179.

Kim, D. H., Sarbassov, D. D., Ali, S. M., King, J. E., Latek, R. R., Erdjument-Bromage, H., . . . Sabatini, D. M. (2002). mTOR interacts with raptor to form a nutrient-sensitive complex that signals to the cell growth machinery. *Cell, 110*, 163–175.

Kim, J., Kundu, M., Viollet, B., & Guan, K. L. (2011). AMPK and mTOR regulate autophagy through direct phosphorylation of Ulk1. *Nature Cell Biology, 13*, 132–141.

Kimura, K. D., Tissenbaum, H. A., Liu, Y., & Ruvkun, G. (1997). daf-2, an insulin receptor-like gene that regulates longevity and diapause in *Caenorhabditis elegans*. *Science, 277*, 942–946.

Kippin, T. E., Martens, D. J., & van der Kooy, D. (2005). p21 loss compromises the relative quiescence of forebrain stem cell proliferation leading to exhaustion of their proliferation capacity. *Genes & Development, 19*, 756–767.

Koo, S. H., Flechner, L., Qi, L., Zhang, X., Screaton, R. A., Jeffries, S., . . . Montminy, M. (2005). The CREB coactivator TORC2 is a key regulator of fasting glucose metabolism. *Nature, 437*, 1109–1111.

Kops, G. J., de Ruiter, N. D., De Vries-Smits, A. M., Powell, D. R., Bos, J. L., & Burgering, B. M. (1999). Direct control of the Forkhead transcription factor AFX by protein kinase B. *Nature, 398*, 630–634.

Kwon, E. S., Narasimhan, S. D., Yen, K., & Tissenbaum, H. A. (2010). A new DAF-16 isoform regulates longevity. *Nature, 466*, 498–502.

Lamming, D. W., Ye, L., Katajisto, P., Goncalves, M. D., Saitoh, M., Stevens, D. M., . . . Baur, J. A. (2012). Rapamycin-induced insulin resistance is mediated by mTORC2 loss and uncoupled from longevity. *Science, 335*, 1638–1643.

Lapasset, L., Milhavet, O., Prieur, A., Besnard, E., Babled, A., Ait-Hamou, N., . . . Lemaitre, J. M. (2011). Rejuvenating senescent and centenarian human cells by reprogramming through the pluripotent state. *Genes & Development, 25*, 2248–2253.

Lapierre, L. R., De Magalhaes Filho, C. D., McQuary, P. R., Chu, C. C., Visvikis, O., Chang, J. T., . . . Hansen, M. (2013). The TFEB orthologue HLH-30 regulates autophagy and modulates longevity in *Caenorhabditis elegans*. *Nature Communications, 4*, 2267.

Laplante, M., & Sabatini, D. M. (2012). mTOR signaling in growth control and disease. *Cell, 149*, 274-293.

Lee, S. S., Kennedy, S., Tolonen, A. C., & Ruvkun, G. (2003). DAF-16 target genes that control *C. elegans* life-span and metabolism. *Science, 300*, 644–647.

Lee, Y. L., Peng, Q., Fong, S. W., Chen, A. C., Lee, K. F., Ng, E. H., . . . Yeung, W. S. (2012). Sirtuin 1 facilitates generation of induced pluripotent stem cells from mouse embryonic fibroblasts through the miR-34a and p53 pathways. *PLoS One, 7*, e45633.

Leko, V., Varnum-Finney, B., Li, H., Gu, Y., Flowers, D., Nourigat, C., . . . Bedalov, A. (2012). SIRT1 is dispensable for function of hematopoietic stem cells in adult mice. *Blood, 119*, 1856–1860.

Li, Y., Wang, W. J., Cao, H., Lu, J., Wu, C., Hu, F. Y., . . . Tian, X. L. (2009). Genetic association of FOXO1A and FOXO3A with longevity trait in Han Chinese populations. *Human Molecular Genetics*, *18*, 4897–4904.

Libina, N., Berman, J. R., & Kenyon, C. (2003). Tissue-specific activities of *C. elegans* DAF-16 in the regulation of lifespan. *Cell*, *115*, 489–502.

Lin, K., Dorman, J. B., Rodan, A., & Kenyon, C. (1997). daf-16: An HNF-3/forkhead family member that can function to double the life-span of *Caenorhabditis elegans*. *Science*, *278*, 1319–1322.

Lin, S. J., Defossez, P. A., & Guarente, L. (2000). Requirement of NAD and SIR2 for life-span extension by calorie restriction in *Saccharomyces cerevisiae*. *Science*, *289*, 2126–2128.

Liu, B., Ghosh, S., Yang, X., Zheng, H., Liu, X., Wang, Z., . . . Zhou, Z. (2012). Resveratrol rescues SIRT1-dependent adult stem cell decline and alleviates progeroid features in laminopathy-based progeria. *Cell Metabolism*, *16*, 738–750.

Liu, Y., Dentin, R., Chen, D., Hedrick, S., Ravnskjaer, K., Schenk, S., . . . Montminy, M. (2008). A fasting inducible switch modulates gluconeogenesis via activator/coactivator exchange. *Nature*, *456*, 269–273.

Lu, J. Y., Lin, Y. Y., Sheu, J. C., Wu, J. T., Lee, F. J., Chen, Y., . . . Boeke, J. D. (2011). Acetylation of yeast AMPK controls intrinsic aging independently of caloric restriction. *Cell*, *146*, 969–979.

Luo, J., Nikolaev, A. Y., Imai, S., Chen, D., Su, F., Shiloh, A., . . . Gu, W. (2001). Negative control of p53 by Sir2alpha promotes cell survival under stress. *Cell*, *107*, 137–148.

Ma, X. M., & Blenis, J. (2009). Molecular mechanisms of mTOR-mediated translational control. *Nature Reviews & Molecular Cell Biology*, *10*, 307–318.

Magri, L., Cambiaghi, M., Cominelli, M., Alfaro-Cervello, C., Cursi, M., Pala, M., . . . Galli, R. (2011). Sustained activation of mTOR pathway in embryonic neural stem cells leads to development of tuberous sclerosis complex-associated lesions. *Cell Stem Cell*, *9*, 447–462.

Mair, W., & Dillin, A. (2008). Aging and survival: The genetics of life span extension by dietary restriction. *Annual Review of Biochemistry*, *77*, 727–754.

Mair, W., Morantte, I., Rodrigues, A. P., Manning, G., Montminy, M., Shaw, R. J., & Dillin, A. (2011). Lifespan extension induced by AMPK and calcineurin is mediated by CRTC-1 and CREB. *Nature*, *470*, 404–408.

Mair, W., Panowski, S. H., Shaw, R. J., & Dillin, A. (2009). Optimizing dietary restriction for genetic epistasis analysis and gene discovery in *C. elegans*. *PLoS One*, *4*, e4535.

Manning, B. D., Tee, A. R., Logsdon, M. N., Blenis, J., & Cantley, L. C. (2002). Identification of the tuberous sclerosis complex-2 tumor suppressor gene product tuberin as a target of the phosphoinositide 3-kinase/akt pathway. *Molecular Cell*, *10*, 151–162.

Martin-Montalvo, A., Mercken, E. M., Mitchell, S. J., Palacios, H. H., Mote, P. L., Scheibye-Knudsen, M., . . . de Cabo, R. (2013). Metformin improves healthspan and lifespan in mice. *Nature Communications*, *4*, 2192.

McBurney, M. W., Yang, X., Jardine, K., Bieman, M., Th'ng, J., & Lemieux, M. (2003). The absence of SIR2alpha protein has no effect on global gene silencing in mouse embryonic stem cells. *Molecular Cancer Research, 1*, 402–409.

Medvedik, O., Lamming, D. W., Kim, K. D., & Sinclair, D. A. (2007). MSN2 and MSN4 link calorie restriction and TOR to sirtuin-mediated lifespan extension in *Saccharomyces cerevisiae*. *PLoS Biology, 5*, e261.

Mihaylova, M. M., & Shaw, R. J. (2011). The AMPK signalling pathway coordinates cell growth, autophagy and metabolism. *Nature Cell Biology, 13*, 1016–1023.

Mihaylova, M. M., Vasquez, D. S., Ravnskjaer, K., Denechaud, P. D., Yu, R. T., Alvarez, J. G., . . . Shaw, R. J. (2011). Class IIa histone deacetylases are hormone-activated regulators of FOXO and mammalian glucose homeostasis. *Cell, 145*, 607–621.

Milne, J. C., Lambert, P. D., Schenk, S., Carney, D. P., Smith, J. J., Gagne, D. J., . . . Westphal, C. H. (2007). Small molecule activators of SIRT1 as therapeutics for the treatment of type 2 diabetes. *Nature, 450*, 712–716.

Minor, R. K., Baur, J. A., Gomes, A. P., Ward, T. M., Csiszar, A., Mercken, E. M., . . . de Cabo, R. (2012). SRT1720 improves survival and healthspan of obese mice. *Scientific Reports, 1*, 70.

Miyamoto, K., Araki, K. Y., Naka, K., Arai, F., Takubo, K., Yamazaki, S., . . . Hirao, A. (2007). FOXO3a is essential for maintenance of the hematopoietic stem cell pool. *Cell Stem Cell, 1*, 101–112.

Morshead, C. M., Reynolds, B. A., Craig, C. G., McBurney, M. W., Staines, W. A., Morassutti, D., . . . van der Kooy, D. (1994). Neural stem cells in the adult mammalian forebrain: A relatively quiescent subpopulation of subependymal cells. *Neuron, 13*, 1071–1082.

Motta, M. C., Divecha, N., Lemieux, M., Kamel, C., Chen, D., Gu, W., . . . Guarente, L. (2004). Mammalian SIRT1 represses forkhead transcription factors. *Cell, 116*, 551–563.

Mouchiroud, L., Houtkooper, R. H., Moullan, N., Katsyuba, E., Ryu, D., Cantó, C., . . . Auwerx, J. (2013). The NAD(+)/Sirtuin Pathway Modulates Longevity through Activation of Mitochondrial UPR and FOXO Signaling. *Cell, 154*, 430–441.

Murakami, M., Ichisaka, T., Maeda, M., Oshiro, N., Hara, K., Edenhofer, F., . . . Yamanaka, S. (2004). mTOR is essential for growth and proliferation in early mouse embryos and embryonic stem cells. *Molecular & Cellular Biology, 24*, 6710–6718.

Murphy, C. T., Lee, S. J., & Kenyon, C. (2007). Tissue entrainment by feedback regulation of insulin gene expression in the endoderm of *Caenorhabditis elegans*. *Proceedings of the National Academy of Sciences of the United States of America, 104*, 19046–19050.

Murphy, C. T., McCarroll, S. A., Bargmann, C. I., Fraser, A., Kamath, R. S., Ahringer, J., . . . Kenyon, C. (2003). Genes that act downstream of DAF-16 to influence the lifespan of *Caenorhabditis elegans*. *Nature, 424*, 277–283.

Nakada, D., Saunders, T. L., & Morrison, S. J. (2010). Lkb1 regulates cell cycle and energy metabolism in haematopoietic stem cells. *Nature, 468*, 653–658.

Nakagawa, T., & Guarente, L. (2011). Sirtuins at a glance. *Journal of Cell Science, 124*, 833–838.

Nakahata, Y., Kaluzova, M., Grimaldi, B., Sahar, S., Hirayama, J., Chen, D., . . . Sassone-Corsi, P. (2008). The NAD+-dependent deacetylase SIRT1 modulates CLOCK-mediated chromatin remodeling and circadian control. *Cell, 134*, 329–340.

Narala, S. R., Allsopp, R. C., Wells, T. B., Zhang, G., Prasad, P., Coussens, M. J., . . . Vaziri, H. (2008). SIRT1 acts as a nutrient-sensitive growth suppressor and its loss is associated with increased AMPK and telomerase activity. *Molecular Biology of the Cell, 19*, 1210–1219.

Oberdoerffer, P., Michan, S., McVay, M., Mostoslavsky, R., Vann, J., Park, S. K., . . . Sinclair, D. A. (2008). SIRT1 redistribution on chromatin promotes genomic stability but alters gene expression during aging. *Cell, 135*, 907–918.

Ogg, S., Paradis, S., Gottlieb, S., Patterson, G. I., Lee, L., Tissenbaum, H. A., & Ruvkun, G. (1997). The Fork head transcription factor DAF-16 transduces insulin-like metabolic and longevity signals in *C. elegans. Nature, 389*, 994–999.

Oh, S. W., Mukhopadhyay, A., Dixit, B. L., Raha, T., Green, M. R., & Tissenbaum, H. A. (2006). Identification of direct DAF-16 targets controlling longevity, metabolism and diapause by chromatin immunoprecipitation. *Nature Genetics, 38*, 251–257.

Onken, B., & Driscoll, M. (2010). Metformin induces a dietary restriction-like state and the oxidative stress response to extend *C. elegans* Healthspan via AMPK, LKB1, and SKN-1. *PLoS One, 5*, e8758.

Ortega-Molina, A., Efeyan, A., Lopez-Guadamillas, E., Muñoz-Martin, M., Gómez-López, G., Cañamero, M., . . . Serrano, M. (2012). Pten positively regulates brown adipose function, energy expenditure, and longevity. *Cell Metabolism, 15*, 382–394.

Ou, X., Chae, H. D., Wang, R. H., Shelley, W. C., Cooper, S., Taylor, T., . . . Broxmeyer, H. E. (2010). SIRT1 deficiency compromises mouse embryonic stem cell hematopoietic differentiation, and embryonic and adult hematopoiesis in the mouse. *Blood, 117*, 440–450.

Paik, J. H., Ding, Z., Narurkar, R., Ramkissoon, S., Muller, F., Kamoun, W. S., . . . DePinho, R. A. (2009). FOXOs cooperatively regulate diverse pathways governing neural stem cell homeostasis. *Cell Stem Cell, 5*, 540–553.

Panopoulos, A. D., Yanes, O., Ruiz, S., Kida, Y. S., Diep, D., Tautenhahn, R., . . . Izpisua Belmonte, J. C. (2012). The metabolome of induced pluripotent stem cells reveals metabolic changes occurring in somatic cell reprogramming. *Cell Research, 22*, 168–177.

Panowski, S. H., Wolff, S., Aguilaniu, H., Durieux, J., & Dillin, A. (2007). PHA-4/Foxa mediates diet-restriction-induced longevity of *C. elegans. Nature, 447*, 550–555.

Paradis, S., Ailion, M., Toker, A., Thomas, J. H., & Ruvkun, G. (1999). A PDK1 homolog is necessary and sufficient to transduce AGE-1 PI3 kinase signals that regulate diapause in *Caenorhabditis elegans. Genes & Development, 13*, 1438–1452.

Paradis, S., & Ruvkun, G. (1998). *Caenorhabditis elegans* Akt/PKB transduces insulin receptor-like signals from AGE-1 PI3 kinase to the DAF-16 transcription factor. *Genes & Development, 12*, 2488–2498.

Pawlikowska, L., Hu, D., Huntsman, S., Sung, A., Chu, C., Chen, J., . . . Ziv, E. (2009). Association of common genetic variation in the insulin/IGF1 signaling pathway with human longevity. *Aging Cell, 8*, 460–472.

Pearson, K. J., Baur, J. A., Lewis, K. N., Peshkin, L., Price, N. L., Labinskyy, N., . . . de Cabo, R. (2008). Resveratrol delays age-related deterioration and mimics transcriptional aspects of dietary restriction without extending life span. *Cell Metabolism*, *8*, 157–168.

Peña-Llopis, S., Vega-Rubin-de-Celis, S., Schwartz, J. C., Wolff, N. C., Tran, T. A., Zou, L., . . . Brugarolas, J. (2011). Regulation of TFEB and V-ATPases by mTORC1. *The EMBO Journal*, *30*, 3242–3258.

Peterson, T. R., Sengupta, S. S., Harris, T. E., Carmack, A. E., Kang, S. A., Balderas, E., . . . Sabatini, D. M. (2011). mTOR complex 1 regulates lipin 1 localization to control the SREBP pathway. *Cell*, *146*, 408–420.

Potter, C. J., Pedraza, L. G., & Xu, T. (2002). Akt regulates growth by directly phosphorylating Tsc2. *Nature Cell Biology*, *4*, 658–665.

Prozorovski, T., Schulze-Topphoff, U., Glumm, R., Baumgart, J., Schröter, F., Ninnemann, O., . . . Aktas, O. (2008). *Sirt1* contributes critically to the redox-dependent fate of neural progenitors. *Nature Cell Biology*, *10*, 385–394.

Puig, O., Marr, M. T., Ruhf, M. L., & Tjian, R. (2003). Control of cell number by *Drosophila* FOXO: Downstream and feedback regulation of the insulin receptor pathway. *Genes & Development*, *17*, 2006–2020.

Rafalski, V. A., Ho, P. P., Brett, J. O., Ucar, D., Dugas, J. C., Pollina, E. A., . . . Brunet, A. (2013). Expansion of oligodendrocyte progenitor cells following SIRT1 inactivation in the adult brain. *Nature Cell Biology*, *15*, 614–624.

Rando, T. A., & Chang, H. Y. (2012). Aging, rejuvenation, and epigenetic reprogramming: Resetting the aging clock. *Cell*, *148*, 46–57.

Rathbone, C. R., Booth, F. W., & Lees, S. J. (2009). *Sirt1* increases skeletal muscle precursor cell proliferation. *European Journal of Cell Biology*, *88*, 35–44.

Renault, V. M., Rafalski, V. A., Morgan, A. A., Salih, D. A., Brett, J. O., Webb, A. E., . . . Brunet, A. (2009). FOXO3 regulates neural stem cell homeostasis. *Cell Stem Cell*, *5*, 527–539.

Riedel, C. G., Dowen, R. H., Lourenco, G. F., Kirienko, N. V., Heimbucher, T., West, J. A., . . . Ruvkun, G. (2013). DAF-16 employs the chromatin remodeller SWI/SNF to promote stress resistance and longevity. *Nature Cell Biology*, *15*, 491–501.

Robida-Stubbs, S., Glover-Cutter, K., Lamming, D. W., Mizunuma, M., Narasimhan, S. D., Neumann-Haefelin, E., . . . Blackwell, T. K. (2012). TOR signaling and rapamycin influence longevity by regulating SKN-1/Nrf and DAF-16/FOXO. *Cell Metabolism*, *15*, 713–724.

Roczniak-Ferguson, A., Petit, C. S., Froehlich, F., Qian, S., Ky, J., Angarola, B., . . . Ferguson, S. M. (2012). The transcription factor TFEB links mTORC1 signaling to transcriptional control of lysosome homeostasis. *Science Signaling*, *5*, ra42.

Rodgers, J. T., Lerin, C., Gerhart-Hines, Z., & Puigserver, P. (2008). Metabolic adaptations through the PGC-1 alpha and SIRT1 pathways. *FEBS Letters*, *582*, 46–53.

Rogina, B., & Helfand, S. L. (2004). Sir2 mediates longevity in the fly through a pathway related to calorie restriction. *Proceedings of the National Academy of Sciences of the United States of America*, *101*, 15998–16003.

Ruckh, J. M., Zhao, J. W., Shadrach, J. L., van Wijngaarden, P., Rao, T. N., Wagers, A. J., & Franklin, R. J. (2012). Rejuvenation of regeneration in the aging central nervous system. *Cell Stem Cell*, *10*, 96–103.

Sabatini, D. M., Erdjument-Bromage, H., Lui, M., Tempst, P., & Snyder, S. H. (1994). RAFT1: A mammalian protein that binds to FKBP12 in a rapamycin-dependent fashion and is homologous to yeast TORs. *Cell*, *78*, 35–43.

Sampath, P., Pritchard, D. K., Pabon, L., Reinecke, H., Schwartz, S. M., Morris, D. R., & Murry, C. E. (2008). A hierarchical network controls protein translation during murine embryonic stem cell self-renewal and differentiation. *Cell Stem Cell*, *2*, 448–460.

Sancak, Y., Bar-Peled, L., Zoncu, R., Markhard, A. L., Nada, S., & Sabatini, D. M. (2010). Ragulator-Rag complex targets mTORC1 to the lysosomal surface and is necessary for its activation by amino acids. *Cell*, *141*, 290–303.

Sancak, Y., Peterson, T. R., Shaul, Y. D., Lindquist, R. A., Thoreen, C. C., Bar-Peled, L., & Sabatini, D. M. (2008). The Rag GTPases bind raptor and mediate amino acid signaling to mTORC1. *Science*, *320*, 1496–1501.

Sarbassov, D. D., Ali, S. M., Kim, D. H., Guertin, D. A., Latek, R. R., Erdjument-Bromage, H., . . . Sabatini, D. M. (2004). Rictor, a novel binding partner of mTOR, defines a rapamycin-insensitive and raptor-independent pathway that regulates the cytoskeleton. *Current Biology*, *14*, 1296–1302.

Sarbassov, D. D., Guertin, D. A., Ali, S. M., & Sabatini, D. M. (2005). Phosphorylation and regulation of Akt/PKB by the rictor-mTOR complex. *Science*, *307*, 1098–1101.

Satoh, A., Brace, C. S., Rensing, N., Cliften, P., Wozniak, D. F., Herzog, E. D., . . . Imai, S. (2013). *Sirt1* extends life span and delays aging in mice through the regulation of Nk2 homeobox 1 in the DMH and LH. *Cell Metabolism*, *18*(3), 416–430.

Saunders, L. R., Sharma, A. D., Tawney, J., Nakagawa, M., Okita, K., Yamanaka, S., . . . Verdin, E. (2010). miRNAs regulate SIRT1 expression during mouse embryonic stem cell differentiation and in adult mouse tissues. *Aging (National Institute on Neurological Disorders and Stroke)*, *2*, 415–431.

Schieke, S. M., Ma, M., Cao, L., McCoy, J. P., Jr., Liu, C., Hensel, N. F., . . . Finkel, T. (2008). Mitochondrial metabolism modulates differentiation and teratoma formation capacity in mouse embryonic stem cells. *Journal of Biological Chemistry*, *283*, 28506–28512.

Selman, C., Lingard, S., Choudhury, A. I., Batterham, R. L., Claret, M., Clements, M., . . . Withers, D. J. (2008). Evidence for lifespan extension and delayed age-related biomarkers in insulin receptor substrate 1 null mice. *FASEB Journal*, *22*, 807–818.

Selman, C., Tullet, J. M., Wieser, D., Irvine, E., Lingard, S. J., Choudhury, A. I., . . . Withers, D. J. (2009). Ribosomal protein S6 kinase 1 signaling regulates mammalian life span. *Science*, *326*, 140–144.

Sengupta, S., Peterson, T. R., Laplante, M., Oh, S., & Sabatini, D. M. (2010). mTORC1 controls fasting-induced ketogenesis and its modulation by ageing. *Nature*, *468*, 1100–1104.

Settembre, C., Zoncu, R., Medina, D. L., Vetrini, F., Erdin, S., Huynh, T., . . . Ballabio, A. (2012). A lysosome-to-nucleus signalling mechanism senses and regulates the lysosome via mTOR and TFEB. *EMBO Journal*, *31*, 1095–1108.

Sharma, A., Diecke, S., Zhang, W. Y., Lan, F., He, C., Mordwinkin, N. M., . . . Wu, J. C. (2013). The role of SIRT6 protein in aging and reprogramming of human induced pluripotent stem cells. *Journal of Biological Chemistry*, *288*, 18439–18447.

Shaw, R. J., Lamia, K. A., Vasquez, D., Koo, S. H., Bardeesy, N., Depinho, R. A., . . . Cantley, L. C. (2005). The kinase LKB1 mediates glucose homeostasis in liver and therapeutic effects of metformin. *Science*, *310*, 1642–1646.

Singh, S. K., Williams, C. A., Klarmann, K., Burkett, S. S., Keller, J. R., & Oberdoerffer, P. (2013). *Sirt1* ablation promotes stress-induced loss of epigenetic and genomic hematopoietic stem and progenitor cell maintenance. *Journal of Experimental Medicine*, *210*, 987–1001.

Slack, C., Foley, A., & Partridge, L. (2012). Activation of AMPK by the putative dietary restriction mimetic metformin is insufficient to extend lifespan in *Drosophila*. *PLoS One*, *7*, e47699.

Soerensen, M., Dato, S., Christensen, K., McGue, M., Stevnsner, T., Bohr, V. A., & Christiansen, L. (2010). Replication of an association of variation in the FOXO3A gene with human longevity using both case-control and longitudinal data. *Aging Cell*, *9*, 1010–1017.

Soukas, A. A., Kane, E. A., Carr, C. E., Melo, J. A., & Ruvkun, G. (2009). Rictor/TORC2 regulates fat metabolism, feeding, growth, and life span in *Caenorhabditis elegans*. *Genes & Development*, *23*, 496–511.

Stenesen, D., Suh, J. M., Seo, J., Yu, K., Lee, K. S., Kim, J. S., . . . Graff, J. M. (2013). Adenosine nucleotide biosynthesis and AMPK regulate adult life span and mediate the longevity benefit of caloric restriction in flies. *Cell Metabolism*, *17*, 101–112.

Suh, Y., Atzmon, G., Cho, M. O., Hwang, D., Liu, B., Leahy, D. J., . . . Cohen, P. (2008). Functionally significant insulin-like growth factor I receptor mutations in centenarians. *Proceedings of the National Academy of Sciences of the United States of America*, *105*, 3438–3442.

Tanner, K. G., Landry, J., Sternglanz, R., & Denu, J. M. (2000). Silent information regulator 2 family of NAD- dependent histone/protein deacetylases generates a unique product, 1-O-acetyl-ADP-ribose. *Proceedings of the National Academy of Sciences of the United States of America*, *97*, 14178–14182.

Tatar, M., Kopelman, A., Epstein, D., Tu, M. P., Yin, C. M., & Garofalo, R. S. (2001). A mutant *Drosophila* insulin receptor homolog that extends life-span and impairs neuroendocrine function. *Science*, *292*, 107–110.

Timmers, S., Konings, E., Bilet, L., Houtkooper, R. H., van de Weijer, T., Goossens, G. H., . . . Schrauwen, P. (2011). Calorie restriction-like effects of 30 days of resveratrol supplementation on energy metabolism and metabolic profile in obese humans. *Cell Metabolism*, *14*, 612–622.

Tissenbaum, H. A., & Guarente, L. (2001). Increased dosage of a sir-2 gene extends lifespan in *Caenorhabditis elegans*. *Nature*, *410*, 227–230.

Tothova, Z., Kollipara, R., Huntly, B. J., Lee, B. H., Castrillon, D. H., Cullen, D. E., . . . Gilliland, D. G. (2007). FOXOs are critical mediators of hematopoietic stem cell resistance to physiologic oxidative stress. *Cell*, *128*, 325–339.

Tullet, J. M., Hertweck, M., An, J. H., Baker, J., Hwang, J. Y., Liu, S., . . . Blackwell, T. K. (2008). Direct inhibition of the longevity-promoting factor SKN-1 by insulin-like signaling in *C. elegans*. *Cell, 132*, 1025–1038.

Vaquero, A., Scher, M., Lee, D., Erdjument-Bromage, H., Tempst, P., & Reinberg, D. (2004). Human SIRT1 interacts with histone H1 and promotes formation of facultative heterochromatin. *Molecular Cell, 16*, 93–105.

Varum, S., Rodrigues, A. S., Moura, M. B., Momcilovic, O., Easley, C. A., IV, Ramalho-Santos, J., . . . Schatten, G. (2011). Energy metabolism in human pluripotent stem cells and their differentiated counterparts. *PLoS One, 6*, e20914.

Vaziri, H., Dessain, S. K., Ng Eaton, E., Imai, S. I., Frye, R. A., Pandita, T. K., . . . Weinberg, R. A. (2001). hSIR2(SIRT1) functions as an NAD-dependent p53 deacetylase. *Cell, 107*, 149–159.

Vazquez-Martin, A., Cufi, S., Lopez-Bonet, E., Corominas-Faja, B., Oliveras-Ferraros, C., Martin-Castillo, B., & Menendez, J. A. (2012). Metformin limits the tumourigenicity of iPS cells without affecting their pluripotency. *Scientific Reports, 2*, 964.

Vazquez-Martin, A., Vellon, L., Quirós, P. M., Cufi, S., Ruiz de Galarreta, E., Oliveras-Ferraros, C., . . . Menendez, J. A. (2012). Activation of AMP-activated protein kinase (AMPK) provides a metabolic barrier to reprogramming somatic cells into stem cells. *Cell Cycle, 11*, 974–989.

Vellai, T., Takacs-Vellai, K., Zhang, Y., Kovacs, A. L., Orosz, L., & Muller, F. (2003). Genetics: Influence of TOR kinase on lifespan in *C. elegans*. *Nature, 426*, 620.

Vilchez, D., Boyer, L., Lutz, M., Merkwirth, C., Morantte, I., Tse, C., . . . Dillin, A. (2013). FOXO4 is necessary for neural differentiation of human embryonic stem cells. *Aging Cell, 12*(3), 518–522.

Vilchez, D., Boyer, L., Morantte, I., Lutz, M., Merkwirth, C., Joyce, D., . . . Dillin, A. (2012). Increased proteasome activity in human embryonic stem cells is regulated by PSMD11. *Nature, 489*, 304–308.

Vilchez, D., Morantte, I., Liu, Z., Douglas, P. M., Merkwirth, C., Rodrigues, A. P., . . . Dillin, A. (2012). RPN-6 determines *C. elegans* longevity under proteotoxic stress conditions. *Nature, 489*, 263–268.

Villeda, S. A., Luo, J., Mosher, K. I., Zou, B., Britschgi, M., Bieri, G., . . . Wyss-Coray, T. (2011). The ageing systemic milieu negatively regulates neurogenesis and cognitive function. *Nature, 477*, 90–94.

Wang, Y., Tian, C., & Zheng, J. C. (2013). FOXO3a contributes to the reprogramming process and the differentiation of induced pluripotent stem cells. *Stem Cells Development*, 22(22), 2954–2963.

Wang, Y., & Tissenbaum, H. A. (2006). Overlapping and distinct functions for a *Caenorhabditis elegans* SIR2 and DAF-16/FOXO. *Mechanisms of Ageing & Development, 127*, 48–56.

Warr, M. R., Binnewies, M., Flach, J., Reynaud, D., Garg, T., Malhotra, R., . . . Passegue, E. (2013). FOXO3A directs a protective autophagy program in haematopoietic stem cells. *Nature, 494*(7437), 323–327.

Webb, A. E., Pollina, E. A., Vierbuchen, T., Urbán, N., Ucar, D., Leeman, D. S., . . . Brunet, A. (2013). FOXO3 shares common targets with ASCL1 genome-wide and inhibits ASCL1-dependent neurogenesis. *Cell Reports*, *4*(3), 477–491.

Willcox, B. J., Donlon, T. A., He, Q., Chen, R., Grove, J. S., Yano, K., . . . Curb, J. D. (2008). FOXO3A genotype is strongly associated with human longevity. *Proceedings of the National Academy of Sciences of the United States of America*, *105*, 13987–13992.

Wolkow, C. A., Kimura, K. D., Lee, M. S., & Ruvkun, G. (2000). Regulation of *C. elegans* life-span by insulinlike signaling in the nervous system. *Science*, *290*, 147–150.

Wood, J. G., Rogina, B., Lavu, S., Howitz, K., Helfand, S. L., Tatar, M., & Sinclair, D. (2004). Sirtuin activators mimic caloric restriction and delay ageing in metazoans. *Nature*, *430*, 686–689.

Yilmaz, Ö. H., Katajisto, P., Lamming, D. W., Gültekin, Y., Bauer-Rowe, K. E., Sengupta, S., . . . Sabatini, D. M. (2012). mTORC1 in the Paneth cell niche couples intestinal stem-cell function to calorie intake. *Nature*, *486*, 490–495.

Yu, Y., Liang, D., Tian, Q., Chen, X., Jiang, B., Chou, B. K., . . . Wang, G. (2013). Stimulation of somatic cell reprogramming by eras-akt-FOXO1 signaling axis. *Stem Cells*. Advance online publication. http://dx.doi.org/10.1002/stem.1447

Zhang, P., Judy, M., Lee, S. J., & Kenyon, C. (2013). Direct and indirect gene regulation by a life-extending FOXO protein in *C. elegans*: Roles for GATA factors and lipid gene regulators. *Cell Metabolism*, *17*, 85–100.

Zhang, X., Yalcin, S., Lee, D. F., Yeh, T. Y., Lee, S. M., Su, J., . . . Ghaffari, S. (2011). FOXO1 is an essential regulator of pluripotency in human embryonic stem cells. *Nature Cell Biology*, *13*, 1092–1099.

Zhou, J., Su, P., Wang, L., Chen, J., Zimmermann, M., Genbacev, O., . . . Wang, F. (2009). mTOR supports long-term self-renewal and suppresses mesoderm and endoderm activities of human embryonic stem cells. *Proceedings of the National Academy of Sciences of the United States of America*, *106*, 7840–7845.

Zid, B. M., Rogers, A. N., Katewa, S. D., Vargas, M. A., Kolipinski, M. C., Lu, T. A., . . . Kapahi, P. (2009). 4E-BP extends lifespan upon dietary restriction by enhancing mitochondrial activity in *Drosophila*. *Cell*, *139*, 149–160.

CHAPTER 2

Essential Genes and Lifespan

Sean P. Curran

ABSTRACT

Recent work in *Caenorhabditis elegans* has identified a class of longevity regulators that play essential roles in organismal development. These loci are particularly exciting because they represent some of the most well-conserved genes across phylogeny. The paradoxical relationship between the essentiality of these genes in the developmental progression toward adulthood and apparent obstruction to longevity in old age is reminiscent of the scenario described in the theory of antagonistic pleiotropy. Despite the complexity of the opposing roles of these genes, their potent effects on lifespan and the rate of aging, and their conserved functions across eukaryotes make them attractive targets for future mechanistic studies in mammals.

Essential genes define a conceptual framework for the minimal genome that can support cellular function. The concept of a minimalistic composition of a genome arose from the observation that many genes can be abolished without a noticeable influence on cellular function, suggesting that they are not necessary for survival (Hutchison et al., 1999). The essential genome comprises genetic loci that are lethal when absent. Lucien Cuénot (1905) first described such loci when he discovered the inability to obtain mice that were homozygous for yellow coat color. Castle and Little (1910) further analyzed this phenotype in the early 1900s when they observed that 25% of the litter did not make it past embryogenesis, confirming the lethality of the locus.

The study of essential genes is inherently difficult; however, the advent of RNA interference (RNAi) has allowed researchers to reduce the expression of any

http://dx.doi.org/10.1891/0198-8794.34.41

gene without completely abolishing it from the genome (Grishok et al., 2001; Timmons, Court, & Fire, 2001). Thus, the cellular and organismal functions of such genes can be revealed by extrapolating from the phenotypes associated with such knockdowns (Kamath & Ahringer, 2003). As such, many genome-wide RNAi screens have been performed, searching for specific phenotypes—such as adiposity (Ashrafi et al., 2003), genome maintenance (Pothof et al., 2003), development (Kamath et al., 2003), and lifespan (Dillin et al., 2002; Hamilton et al., 2005; Hansen, Hsu, Dillin, & Kenyon, 2005; S. S. Lee et al., 2003; Samuelson, Carr, & Ruvkun, 2007)—because each gene is independently knocked down.

This chapter will discuss the role of essential genes on the aging process. Of course, as would be expected, many essential genes are absolutely required from birth to death. However, work over the last decade has uncovered the surprising finding that many essential genes can be turned off in adulthood, and this can lead to a longevity state (see Figure 2.1; Curran & Ruvkun, 2007). Network analyses have also revealed a link between aging-related genes and development; known longevity-associated genes (LAGs) are enriched for essential genes or those required for development, and essential genes are equally enriched for LAGs (Budovsky et al., 2009; Curran & Ruvkun, 2007; de Magalhães & Toussaint, 2004; Tacutu, Budovsky, Wolfson, & Fraifeld, 2010; Tacutu, Budovsky, Yanai, & Fraifeld, 2011).

DEVELOPMENTAL ARREST AS A SURROGATE FOR LONGEVITY MUTANTS

Caenorhabditis elegans has proven to yield some of the most significant advances toward our understanding of the molecular and genetic determinants of lifespan and the rate of aging (M. Hansen, Flatt, & Aguilaniu, 2013; Kenyon, 2005; Wolff & Dillin, 2006). *C. elegans* is an attractive model for aging studies because it was the first multicellular organism to have its genome fully sequenced (*C. elegans* Sequencing Consortium, 1998), follows a simple and developmentally invariant body plan consisting of 959 somatic cells (Brenner, 1974; Ellis & Horvitz, 1986; Sulston & Brenner, 1974), utilizes a short developmental period (egg to adult in ~3 days), and lives a short reproducible lifespan of 2–3 weeks (M. R. Klass, 1983; M. Klass & Hirsh, 1976). Longevity genes and genes essential for development share a technical difficulty in a researcher's ability to isolate and study them tractably (Edgley, Baillie, Riddle, & Rose, 1995; Herman, Albertson, & Brenner, 1976; Johnson & Wood, 1982). Phenotypically, it is impossible, at the time of identification, to maintain either type of mutant because once longevity mutants are discovered, the long-lived organism has well surpassed its reproductive period, whereas mutations in essential genes prohibit an organism

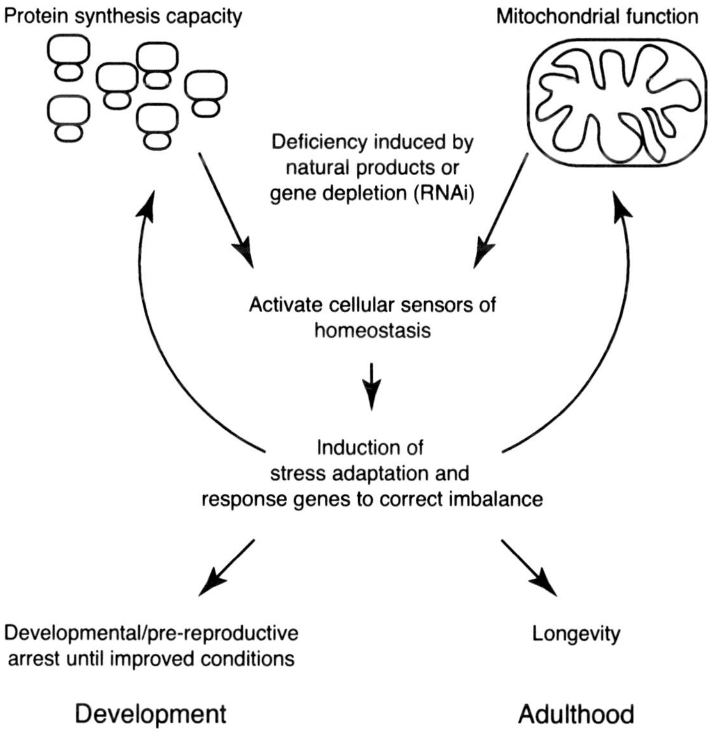

FIGURE 2.1 Model of arrest and longevity.

from ever making it to adulthood. As such, the first genetic mutants that were identified as long-lived were not isolated based on longevity but rather through changes in the ability to enter an alternative developmental state called *dauer* (Cassada & Russell, 1975; Golden & Riddle, 1984; Gottlieb & Ruvkun, 1994; Kenyon, Chang, Gensch, Rudner, & Tabtiang, 1993; Klass, 1983; Larsen, Albert, & Riddle, 1995).

The dauer state was first characterized by Michael Klass and David Hirsh in 1976 and was defined as nonaging by these researchers (Klass & Hirsh, 1976). Dauers, like most organisms that have exceptional longevity, are genetically primed to resist intracellular and extracellular insults encountered by the organism. These mutants came in two distinct classes: dauer formation-constitutive (Daf-c) and dauer formation-defective (Daf-d). The Daf-c genetic mutants, as their name implies, form dauers even in the absence of environmental cues that typically drive the dauer decision and maintain the dauer state even under developmentally favorable conditions. Intriguingly, the genetic pathways that regulate the dauer decision were subsequently shown to also act in adulthood and could potently regulate adult lifespan (Gottlieb & Ruvkun, 1994; Kenyon et al., 1993). Seminal work by the laboratories of Tom Johnson, Cynthia Kenyon, and Gary Ruvkun beautifully demonstrated that although early inactivation of this pathway could trap animals in the dauer state, thus preventing them from ever reaching adulthood, late inactivation could potently increase lifespan (Dorman, Albinder, Shroyer, & Kenyon, 1995; Gottlieb & Ruvkun, 1994; Larsen et al., 1995; Murakami & Johnson, 1996; Tissenbaum & Ruvkun, 1998; Wood & Johnson, 1994). As such, this was the first example of a genetic program that could regulate development that also affected adult lifespan. The Ruvkun and Kenyon laboratories also cloned and demonstrated that these mutations were in components of the mammalian insulin/IGF1-like signaling cascade (Kimura, Tissenbaum, Liu, & Ruvkun, 1997; Morris, Tissenbaum, & Ruvkun, 1996; Ogg et al., 1997; Paradis, Ailion, Toker, Thomas, & Ruvkun, 1999; Paradis & Ruvkun, 1998; Tissenbaum & Ruvkun, 1998). Subsequently, this highly conserved nutrient signaling pathway has been shown to modulate adult lifespan across phylogeny, including yeast, flies, mice, and potentially even humans (Longo & Finch, 2003).

RNAi DRIVES THE DISCOVERY OF ESSENTIAL LONGEVITY GENES

The discovery of RNAi as a methodology that allowed the research to specifically knockdown the expression of any gene in *C. elegans* accelerated the discovery of genes that could impact the rate of aging. RNAi in *C. elegans* is remarkably simple because it uses the standard laboratory food source, *Escherichia coli* (Timmons et al., 2001). In brief, these bacteria are designed to generate double stranded RNA specific for each gene coded for in the *C. elegans* genome. Individual bacteria strains have been generated to target nearly every single gene. Worms are then allowed to feed on each bacterial strain, where they ingest the double stranded RNA, which triggers the destruction of the specific mRNA.

Genome-wide RNAi screens, where worms are allowed to feed on each RNAi clone, have been performed and have identified hundreds of genes that can influence lifespan (Dillin et al., 2002; Hamilton et al., 2005; Hansen et al., 2005; S. S. Lee et al., 2003). These genes represent unique functional pathways that impact multiple aspects of cellular biology. Intriguingly, multiple genome-wide RNAi screens have been performed but yielded very few overlapping genes (S. S. Lee, 2006). The functional classes of genes, however, were similarly represented among these replicates. Most notable among these functional groups are genes involved in mitochondrial function, endocrine signaling, reproduction, and loci that mimic caloric restriction when inactivated.

These initial screens inactivated each gene from the earliest larval stage during development and then looked for adult lifespan phenotypes. Despite the large number of genes identified in these large-scale approaches, this methodology prevented the identification of developmental genes that could impact lifespan because early inactivation of these essential genes leads to pleiotropic phenotypes that prevent the animal from ever reaching adulthood. Therefore, postdevelopmental RNAi approaches were developed to begin the inactivation of these essential genes after the animals completed development (Curran & Ruvkun, 2007). This approach proved fruitful because screening the postdevelopmental knockdown of 2,700 essential genes identified 64 developmental genes (~2.4%) that could extend adult lifespan. This enrichment of longevity genes in the pool of essential genes was a significant increase in frequency as compared to the previous whole life, genome-wide RNAi screens that identified 89 out of 16,000 genes or 0.6% that could increase lifespan. A similar screen was performed in the Kapahi laboratory, challenging worms with RNAi targeting 57 essential genes (Chen, Pan, Palter, & Kapahi, 2007). Only 4 genes were identified in both screens: 1 translation factor, *eIF3f*; and 3 mitochondrial genes, *F59C6.5*, *spg7*, and *atp3*. The lack of overlap is likely caused by the different number of RNAi clones sampled in the two screens and the fact that Curran and Ruvkun (2007) used a worm strain with enhanced sensitivity to RNAi (Kennedy, Wang, & Ruvkun, 2004; Simmer et al., 2002). However, like the previous genome-wide RNAi screens, both screens uncovered similar functional classes of genes including protein synthesis, mitochondrial respiration, and mRNA processing (Yanos, Bennett, & Kaeberlein, 2012).

The unbiased identification of the involvement of essential protein synthesis pathways on lifespan is further supported by directed studies from the Kenyon, Tavernarakis, and Kapahi laboratories, which collectively demonstrated that reduced translation leads to longevity (Hansen et al., 2007; Hipkiss, 2007; Pan et al., 2007; Syntichaki, Troulinaki, & Tavernarakis, 2007). Mitochondrial function is a well-established regulator of lifespan (Chen et al., 2007; Curran & Ruvkun, 2007; Dillin et al., 2002; Durieux, Wolff, & Dillin, 2011; Hekimi & Guarente, 2003; Larsen & Clarke, 2002; S. S. Lee et al., 2003; Lemire, Behrendt, DeCorby, & Gaskova, 2009; Paek et al., 2012; Rea & Johnson, 2003). The slowed metabolism and diminished production of ATP through mitochondrial deficiency is thought to slow the aging process as predicted by the rate of living theory of aging by Raymond Pearl in 1928 (Pearl, 1928; Speakman, Selman, McLaren, & Harper, 2002). Although primarily regarded as the major contributor of cellular energy, mitochondria are also generators of reactive oxygen species (ROS). ROS play a complicated role in the aging process (S. J. Lee, Hwang, & Kenyon, 2010; Yang & Hekimi, 2010; Zarse et al., 2012). Too much ROS can lead to cellular damage and increased rates of aging, whereas low levels of ROS have proven to be beneficial and can induce genetically coded cytoprotective pathways, which may contribute to the longevity phenotype (An et al., 2005; Durieux et al., 2011; Nargund, Pellegrino, Fiorese, Baker, & Haynes, 2012; Paek et al., 2012; Park, Tedesco, & Johnson, 2009).

An analysis of the essential longevity genes reveals that many use the transcription factor DAF-16/FOXO, which is central to the insulin/IGF1 pathway (Johnson et al., 2002; R. Y. Lee, Hench, & Ruvkun, 2001; S. S. Lee, Kennedy, Tolonen, & Ruvkun, 2003; Libina, Berman, & Kenyon, 2003; Lin, Dorman, Rodan, & Kenyon, 1997; Murphy et al., 2003; Ogg, et al., 1997). Notably, inactivation of the mitochondrial and protein synthesis genes was capable of increasing lifespan independent of this canonical mechanism (Chen et al., 2007; Curran & Ruvkun, 2007). Intriguingly, although DAF-16 was dispensable for the longevity phenotype, inactivation of the protein synthesis machinery was still capable of inducing DAF-16 nuclear localization and activity as measured by the expression of the DAF-16 target gene *sod-3*. The downstream factors that respond to the diminished protein synthesis capacity and facilitate the longevity phenotype remain elusive.

Network biology has become a proven approach to understanding complex biological systems and phenotypes such as aging. Networks have been built from essentially all biological relevant and well-annotated pathways. Because most biological systems are often executed by protein complexes, it seemed reasonable to assume that the protein–protein interactors of the essential longevity regulators would also participate in the regulation of lifespan. Tacutu et al. (2012) developed an intricate interaction map of the known LAGs from yeast, worms, and humans and then interrogated the first-order interactors for longevity phenotypes. The results of this analysis confirmed that the human and worm longevity networks were functionally relevant and could be used as a powerful tool to predict new longevity modulators (see Figure 2.1). Despite the fact that the new essential longevity modulators identified by this methodology were only modestly capable of altering life expectancy, the design of this approach was to uncover regulatory and peripheral components of longevity-effecting complexes. It is plausible that the initial screens of the essential genome picked up the strongest hits and that the new genes represent modifiers of core longevity pathways. Approximately 25% of the LAGs identified in the worm are interconnected, in comparison to a randomized selection of genes of the same size where ~5% are interconnected. As more LAGs are added into the network, the interconnectivity changes with it. Importantly, 66% of the newly identified LAGs derived from initial bioinformatics analysis are connected to at least one prominent lifespan modulator (*daf-2*, *bar-1*, and *clk-2*). Moreover, five genes from this analysis are connected to all three of these pathways. This initial work that integrates computational and molecular approaches to the identification of longevity networks can now be applied across diverse organisms as soon as relevant networks are constructed.

TARGETING ESSENTIAL PATHWAYS IN NATURE

Complete loss of function of an essential gene during development typically results in death. However, in the case of RNAi, essential genes can be simply knocked down, leaving a small amount of normal gene activity remaining. In many cases, early knock-down of essential genes results in a developmental arrest phenotype in an immature state (Kamath et al., 2003; Simmer et al., 2002; Tewari et al., 2004; Timmons et al., 2001). This prereproductive arrest could provide an advantageous adaptive mechanism, which contributes to evolutionary success. Indeed, the Insulin/IGF1 signaling pathway represents the classical example of this adaptive arrest pathway (Arantes-Oliveira, Berman, & Kenyon, 2003). As previously discussed, mutations in *daf-2* (insulin/IGF1 receptor), which can lead to longevity in adulthood, result in constitutive arrest in the dauer stage if the inactivation occurs in development. Similarly, mutations in *daf-16* (FOXO transcription factor), which have a short adult lifespan, also fail to arrest at the dauer stage, as well as L1 larvae, in the absence of food (Baugh & Sternberg, 2006; Vowels & Thomas, 1992). Although there are exceptions to the rule, collectively, a clear trend emerges where mutants that are more prone to arrest are long-lived, whereas mutations that suppress the ability to arrest are short-lived (Antebi, Culotti, & Hedgecock, 1998; Cassada & Russell, 1975; Dorman et al., 1995; Golden & Riddle, 1984; Gottlieb & Ruvkun, 1994; Kenyon et al., 1993; Kimura et al., 1997; Klass, 1983; Larsen, 1993; Larsen et al., 1995; Murakami & Johnson, 1996; Ogg et al., 1997; Tissenbaum & Ruvkun, 1998; Vowels & Thomas, 1992). Why would arrest correlate with longevity? We can gain insight into this question when we consider the case of the dauer pathway. The environmental triggers that influence dauer entry and exit are abundance of food, population density, and temperature. These three conditions have a direct impact on the evolutionary success of an animal or, in other words, the ability of an animal to successfully pass genetic material to the next generation. Prereproductive arrest in an environment of low food, crowding, and high temperature can facilitate the initiation of a biological "pause button" where an animal can wait until conditions improve before initiating reproduction, thus increasing the chances of success of its progeny.

Similarly, early inactivation of many other essential genes leads to highly penetrant arrest at various larval stages (Curran & Ruvkun, 2007; Melo & Ruvkun, 2012; Shore & Ruvkun, 2013). Unlike the insulin/IGF1 pathway mutants, these animals don't form dauers but can survive in the arrested state for extended periods, far beyond the normal 2- to 3-week lifespan of a normal animal but shorter than dauer diapause. Similarly, to the insulin/IGF1 pathway mutants, induction of the arrested state and survival in that state was modulated by DAF-16/FOXO. This provides an intriguing hypothesis that animals have the capacity to trigger developmental arrest to help ensure survival.

The ability to survive for extended periods in less than ideal environmental conditions requires the activation of cellular proactive mechanisms including but not limited to electrophile response pathways, protein folding chaperones and proteases, metabolic adaptation mechanisms, and DNA damage and repair pathways (Hwang, Jeong, & Lee, 2012; Kaeberlein, 2012; Yanos et al., 2012). Many of these pathways that ensure the successful arrest and recovery when essential genes are inactivated early are also induced in conditions that lead to long-lived adults. As such, it would seem that the longevity associated with adult-specific inactivation of essential genes results from hijacking well-established and highly regulated developmental pathways.

In the case of *C. elegans*, the idea of targeting essential development pathways was not first attempted in the laboratory, but instead represents an ancient battle between microorganisms in the wild. Components of the protein synthesis machinery were among the pathways that most potently induced developmental arrest and longevity. Translation is one of the major targets of antibiotics, which are manufactured by fungi and other microbes that *C. elegans* can encounter in the environment (Huss et al., 2002; Tercero, Espinosa, Lacalle, & Jiménez, 1996). As larvae move into an environment with high levels of antibiotic, signaling pathways, including those that converge upon DAF-16/FOXO, are engaged to trigger developmental arrest and xenobiotic detoxification. This induced arrest would facilitate protection until the animal could escape the antibiotic and then resume reproductive development. As such, in the laboratory, RNAi inactivation of the ribosome and translational machinery may mimic the translational deficiency sensed in the presence of antibiotics in the wild. These studies are particularly exciting because they suggest that an organismal protective mechanism can be induced by exposure to small molecules that target specific cellular targets. Compounds developed to activate these pathways without other pleiotropic side effects could become pharmacological factors to suppress age-related deficiencies.

THE DISPENSABILITY OF ESSENTIAL GENE PARADOX

Despite decades of fantastic work and discoveries, the biological basis of aging and longevity is unknown. Multiple theories have been proposed to explain the process of aging (Finch, 1993). However, alone, none of these current theories can satisfactorily define this exceptionally complicated phenomenon.

It might seem ironic that lifespan can be extended in *C. elegans* by disruption of essential cellular processes, such as insulin/IGF1 signaling, mitochondrial function, and disruption of protein synthesis. Each of these deficiencies evokes a cellular stress response that likely evokes a hormetic mechanism that leads to a longevity promoting physiological state. Hormesis is defined by the observation that minor exposure to stress induces a stress response that can persist beyond conquering the perceived stress. This lingering response leads to a stronger physiologic state (Neafsey, 1990; Neafsey, Boxenbaum, Ciraulo, & Fournier, 1988). This idea of hormesis was recently tested and confirmed a conserved cytoprotective regulatory cascade that is critical for stress tolerance and the extension of lifespan induced by perturbing these essential cellular pathways (Shore & Ruvkun, 2013). Importantly, this pathway has little effect on normal longevity and appears specific to maintaining arrest and a long-lived state. An examination of the overlapping regulatory signals and the synergistic additivity between these distinct pathways with regard to the hormesis model has yet to be studied, but perhaps if a little stress indeed makes you stronger, then a tiny bit of different stresses can make you the strongest.

The postdevelopmental inactivation of essential genes by RNAi is among the most potent interventions to increase the lifespan and health span of *C. elegans* (Chen et al., 2007; Curran & Ruvkun, 2007; M. Hansen et al., 2007; Melo & Ruvkun, 2012; Pan et al., 2007; Syntichaki et al., 2007; Tacutu et al., 2012). The identification of these essential modulators of lifespan provides experimental support for the theory of antagonistic pleiotropy, first proposed by George Williams in 1957 (Williams, 1957). By definition, the term *antagonistic pleiotropy* seems perfect for these essential genes that influence lifespan. They are pleiotropic because a single gene can impact more than one phenotype (development and lifespan) and antagonistic as the normal role of these genes is beneficial in the context of development but detrimental for longevity. The theory of antagonistic pleiotropy provides the framework for how essential genes that have such a strong effect on lifespan have been selected for across evolutionary time; the selection occurs on the level of the developmental role. In other words, the beneficial effects of the gene early in life have a larger impact on fitness. There are multiple examples of this in human physiology as well. Testosterone levels in men can lead to increased fitness early in life, but lead to a higher risk of prostate cancer in old age (Gann, Hennekens, Ma, Longcope, & Stampfer, 1996). The tumor suppressor p53 can confer protection against cancer by blocking the proliferation of abnormal cells. However, blockage of proliferation in stem cells can inhibit tissue repair and homeostasis, which accelerates the rate of aging (Ungewitter & Scrable, 2009). Similarly, apolipoprotein E4 has been linked to the development of Alzheimer's disease but may actually be beneficial for younger populations (Tuminello & Han, 2011).

The essential genes and pathways previously discussed have many similar characteristics. Early use of these genes provides the molecular basis of rapid development through reproduction, but postreproductively their continued activity is detrimental. For example, in *C. elegans*, with age, when sperm becomes depleted oocytes still accumulate and densely pack within the germline and yolk proteins can be found in inappropriate tissues because of failed localization, cuticle overgrowth causes blebbing and hypodermal tissue irregularities, and lipids are deposited inappropriately in the body wall muscle cells (Herndon et al., 2002; Jud et al., 2008). RNAi inactivation of the factors that control these biological functions, during adulthood, can alleviate the adult-specific detrimental effects.

Intriguingly, the Kenyon and Lithgow laboratories looked at the composition of protein aggregates, whose size and number increase with age, and identified the protein products of many essential genes (David et al., 2010; Reis-Rodrigues et al., 2012). The presence of these proteins in these aggregates may represent the cell's attempt to sequester essential players that have outlived their cellular usefulness to inactivate them. This finding begs the question, however, of how postdevelopmental RNAi of essential genes increases lifespan. Is it the reduced biochemical activity of these proteins during adulthood that signals a stress response or is it simply a reduction in the abundance of these proteins, which alleviates the need to inactivate and corral them, allowing cellular resources to be directed elsewhere. The future identification of chemical inhibitors of the biochemical function of essential pathways will help to clarify this distinction.

Consistent with the idea that the continued activity of essential genes in adulthood contributes to the aging process, a recently proposed new theory was conceived by Blagosklonny that introduces the proposition that aging is caused by hyperfunction (Blagosklonny, 2012; Gems & de la Guardia, 2013). Hyperfunction is the overactivity of developmental processes during adulthood. Most of these processes are representatives of biosynthetic pathways that contribute to development as well as reproduction. This new theory supports the notion that aging is actually programmed, in that the degree of hyperfunction can lead to hypertrophy-associated pathologies, which cause the age increase in death, and this rate is set by the activity of essential and developmental genes.

PERSPECTIVES

Essential genes are of particular interest because throughout evolution their functions have been maintained and they represent a set of the most conserved genes from yeast to man. These genes have evolved to facilitate the smooth progression through development, expediting the time to reproductive maturity, and ensuring the faithful transmission of genetic information to the next generation.

Conceptually, evolution had no reason to develop an off switch for these essential genes because this would oppose a pathway designed to increase fitness. In addition, the detrimental effects of these genes are not apparent until the postreproductive period, where selective pressure is diminished. In *C. elegans*, it has become increasingly clear that regulating the expression of these essential genes postdevelopmentally provides a clear survival advantage. Although a more thorough understanding of the mechanisms underlying the increased longevity resulting from essential gene perturbation in adulthood is needed, the high degree of conservation of these targets, in both structure and function, should perhaps prioritize them for translational studies in humans.

ACKNOWLEDGMENTS

Special thanks to Dr. Shanshan Pang, PhD and Jacqueline Lo for thoughtful discussions. S.P.C. is Ellison Medical Foundation New Scholar in Aging.

REFERENCES

An, J. H., Vranas, K., Lucke, M., Inoue, H., Hisamoto, N., Matsumoto, K., & Blackwell, T. K. (2005). Regulation of the *Caenorhabditis elegans* oxidative stress defense protein SKN-1 by glycogen synthase kinase-3. *Proceedings of the National Academy of Sciences of the United States of America*, *102*(45), 16275–16280.

Antebi, A., Culotti, J. G., & Hedgecock, E. M. (1998). daf-12 regulates developmental age and the dauer alternative in *Caenorhabditis elegans*. *Development*, *125*(7), 1191–1205.

Arantes-Oliveira, N., Berman, J. R., & Kenyon, C. (2003). Healthy animals with extreme longevity. *Science*, *302*(5645), 611.

Ashrafi, K., Chang, F. Y., Watts, J. L., Fraser, A. G., Kamath, R. S., Ahringer, J., & Ruvkun, G. (2003). Genome-wide RNAi analysis of *Caenorhabditis elegans* fat regulatory genes. *Nature*, *421*(6920), 268–272. http://dx.doi.org/10.1038/nature01279

Baugh, L., & Sternberg, P. (2006). DAF-16/FOXO regulates transcription of cki-1/Cip/Kip and repression of lin-4 during *C. elegans* L1 arrest. *Current Biology*, *16*(8), 780–785. http://dx.doi.org/10.1016/j.cub.2006.03.021

Blagosklonny, M. V. (2012). Answering the ultimate question "what is the proximal cause of aging?" *Aging*, *4*(12), 861–877.

Brenner, S. (1974). The genetics of *Caenorhabditis elegans*. *Genetics*, *77*(1), 71–94.

Budovsky, A., Tacutu, R., Yanai, H., Abramovich, A., Wolfson, M., & Fraifeld, V. (2009). Common gene signature of cancer and longevity. *Mechanisms of Ageing & Development*, *130*(1–2), 33–39. http://dx.doi.org/10.1016/j.mad.2008.04.002

C. elegans Sequencing Consortium. (1998). Genome sequence of the nematode *C. elegans*: A platform for investigating biology. *Science*, *282*(5396), 2012–2018.

Cassada, R., & Russell, R. (1975). The dauerlarva, a post-embryonic developmental variant of the nematode *Caenorhabditis elegans*. *Developmental Biology*, *46*(2), 326–342.

Castle, W. E., & Little, C. C. (1910). On a modified Mendelian ratio among yellow mice. *Science*, *32*(833), 868–870. http://dx.doi.org/10.1126/science.32.833.868

Chen, D., Pan, K. Z., Palter, J. E., & Kapahi, P. (2007). Longevity determined by developmental arrest genes in *Caenorhabditis elegans*. *Aging cell*, *6*(4), 525–533. http://dx.doi.org/10.1111/j.1474-9726.2007.00305.x

Cuénot, L. (1905). Les races pures et leurs combinaisons chez les souris. *Archives de Zoologie Experimentale et Generale*, *4*, 123–132.

Curran, S., & Ruvkun, G. (2007). Lifespan regulation by evolutionarily conserved genes essential for viability. *PLoS Genetics*, *3*(4), e56. http://dx.doi.org/10.1371/journal.pgen.0030056

David, D. C., Ollikainen, N., Trinidad, J. C., Cary, M. P., Burlingame, A. L., & Kenyon, C. (2010). Widespread protein aggregation as an inherent part of aging in *C. elegans*. *PLoS Biology*, *8*(8), e1000450. http://dx.doi.org/10.1371/journal.pbio.1000450

de Magalhães, J. P., & Toussaint, O. (2004). GenAge: A genomic and proteomic network map of human ageing. *FEBS Letters*, *571*(1–3), 243–247. http://dx.doi.org/10.1016/j.febslet.2004.07.006

Dillin, A., Hsu, A., Arantes-Oliveira, N., Lehrer-Graiwer, J., Hsin, H., Fraser, A., . . . Kenyon, C. (2002). Rates of behavior and aging specified by mitochondrial function during development. *Science*, *298*(5602), 2398–2401. http://dx.doi.org/10.1126/science.1077780

Dorman, J. B., Albinder, B., Shroyer, T., & Kenyon, C. (1995). The age-1 and daf-2 genes function in a common pathway to control the lifespan of *Caenorhabditis elegans*. *Genetics*, *141*(4), 1399–1406.

Durieux, J., Wolff, S., & Dillin, A. (2011). The cell-non-autonomous nature of electron transport chain-mediated longevity. *Cell*, *144*(1), 79–91. http://dx.doi.org10.1016/j.cell.2010.12.016

Edgley, M. L., Baillie, D. L., Riddle, D. L., & Rose, A. M. (1995). Genetic balancers. [Review]. *Methods in Cell Biology*, *48*, 147–184.

Ellis, H. M., & Horvitz, H. R. (1986). Genetic control of programmed cell death in the nematode *C. elegans*. *Cell*, *44*(6), 817–829.

Finch, C. E. (1993). FRAR course on laboratory approaches to aging. Theories of aging. [Review]. *Aging*, *5*(4), 277–289.

Gann, P. H., Hennekens, C. H., Ma, J., Longcope, C., & Stampfer, M. J. (1996). Prospective study of sex hormone levels and risk of prostate cancer. *Journal of the National Cancer Institute*, *88*(16), 1118–1126.

Gems, D., & de la Guardia, Y. (2013). Alternative perspectives on aging in *Caenorhabditis elegans*: Reactive oxygen species or hyperfunction? *Antioxidants & Redox Signaling*, *19*(3), 321–329. http://dx.doi.org/10.1089/ars.2012.4840

Golden, J. W., & Riddle, D. L. (1984). The *Caenorhabditis elegans* dauer larva: Developmental effects of pheromone, food, and temperature. *Developmental Biology*, *102*(2), 368–378.

Gottlieb, S., & Ruvkun, G. (1994). daf-2, daf-16 and daf-23: Genetically interacting genes controlling Dauer formation in *Caenorhabditis elegans*. *Genetics*, *137*(1), 107–120.

Grishok, A., Pasquinelli, A. E., Conte, D., Li, N., Parrish, S., Ha, I., . . . Mello, C. C. (2001). Genes and mechanisms related to RNA interference regulate expression of the small temporal RNAs that control *C. elegans* developmental timing. *Cell*, *106*(1), 23–34.

Hamilton, B., Dong, Y., Shindo, M., Liu, W., Odell, I., Ruvkun, G., & Lee, S. S. (2005). A systematic RNAi screen for longevity genes in *C. elegans*. *Genes Dev*, *19*(13), 1544–1555.

Hansen, M., Flatt, T., & Aguilaniu, H. (2013). Reproduction, fat metabolism, and life span: What is the connection? *Cell Metabolism*, *17*(1), 10–19. http://dx.doi.org/10.1016/j.cmet.2012.12.003

Hansen, M., Hsu, A. L., Dillin, A., & Kenyon, C. (2005). New genes tied to endocrine, metabolic, and dietary regulation of lifespan from a *Caenorhabditis elegans* genomic RNAi screen. *PLoS Genetics*, *1*(1), e17.

Hansen, M., Taubert, S., Crawford, D., Libina, N., Lee, S., & Kenyon, C. (2007). Lifespan extension by conditions that inhibit translation in *Caenorhabditis elegans*. *Aging Cell*, *6*(1), 95–110. http://dx.doi.org/10.1111/j.1474-9726.2006.00267.x

Hekimi, S., & Guarente, L. (2003). Genetics and the specificity of the aging process. *Science*, *299*(5611), 1351–1354.

Herman, R. K., Albertson, D. G., & Brenner, S. (1976). Chromosome rearrangements in *Caenorhabditis elegans*. *Genetics*, *83*(1), 91–105.

Herndon, L. A., Schmeissner, P. J., Dudaronek, J. M., Brown, P. A., Listner, K. M., Sakano, Y., . . . Driscoll, M. (2002). Stochastic and genetic factors influence tissue-specific decline in ageing *C. elegans*. *Nature*, *419*(6909), 808–814. http://dx.doi.org/10.1038/nature01135

Hipkiss, A. R. (2007). On why decreasing protein synthesis can increase lifespan. *Mechanisms of Ageing & Development*, *128*(5–6), 412–414. http://dx.doi.org/10.1016/j.mad.2007.03.002

Huss, M., Ingenhorst, G., König, S., Gassel, M., Dröse, S., Zeeck, A., . . . Wieczorek, H. (2002). Concanamycin A, the specific inhibitor of V-ATPases, binds to the V(o) subunit c. *Journal of Biological Chemistry*, *277*(43), 40544–40548.

Hutchison, C. A., Peterson, S. N., Gill, S. R., Cline, R. T., White, O., Fraser, C. M., . . . Venter, J. C. (1999). Global transposon mutagenesis and a minimal *Mycoplasma* genome. *Science*, *286*(5447), 2165–2169.

Hwang, A. B., Jeong, D. E., & Lee, S. J. (2012). Mitochondria and organismal longevity. *Current Genomics*, *13*(7), 519–532. http://dx.doi.org/10.2174/138920212803251427

Johnson, T. E., Henderson, S., Murakami, S., de Castro, E., de Castro, S. H., Cypser, J., . . . Link, C. (2002). Longevity genes in the nematode *Caenorhabditis elegans* also mediate increased resistance to stress and prevent disease. [Review]. *Journal of Inherited Metabolic Disease*, *25*(3), 197–206.

Johnson, T. E., & Wood, W. B. (1982). Genetic analysis of life-span in *Caenorhabditis elegans*. *Proceedings of the National Academy of Sciences of the United States of America*, *79*(21), 6603–6607.

Jud, M. C., Czerwinski, M. J., Wood, M. P., Young, R. A., Gallo, C. M., Bickel, J. S., . . . Schisa, J. A. (2008). Large P body-like RNPs form in *C. elegans* oocytes in response to arrested ovulation, heat shock, osmotic stress, and anoxia and are regulated by the major sperm protein pathway. *Developmental Biology*, *318*(1), 38–51. http://dx.doi.org/10.1016/j.ydbio.2008.02.059

Kaeberlein, M. (2012). Genomics and genetics of aging. *Current Genomics*, *13*(7), 499. http://dx.doi.org/10.2174/138920212803251409

Kamath, R. S., & Ahringer, J. (2003). Genome-wide RNAi screening in *Caenorhabditis elegans*. *Methods*, *30*(4), 313–321.

Kamath, R. S., Fraser, A. G., Dong, Y., Poulin, G., Durbin, R., Gotta, M., . . . Ahringer, J. (2003). Systematic functional analysis of the *Caenorhabditis elegans* genome using RNAi. *Nature*, *421*(6920), 231–237. http://dx.doi.org/10.1038/nature01278

Kennedy, S., Wang, D., & Ruvkun, G. (2004). A conserved siRNA-degrading RNase negatively regulates RNA interference in *C. elegans*. *Nature*, *427*(6975), 645–649.

Kenyon, C. (2005). The plasticity of aging: Insights from long-lived mutants. *Cell*, *120*(4), 449–460.

Kenyon, C., Chang, J., Gensch, E., Rudner, A., & Tabtiang, R. (1993). A *C. elegans* mutant that lives twice as long as wild type. *Nature*, *366*(6454), 461–464.

Kimura, K. D., Tissenbaum, H. A., Liu, Y., & Ruvkun, G. (1997). daf-2, an insulin receptor-like gene that regulates longevity and diapause in *Caenorhabditis elegans*. *Science*, *277*(5328), 942–946.

Klass, M. R. (1983). A method for the isolation of longevity mutants in the nematode *Caenorhabditis elegans* and initial results. *Mechanisms of Ageing & Development*, *22*(3–4), 279–286.

Klass, M., & Hirsh, D. (1976). Non-ageing developmental variant of *Caenorhabditis elegans*. *Nature*, *260*(5551), 523–525.

Larsen, P. L. (1993). Aging and resistance to oxidative damage in *Caenorhabditis elegans*. *Proceedings of the National Academy of Sciences of the United States of America*, *90*(19), 8905–8909.

Larsen, P., Albert, P., & Riddle, D. (1995). Genes that regulate both development and longevity in *Caenorhabditis elegans*. *Genetics*, *139*(4), 1567–1583.

Larsen, P. L., & Clarke, C. F. (2002). Extension of life-span in *Caenorhabditis elegans* by a diet lacking coenzyme Q. *Science*, *295*(5552), 120–123.

Lee, R. Y., Hench, J., & Ruvkun, G. (2001). Regulation of *C. elegans* DAF-16 and its human ortholog FKHRL1 by the daf-2 insulin-like signaling pathway. *Current Biology*, *11*(24), 1950–1957.

Lee, S. J., Hwang, A. B., & Kenyon, C. (2010). Inhibition of respiration extends *C. elegans* life span via reactive oxygen species that increase HIF-1 activity. *Current Biology*, *20*(23), 2131–2136. http://dx.doi.org/10.1016/j.cub.2010.10.057

Lee, S. S. (2006). Whole genome RNAi screens for increased longevity: Important new insights but not the whole story. *Experimental Gerontolgy*, *41*(10), 968–973.

Lee, S. S., Kennedy, S., Tolonen, A. C., & Ruvkun, G. (2003). DAF-16 target genes that control *C. elegans* life-span and metabolism. *Science*, *300*(5619), 644–647.

Lee, S. S., Lee, R. Y., Fraser, A. G., Kamath, R. S., Ahringer, J., & Ruvkun, G. (2003). A systematic RNAi screen identifies a critical role for mitochondria in *C. elegans* longevity. *Nature Genetics*, *33*(1), 40–48.

Lemire, B. D., Behrendt, M., DeCorby, A., & Gaskova, D. (2009). *C. elegans* longevity pathways converge to decrease mitochondrial membrane potential. *Mechanisms of Ageing & Development*, *130*(7), 461–465. http://dx.doi.org/10.1016/j.mad.2009.05.001

Libina, N., Berman, J., & Kenyon, C. (2003). Tissue-specific activities of *C. elegans* DAF-16 in the regulation of lifespan. *Cell*, *115*(4), 489–502.

Lin, K., Dorman, J. B., Rodan, A., & Kenyon, C. (1997). daf-16: An HNF-3/forkhead family member that can function to double the life-span of *Caenorhabditis elegans*. *Science*, *278*(5341), 1319–1322.

Longo, V. D., & Finch, C. E. (2003). Evolutionary medicine: From dwarf model systems to healthy centenarians? *Science*, *299*(5611), 1342–1346.

Melo, J. A., & Ruvkun, G. (2012). Inactivation of conserved *C. elegans* genes engages pathogen- and xenobiotic-associated defenses. *Cell*, *149*(2), 452–466. http://dx.doi.org/10.1016/j.cell.2012.02.050

Morris, J. Z., Tissenbaum, H. A., & Ruvkun, G. (1996). A phosphatidylinositol-3-OH kinase family member regulating longevity and diapause in *Caenorhabditis elegans*. *Nature*, *382*(6591), 536–539.

Murakami, S., & Johnson, T. E. (1996). A genetic pathway conferring life extension and resistance to UV stress in *Caenorhabditis elegans*. *Genetics*, *143*(3), 1207–1218.

Murphy, C. T., McCarroll, S. A., Bargmann, C. I., Fraser, A., Kamath, R. S., Ahringer, J., . . . Kenyon, C. (2003). Genes that act downstream of DAF-16 to influence the lifespan of *Caenorhabditis elegans*. *Nature*, *424*(6946), 277–283.

Nargund, A. M., Pellegrino, M. W., Fiorese, C. J., Baker, B. M., & Haynes, C. M. (2012). Mitochondrial import efficiency of ATFS-1 regulates mitochondrial UPR activation. *Science*, *337*(6094), 587–590. http://dx.doi.org/10.1126/science.1223560

Neafsey, P. J. (1990). Longevity hormesis. A review. *Mechanisms of Ageing & Development*, *51*(1), 1–31.

Neafsey, P. J., Boxenbaum, H., Ciraulo, D. A., & Fournier, D. J. (1988). A Gompertz age-specific mortality rate model of aging, hormesis, and toxicity: Fixed-dose studies. *Drug Metabolism Reviews*, *19*(3–4), 369–401. http://dx.doi.org/10.3109/03602538808994141

Ogg, S., Paradis, S., Gottlieb, S., Patterson, G. I., Lee, L., Tissenbaum, H. A., & Ruvkun, G. (1997). The Forkhead transcription factor DAF-16 transduces insulin-like metabolic and longevity signals in *C. elegans*. *Nature*, *389*(6654), 994–999.

Paek, J., Lo, J. Y., Narasimhan, S. D., Nguyen, T. N., Glover-Cutter, K., Robida-Stubbs, S., . . . Curran, S. P. (2012). Mitochondrial SKN-1/Nrf mediates a conserved starvation response. *Cell Metabolism*, *16*(4), 526–537. http://dx.doi.org/10.1016/j.cmet.2012.09.007

Pan, K., Palter, J., Rogers, A., Olsen, A., Chen, D., Lithgow, G., & Kapahi, P. (2007). Inhibition of mRNA translation extends lifespan in *Caenorhabditis elegans*. *Aging Cell*, *6*(1), 111–119. http://dx.doi.org/10.1111/j.1474-9726.2006.00266.x

Paradis, S., Ailion, M., Toker, A., Thomas, J. H., & Ruvkun, G. (1999). A PDK1 homolog is necessary and sufficient to transduce AGE-1 PI3 kinase signals that regulate diapause in *Caenorhabditis elegans*. *Genes & Development*, *13*(11), 1438–1452.

Paradis, S., & Ruvkun, G. (1998). *Caenorhabditis elegans* Akt/PKB transduces insulin receptor-like signals from AGE-1 PI3 kinase to the DAF-16 transcription factor. *Genes & Development*, *12*(16), 2488–2498.

Park, S. K., Tedesco, P. M., & Johnson, T. E. (2009). Oxidative stress and longevity in *Caenorhabditis elegans* as mediated by SKN-1. *Aging cell*, *8*(3), 258–269. http://dx.doi.org/10.1111/j.1474-9726.2009.00473.x

Pearl, R. (1928). *The rate of living: Being an account of some experimental studies on the biology of life duration*. New York, NY: A.A. Knopf.

Pothof, J., van Haaften, G., Thijssen, K., Kamath, R. S., Fraser, A. G., Ahringer, J., . . . Tijsterman, M. (2003). Identification of genes that protect the *C. elegans* genome against mutations by genome-wide RNAi. *Genes & Development*, *17*(4), 443–448. http://dx.doi.org/10.1101/gad.1060703

Rea, S., & Johnson, T. E. (2003). A metabolic model for life span determination in *Caenorhabditis elegans*. *Development Cells*, *5*(2), 197–203.

Reis-Rodrigues, P., Czerwieniec, G., Peters, T. W., Evani, U. S., Alavez, S., Gaman, E. A., . . . Hughes, R. E. (2012). Proteomic analysis of age-dependent changes in protein solubility identifies genes that modulate lifespan. *Aging Cell*, *11*(1), 120–127. http://dx.doi.org/10.1111/j.1474-9726.2011.00765.x

Samuelson, A. V., Carr, C. E., & Ruvkun, G. (2007). Gene activities that mediate increased life span of *C. elegans* insulin-like signaling mutants. *Genes & Development*, *21*(22), 2976–2994.

Shore, D. E., & Ruvkun, G. (2013). A cytoprotective perspective on longevity regulation. *Trends in Cell Biology*. http://dx.doi.org/10.1016/j.tcb.2013.04.007

Simmer, F., Tijsterman, M., Parrish, S., Koushika, S. P., Nonet, M. L., Fire, A., . . . Plasterk, R. H. (2002). Loss of the putative RNA-directed RNA polymerase RRF-3 makes *C. elegans* hypersensitive to RNAi. *Current Biology*, *12*(15), 1317–1319.

Speakman, J. R., Selman, C., McLaren, J. S., & Harper, E. J. (2002). Living fast, dying when? The link between aging and energetics. *The Journal of Nutrition*, *132*(6, Suppl. 2), 1583S–1597S.

Sulston, J. E., & Brenner, S. (1974). The DNA of *Caenorhabditis elegans*. *Genetics*, *77*(1), 95–104.

Syntichaki, P., Troulinaki, K., & Tavernarakis, N. (2007). eIF4E function in somatic cells modulates ageing in *Caenorhabditis elegans*. *Nature*, *445*(7130), 922–926.

Tacutu, R., Budovsky, A., Wolfson, M., & Fraifeld, V. E. (2010). MicroRNA-regulated protein-protein interaction networks: How could they help in searching for pro-longevity targets? *Rejuvenation Research*, *13*(2–3), 373–377. http://dx.doi.org/10.1089/rej.2009.0980

Tacutu, R., Budovsky, A., Yanai, H., & Fraifeld, V. E. (2011). Molecular links between cellular senescence, longevity and age-related diseases—A systems biology perspective. *Aging*, *3*(12), 1178–1191.

Tacutu, R., Shore, D. E., Budovsky, A., de Magalhães, J. P., Ruvkun, G., Fraifeld, V. E., & Curran, S. P. (2012). Prediction of *C. elegans* longevity genes by human and worm longevity networks. *PloS One*, *7*(10), e48282. http://dx.doi.org/10.1371/journal.pone.0048282

Tercero, J. A., Espinosa, J. C., Lacalle, R. A., & Jiménez, A. (1996). The biosynthetic pathway of the aminonucleoside antibiotic puromycin, as deduced from the molecular analysis of the pur cluster of Streptomyces alboniger. *Journal of Biological Chemistry*, *271*(3), 1579–1590.

Tewari, M., Hu, P. J., Ahn, J. S., Ayivi-Guedehoussou, N., Vidalain, P. O., Li, S., . . . Vidal, M. (2004). Systematic interactome mapping and genetic perturbation analysis of a *C. elegans* TGF-beta signaling network. *Molecular Cell*, *13*(4), 469–482.

Timmons, L., Court, D. L., & Fire, A. (2001). Ingestion of bacterially expressed dsRNAs can produce specific and potent genetic interference in *Caenorhabditis elegans*. *Gene*, *263*(1–2), 103–112.

Tissenbaum, H., & Ruvkun, G. (1998). An insulin-like signaling pathway affects both longevity and reproduction in *Caenorhabditis elegans*. *Genetics*, *148*(2), 703–717.

Tuminello, E. R., & Han, S. D. (2011). The apolipoprotein e antagonistic pleiotropy hypothesis: Review and recommendations. *International Journal of Alzheimer's Disease*, *2011*, 726197. http://dx.doi.org/10.4061/2011/726197

Ungewitter, E., & Scrable, H. (2009). Antagonistic pleiotropy and p53. *Mechanisms of Ageing & Development*, *130*(1–2), 10–17. http://dx.doi.org/10.1016/j.mad.2008.06.002

Vowels, J. J., & Thomas, J. H. (1992). Genetic analysis of chemosensory control of dauer formation in *Caenorhabditis elegans*. *Genetics*, *130*(1), 105–123.

Williams, G. C. (1957). Pleiotropy, natural selection, and the evolution of senescence. *Evolution*, *11*, 398–809.

Wolff, S., & Dillin, A. (2006). The trifecta of aging in *Caenorhabditis elegans*. *Experimental Gerontology*, *41*(10), 894–903.

Wood, W. B., & Johnson, T. E. (1994). Aging. Stopping the clock. *Current Biology*, *4*(2), 151–153.

Yang, W., & Hekimi, S. (2010). A mitochondrial superoxide signal triggers increased longevity in *Caenorhabditis elegans.PLoS Biology*, *8*(12), e1000556. http://dx.doi.org/10.1371/journal.pbio.1000556

Yanos, M. E., Bennett, C. F., & Kaeberlein, M. (2012). Genome-Wide RNAi Longevity Screens in *Caenorhabditis elegans*. *Current Genomics*, *13*(7), 508–518. http://dx.doi.org/10.2174/138920212803251391

Zarse, K., Schmeisser, S., Groth, M., Priebe, S., Beuster, G., Kuhlow, D., . . . Ristow, M. (2012). Impaired insulin/IGF1 signaling extends life span by promoting mitochondrial L-proline catabolism to induce a transient ROS signal. *Cell Metabolism*, *15*(4), 451–465. http://dx.doi.org/10.1016/j.cmet.2012.02.013

CHAPTER 3

Oxygen and Aging

Jason N. Pitt, Scott F. Leiser, and M. Kaeberlein

ABSTRACT

Oxygen is a double-edged sword. Despite the near universal requirement for oxygen for survival and reproduction in animals, oxygen and oxidative metabolism are responsible for the production of reactive oxygen species (ROS), which has, until recently, been considered a cellular toxin and a major cause of aging. Alterations in environmental oxygen can alter rates of aging and ROS production in many organisms. Animals coordinate the cellular response to low oxygen with a conserved hypoxic response mediated by the hypoxia inducible transcription factor, hypoxia-inducible factor (HIF). In addition to hypoxia, HIF has been shown to have roles in aging, cancer, cardiovascular disease, and stem cell maintenance in organisms from worms to humans. Furthermore, HIF has been shown to interact with mechanistic target of rapamycin (mTOR), Sirtuins, and to influence other pathways and interventions known to affect the aging. This chapter focuses on the effects of altered oxygen concentrations on the aging, its similarities to dietary restriction, how mutations in the HIF pathway affect lifespan and health span, and how the HIF pathway interacts with other conserved longevity pathways.

INTRODUCTION

Although the first organisms arose on the planet in the absence of oxygen (O_2), complex animal life did not evolve until oxygen approached present day levels (21 kPa) during the Cambrian some 500 million years ago (Holland, 2006).

http://dx.doi.org/10.1891/0198-8794.34.59

With only one known exception (Danovaro et al., 2010), all extant animals require oxygen to complete their life cycle. More than 90% of the oxygen used by animals is reduced to water in the active site of a single enzyme, cytochrome *c* oxidase, at the terminal step of the electron transport chain in mitochondria (Hochachka & Somero, 2002; Wikström, Krab, & Saraste, 1981). Oxygen's high redox potential and water's low toxicity provide an enormous energetic advantage to organisms capable of oxidative phosphorylation. However, oxidative metabolism is not without its disadvantages. The same high reactivity that powers oxidative phosphorylation can lead to the formation of highly reactive oxygen species (ROS) that can modify cellular macromolecules. Cells have evolved mechanisms to repair the oxidative damage resulting from ROS, but one of the leading theories of how cells age suggests that the cumulative damage caused by ROS on cellular macromolecules is responsible for the various pathologies associated with organismal aging.

The free radical or oxidative stress theory of aging, originally proposed by Harman (1956), provides a mechanistic basis for Pearl's older rate of living theory of aging (Pearl, 1928 and reviewed in Speakman, 2005), which posited that metabolic rate was the key determinant of aging. If the rate of aerobic metabolism was directly proportional to the rate of ROS production, it would explain the observation that smaller animals with higher per gram oxygen consumption age faster than larger animals with slower metabolic rates. Although this had been assumed, current evidence suggests that ROS production may not be directly correlated to metabolic rate (reviewed in Jackson, Pye, & Palomero, 2007; Van Voorhies, 2004). Although the rate of living theory appears to hold true for many animals, there are notable exceptions, primarily birds and bats (Austad & Fischer, 1991). Birds expend approximately 3.5-fold more energy per lifetime per gram of tissue than does a gram of mammal and, within the birds, there is no significant relationship between body size and lifetime energy expenditure (Speakman, 2005). These and other exceptions have cast doubt on the rate of living theory, even though for terrestrial mammals the relationship between lifetime energy expenditure per gram and lifespan holds.

Ambient temperature can strongly affect metabolic rate in all animals. Although this is especially true in poikilothermic animals, even in endothermic homeotherms such as ourselves, metabolic output is affected by ambient temperature (Westerterp-Plantenga, van Marken Lichtenbelt, Strobbe, & Schrauwen, 2002). The effects of temperature on lifespan have been well studied, and in poikilothermic animals, within their physiologically tolerated temperature range, there is clear inverse relationship between lifespan and temperature (Conti, 2008). As temperature drops, O_2 consumption and metabolic rate falls, and there is a concomitant increase in lifespan. In humans too, low core body temperature is the only known variable that is consistently correlated with longevity; however, prospective studies are lacking (Waalen & Buxbaum, 2011). The effects of dietary nutrient availability on both metabolism and aging have also been well studied. Restriction of caloric intake has been shown to reduce body temperature, decrease overall metabolic rate, and increase lifespan (discussed further in the following text). However, equally important for the efficient production of calories by aerobic respiration is the availability of oxygen. But although oxygen has clear effects on metabolism, compared to the effects of temperature and nutrient alterations, far fewer studies have looked at the effects of alterations of oxygen concentration on lifespan.

In this annual review, we focus on how manipulations of oxygen availability and in oxygen consumption influence the aging process; how interventions known to affect aging modulate oxygen consumption; and how genes known to be involved in the cellular utilization of oxygen and cellular response to hypoxia modulate longevity. Regrettably, a comprehensive understanding of oxygen's role in aging has, thus far, failed to emerge. Nevertheless, it is clear that although there may be no single unifying mechanism that ties together how oxygen affects longevity across phyla, oxygen's significance in influencing the rate of the aging process appears universal.

OXYGEN AVAILABILITY MODULATES AGING

Perhaps owing to its ubiquity in air, an underappreciated yet inescapable fact of aerobic metabolism is that, just as organisms require a constant supply of reduced carbon sources to maintain metabolic output, they also require a constant supply of oxygen. Oxygen is poorly soluble in water. At 20 °C and atmospheric pressure, only 9 mg of oxygen dissolves per liter of water. Because physiological demands for oxygen fluctuate in response to an organism's activity levels, the cardiopulmonary and respiratory pigment systems of higher animals evolved to provide tissues with a steady supply of oxygen in response to large energy demands. Even in small animals, like nematodes, which lack circulatory systems and respiratory pigments, and rely on passive diffusion for gas exchange, the rate of oxygen consumption is a key determinant of metabolic rate. The effect of altering the concentration of oxygen on animal survival dates to the discovery of oxygen itself. In 1774, Priestly discovered that burning mercuric oxide in a bell jar allowed an enclosed mouse to live five times longer than controls. The substance produced by this reaction was named oxygen by Lavoisier 3 years later. Lavoisier showed that both respiring rodents and burning lumps of coal consumed oxygen and produced fixed air (CO_2) and heat in proportion to the amount of oxygen provided, and that the only difference between the fire and the rodent was the rate at which the oxygen was consumed (Severinghaus, 2002; Underwood, 1944).

Hyperoxia

Although a small amount of excess oxygen is useful for mice to delay asphyxiation in a bell jar, a lifetime spent in hyperoxia (defined here as O_2 concentrations > 21 kPa) results in a shortened lifespan. Fruit flies exposed to hyperoxia have extremely shortened lifespans (Mockett, Sohal, & Orr, 1999; Rascón & Harrison, 2010; Van Voorhies, 2009) and mammals exposed to hyperoxia at atmospheric pressure die within days, and when exposed to 100% oxygen at higher pressures die in hours (Jamieson, 1989). The toxic effects of oxygen concentrations greater than 21 kPa are thought to result from the production of superoxide and other reactive oxygen species. This hypothesis has been tested directly in the fly where lethality in hyperoxia was mitigated by treatment with antioxidants (Mockett et al., 1999). In this regard, hyperoxia may be considered analogous to an accelerated aging process, which is not surprising given that it was the difference in radiation induced damage in normoxic versus anoxic (no oxygen) cells that lead Harman (1956) to originally propose the free radical theory of aging.

Intriguingly, the effects of hyperoxia on lifespan are not always negative (see Table 3.1). Sohal, Agarwal, Dubey, and Orr (1993) showed that house flies raised in constant hyperoxia live shorter than normoxic controls, but flies exposed to 100% oxygen through day 4 of life and then aged in normoxia live nearly 50% longer than normoxia-only controls. However, in this experiment, the hyperoxia treated flies showed signs of oxidative injury and responded to hyperoxia by decreasing oxygen consumption. Thus, the lifespan extension in this case may actually result from a decreased metabolic rate following hyperoxia-induced injury.

Surprisingly, the nematode *Caenorhabditis elegans*, which is a facilitative anaerobe and can survive days in complete anoxia, can also be grown in 100% O_2 for more than 50 generations with no negative effects on lifespan or reproduction (Van Voorhies & Ward, 2000). This is particularly remarkable given that worms show aerotaxis behaviors that allow them to locate their preferred oxygen concentration, which appears to be around 7 kPa (Chang, Chronis, Karow, Marletta, & Bargmann, 2006). The mechanistic basis of the worm's remarkable survival in hyperoxia appears to be caused by the activity of the Mn superoxide dismutases *sod-2* and *sod-3*. Mutations in these two genes render worms in 98% oxygen dead in 2 days (Y. Honda, Tanaka, & Honda, 2008). Interestingly, 6-day-old control worms exposed to 90% oxygen for 48 hr showed a 1 day increase in mean lifespan (Y. Honda & Honda, 2001). Hyperoxia exposure has been shown to correlate with large increases in SOD activity in worm extracts and resistance to oxidative stress when young animals are exposed; however, 10- and 20-day-old worms fail to adapt to hyperoxia like younger animals (Darr & Fridovich, 1995). This suggests that either dysregulation of redox signaling mechanisms

TABLE 3.1
Effects of Altered Oxygen Concentration on Lifespan

Oxygen Level	Organism	Lifespan Effect at $[O_2]$	Reference
Hypoxia	*Saccharomyces cerevisiae*	Decrease 0 kPa	Koc et al., 2004
	C. elegans	Increase 4 kPa, 1 kPa, and 500 Pa	S. Honda et al., 1993; Leiser et al., 2013; Liu & Cai, 2013; Mehta et al., 2009
	Drosophila melanogaster	Increase 10 kPa Decrease at 2 kPa, Decrease 5 kPa (modulated by DR)	Rascón & Harrison, 2010; Vigne & Frelin, 2006
	Mus musculus	Decrease <8 kPa, Increase in health span in p53–/– 10 kPa	Benderro & Lamanna, 2011; Debonneuil et al, 2006; Sung et al., 2011
	Homo sapiens (cell lines)	Increase 10 kPa	Packer & Fuehr, 1977
Hyperoxia	*C. elegans*	Decrease or increase or no effect varies with time/length of exposure	Y. Honda & Honda, 2001; Van Voorhies & Ward, 2000
	Drosophila melanogaster	Decrease	Mockett, Sohal, & Orr, 1999; Rascón & Harrison, 2010; Van Voorhies, 2009
	Musca domestica	Decrease or increase varies with time/ length of exposure	Sohal et al., 1993
	Mus musculus	Decrease	Jamieson, 1989
High altitude	*Homo sapiens*	Increase in health span	Weinberg et al., 1987

during old age sensitizes worms to oxidative damage or hyperactivation of antioxidant defense systems early in life delays the damaging effects of ROS.

Hypoxia

If hyperoxia generally leads to increased ROS and shortened lifespan, then hypoxia (defined here as O_2 concentrations < 21 kPa) might show the opposite effect. Paradoxically, although some oxygen is required for the production of superoxide, decreasing the availability of oxygen has been shown to increase the production of ROS. In several different cell lines and isolated mitochondria, exposure of cells to hypoxia or hypoxia mimetics leads to elevated ROS levels (Dawson, Gores, Nieminen, Herman, & Lemasters, 1993; Guzy et al., 2005; Mansfield et al., 2005). This effect has been hypothesized to occur because of the slowing of the electron transport chain resulting in the aberrant transfer of electrons to dioxygen upstream of cytochrome *c* oxidase (Turrens, 2003). Although the role of hypoxia-induced ROS in the stabilization of the hypoxia-induced transcription factor hypoxia-inducible factor (HIF; see next section) has been controversial (Hagen, 2012), the role of ROS in the pathogenesis resulting from hypoxia-induced conditions such as ischemic stroke and myocardial infarction is well accepted (Bolli & Marbán, 1999; Dhalla, Elmoselhi, Hata, & Makino, 2000; Lefer & Granger, 2000; Loh, Huang, De Silva, Tan, & Zhu, 2006).

Oxygen levels lower than ambient (10 kPa O_2) have been known since the 1970s to increase the replicative lifespan of cultured human cells (Packer & Fuehr, 1977). Furthermore, low oxygen levels have been shown to be important for stem cell maintenance, and many immortalized tumor lines show low rates of oxygen consumption and high rates of glycolysis (Fehrer et al., 2007). In budding yeast, anoxia appears to decrease replicative lifespan (Koc, Gasch, Rutherford, Kim, & Gladyshev, 2004). *Drosophila* embryos can survive limited anoxia, and in larvae and adults, hypoxia has been shown to both increase and decrease lifespan, depending on the specific oxygen concentration and time of exposure (Foe & Alberts, 1985; Rascón & Harrison, 2010; Van Voorhies, 2009; Vigne & Frelin, 2006). In the mouse, severe hypoxia (<8 kPa O_2) is not consistent with long life, and its negative effects are manifested more rapidly in elderly mice (Benderro & Lamanna, 2011; Debonneuil, Quillard, & Baulieu, 2006). However, p53 null mice show a 50% increase in tumor free survival time when raised in 10 kPa O_2 (Sung et al., 2011), and humans at high altitude show a lower incidence of cardiovascular disease and cancer (Weinberg, Brown, & Hoel, 1987).

It seems clear that like hyperoxia, hypoxia can have both positive and negative effects on health and longevity. Owing to its broad oxygen tolerance and lack of a circulatory system, *C. elegans* has been a particularly useful model system to study the genetic responses to hypoxia and the effects of hypoxia on longevity. Adult worms can survive prolonged anoxia and, interestingly, lifespan-extending mutations in the worm insulin-like receptor *daf2* also lead to increased survival in high temperature hypoxia or extended anoxia (Mendenhall, LaRue, & Padilla, 2006; Scott, Avidan, & Crowder, 2002; Van Voorhies & Ward, 2000). A simple interpretation of this result is that reduced insulin-like signaling pre-conditions animals for decreased oxygen consumption and increased reliance on glycolysis. This hypothesis is supported by work from Padilla's group showing that mutations in the two worm glyceraldehyde-3-phosphate dehydrogenase (GAPDH) genes, *gpd2* and *gpd3*, suppress the resistance of *daf-2* mutants to anoxia (Mendenhall et al., 2006).

Hypoxia has been shown to directly extend lifespan in *C. elegans* (S. Honda, Ishii, Suzuki, & Matsuo, 1993; Leiser, Fletcher, Begun, & Kaeberlein, 2013; Mehta et al., 2009). This extension requires both HIF-1 and the FOXO transcription factor DAF-16, which also mediates the longevity promoting effects of reduced insulin signaling (Kenyon, Chang, Gensch, Rudner, & Tabtiang, 1993; Leiser et al., 2013). Hypoxia leads to a rapid nuclear localization of DAF-16 and transcriptional activation of DAF-16 target genes that are known to promote longevity. Although the mechanism of hypoxia-induced DAF-16 activation in worms is not certain, it has recently been shown that oxidative stress leads to a ROS catalyzed disulfide bond between FOXO and the karyopherin transportin 1 (TNPO1) resulting in FOXO accumulation in the nucleus (Putker et al., 2013). DAF-16::GFP was shown to be localized to the nucleus in vivo in response to paraquat and high temperature treatments, and this required the worm TNPO4 homolog IMB-1. Interestingly, IMB-1 was not required for DAF-16 activation in response to starvation, suggesting that oxidative, temperature, and nutritional stresses may have distinct mechanisms for DAF-16 activation (Putker et al., 2013). However, given that hypoxia is known to increase ROS, it is likely that a similar ROS signaling mechanism is responsible for DAF-16 activation in hypoxia.

Because worms lack physiological mechanisms to respond to altered oxygen supplies, they instead rely on a neurosensory circuit composed of the BAG and URX neurons under the control of a series of soluble guanylate cyclases (sGC) to move to environments that have nontoxic levels of oxygen. Mutations in the guanylate cyclase *gcy-31*, *gcy-33*, *gcy-35*, and *gcy-36* suppress aerotaxis behavior and their misexpression in other neurons is sufficient to induce oxygen sensitive depolarization (Zimmer et al., 2009). Interestingly, Liu and Cai (2013) showed that mild hypoxia extends lifespans in the worm and that this extension relies on sGCs. Perhaps most remarkable was that hyperoxia-sensitive and hypoxia-sensitive neurons had opposite effects on lifespan extension, suggesting that neurosignaling responses rather than metabolic effects may play a role in determining lifespan in altered oxygen environments.

THE ROLE OF THE HYPOXIC RESPONSE IN AGING

In worms, as in other metazoans, the cellular response to hypoxia is mediated largely by the HIF, a transcriptional regulator of hypoxia-responsive genes collectively referred to as the hypoxic response. HIF functions as a heterodimer containing a regulated HIF-α subunit and a constitutive HIF-β subunit (G. L. Wang, Jiang, Rue, & Semenza, 1995). When oxygen is abundant, HIF-α is degraded by the proteasome following hydroxylation by oxygen-dependent proline hydroxylases and ubiquitination by the von Hippel Lindau protein (pVHL; see Figure 3.1). Under hypoxia, these posttranslational modifications are inhibited, and HIF-α becomes stabilized (W. Kim & Kaelin, 2003).

HIF activates various genes related to the systemic and metabolic responses necessary under hypoxia (summarized in Figure 3.2). In both lower (worms)

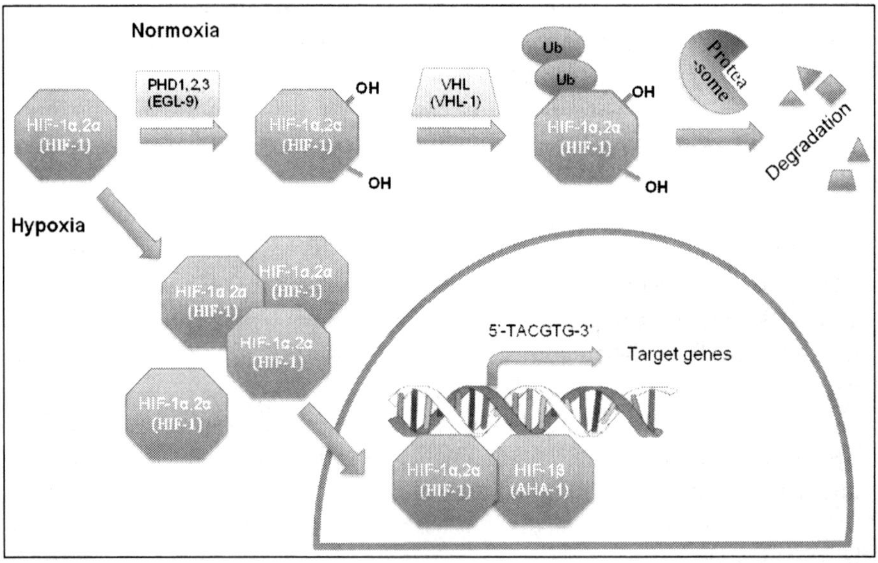

FIGURE 3.1 Model of HIF regulation in normoxia/hypoxia. In normoxia, HIF is continuously expressed but immediately hydroxylated, bound to E3 ubiquitin ligase VHL complex and degraded by the proteasome. In hypoxia, prolyl hydroxylation is blocked, thereby stabilizing HIFα to enter the nucleus where it binds HIF-1β and activates its downstream targets. Mammalian genes are shown with *C. elegans* homologs in parentheses.

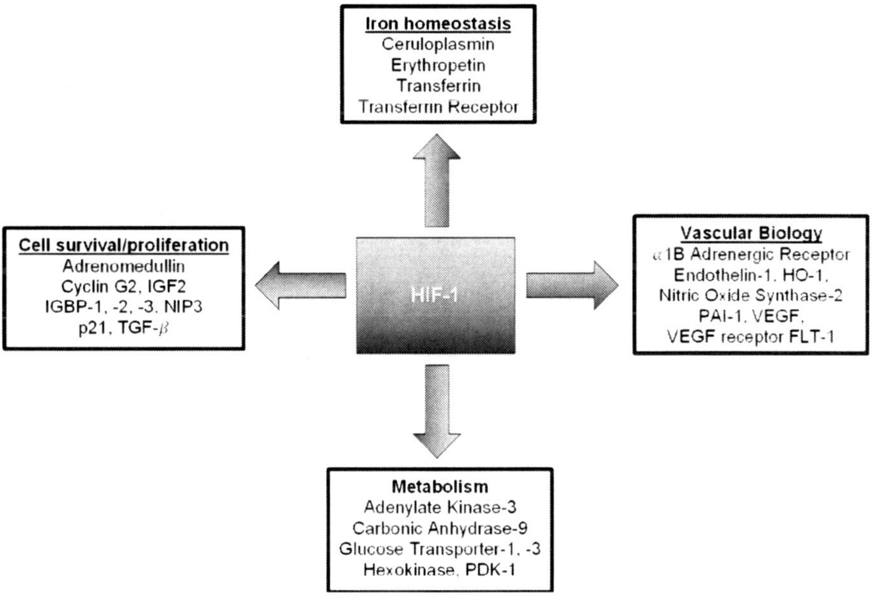

FIGURE 3.2 HIF-1 targets a diverse array of genes responsible for modifying multiple biochemical pathways (reviewed in G. Semenza, 2009).

and higher (mammals) animals, HIF activates genes involved in metabolic modification, including glucose transporters, hexokinases, and carbonic anhydrases (Bishop et al., 2004; G. Semenza, 2002). These genes allow for cells under hypoxia to decrease respiration and increase glycolysis to maintain ATP levels in the cell. Similarly, it is reported that HIF activates multiple genes involved in cell survival, presumably to gain time to reset homeostatic mechanisms (G. Semenza, 2002). In mammals, HIF-modulated genes that are known to be involved in improving vascular biology, including vascular endothelial growth factor (VEGF), platelet derived growth factor (PDGF), and erythropoietin (EPO; G. Semenza, 2002). One of these genes (EPO) and several others (e.g., transferrin, ceruloplasmin) are also involved in iron homeostasis, a role that appears to be conserved from worms to humans. The HIF-iron connection reflects iron's crucial role in both oxygen transport and mitochondrial biochemistry, where HIF is reported to decrease respiration through PDK1 activation (Kirito, Hu, & Komatsu, 2009). Iron is also incorporated into the HIF-regulating prolyl hydroxylases, indicating that iron availability directly regulates HIF activity (McDonough et al., 2006; McNeill et al., 2005). The function of HIF target gene modulation is to promote cellular survival under hypoxic stress. Although cellular survival and adaptation is invaluable when an organism is challenged with environmentally or physiologically induced hypoxia, these same mechanisms can be co-opted by cancer cells to allow enhanced growth and pathogenicity.

HIF-1 has long been known to be involved in diseases of aging, particularly solid tumors that often show stabilization of HIF-1 to promote vascularization and growth under hypoxic conditions. More recently, several studies have pointed to a more fundamental role of HIF-1 as a direct modulator of aging. These studies have demonstrated that HIF-1 can both promote and limit longevity via pathways that are mechanistically distinct in *C. elegans*. In addition to directly modulating aging rate, the hypoxic pathway is also interconnected with other aging pathways, including mTOR, insulin-like signaling, and dietary restriction (discussed further below).

HIF-1 and Aging in *C. elegans*

The *C. elegans* hypoxic response pathway is well characterized through genetic and microarray studies (Bishop et al., 2004; H. Jiang, Guo, & Powell-Coffman, 2001; Shen & Powell-Coffman, 2003). Nematodes have a single HIF-α gene (*hif-1*), and the oxygen-dependent proteasomal degradation of the HIF-1 protein is mediated by a single prolyl hydroxylase (EGL-9) and a single cullin E3 ligase (VHL-1). Both EGL-9 and VHL-1 are necessary for HIF-1 targeted degradation; however, data suggest that EGL-9 and perhaps VHL-1 also individually regulate HIF-1 activity in distinct ways (Shen, Shao, & Powell-Coffman, 2006). Multiple mRNA analyses show that EGL-9 downregulates HIF-1 activity in the absence of VHL-1, and *vhl-1* and *egl-9* transcriptional profiles differ significantly (Bishop et al., 2004; Shao, Zhang, & Powell-Coffman, 2009; Shen et al., 2006).

Mehta et al. (2009) were the first group to establish HIF-1 as a longevity factor by showing that stabilization of HIF-1 through RNAi knockdown of either *egl-9* or *vhl-1*, or by deletion of *vhl-1*, is sufficient to significantly increase the lifespan of adult worms by 30%–50%. Further studies replicated these data using both *vhl-1* mutants (Müller et al., 2009) and HIF-1 transgenic overexpression (Y. Zhang, Shao, Zhai, Shen, & Powell-Coffman, 2009). Notably, loss of VHL-1 protein appeared to improve multiple measures of health span, including resistance to amyloid beta and polyglutamine toxicity, and accumulation of age-associated autofluorescence (Mehta et al., 2009). Also notable, the evidence from these papers suggests that stabilized HIF-1 acts in a pathway independent of insulin-like signaling and dietary restriction (DR), suggesting that the hypoxic response represents a novel longevity pathway.

Soon after the initial publication showing that stabilization of HIF-1 can extend lifespan in *C. elegans*, two groups independently found that deletion of *hif-1* can also increase lifespan in *C. elegans* (D. Chen, Thomas, & Kapahi, 2009;

Y. Zhang et al., 2009). These data initially appeared contradictory to survival data for *hif-1* deletion mutants in Mehta et al. (2009) that showed no significant difference compared to wild-type animals; however, several differences in methodology between the two studies were noted at the time (M. Kaeberlein & Kapahi, 2009). Subsequently, it was determined that the experimental temperature is a critical feature determining the effect of HIF-1 loss on lifespan in *C. elegans*: deletion of *hif-1* extends lifespan at 25 °C but not at lower temperatures, whereas stabilization of HIF-1 through deletion of *vhl-1* extends lifespan robustly throughout the temperature range between 15 °C and 25 °C (other temperatures outside of this range are rarely used for *C. elegans* studies and were not tested; Leiser, Begun, & Kaeberlein, 2011). Apparently, loss of basal levels of HIF-1 activates the FOXO transcription factor, DAF-16, leading to increased lifespan at higher temperature. Interestingly, at 20 °C and 15 °C, *hif-1* mutation was associated with a loss of health span, as measured by an increase in age-related vulval integrity defects, a worm phenotype that in this case may uncouple health span and lifespan.

Since the initial publications on HIF-1 as a longevity factor, multiple studies have provided additional evidence for HIF-1's role in worm aging. A study by Bellier, Chen, Kao, Cinar, & Aroian (2009) found that HIF-1 is necessary for defense against bacterial toxins, and that stabilization of HIF-1 enhanced the resistance to these toxins. A recent study also showed that HIF-1 is necessary for lifespan extension from loss of the nematode folliculin protein, which causes a disease similar to VHL syndrome when mutated in people (Gharbi et al., 2013). Another study from the Lee and Kenyon labs proposed that HIF-1 targets are activated by RNAi or mutation of mitochondrial proteins that extend lifespan, and that HIF-1 is necessary for the extension of lifespan (S.-J. Lee, Hwang, & Kenyon, 2010). Stabilization of HIF-α has also been reported in long-lived MCLK1 heterozygous mutant mice, which contain a defect in a mitochondrial hydroxylase that is necessary for the biosynthesis of ubiquinone (D. Wang, Malo, & Hekimi, 2010; Zheng, Lapointe, & Hekimi, 2010). These results, along with previous evidence that HIF-1 can down-regulate mitochondrial respiration (Tormos & Chandel, 2010) and multiple studies showing that HIF-1 regulates iron homeostasis (possibly through the mitochondria; Ackerman & Gems, 2012; Kirienko et al., 2013), suggest that HIF-1 and mitochondria may function together to modulate aging.

Mammalian HIFs in Aging and Disease

In mammals, the hypoxic response is more elaborate than in *C. elegans*, which contain only one HIF-α gene (HIF-1), one HIF-regulatory prolyl hydroxylase (EGL-9), one HIF-regulatory E3 ligase (VHL-1), and one additional negative regulator (RHY-1; Bishop et al., 2004; Shen, Nettleton, Jiang, Kim, & Powell-Coffman, 2005; Shen et al., 2006). Mammals have at least three HIF-α genes (HIF-1α, HIF-2α, HIF-3α), three prolyl hydroxylases (PHD1, PHD2, PHD3), many potential effectors of HIF function, and as many as 500 predicted transcriptional targets (Benita et al., 2009; Schofield & Ratcliffe, 2004; Yee Koh, Spivak-Kroizman, & Powis, 2008; see Figure 3.1). As is often the case when translating results from invertebrates to mammals, the added complexity of mammalian systems leads to different outcomes. In this regard, it is important to note that stabilization of HIF-α proteins in mammals through loss of VHL protein does not increase longevity but instead leads to a well-characterized cancer syndrome, von Hippel Lindau disease (Kaelin, 2002). It is also important to note that VHL mutations have pleiotropic effects in mammals because VHL has several HIF-independent functions including interactions with MDM2/p53, NF-κB, aPKC, p400/Rb, collagen IV, kinesin 2, and fibronectin (reviewed in Li & Kim, 2011). Knocking out HIF will also not improve mammalian longevity because both HIF-1α and HIF-2α are necessary for development (Iyer et al., 1998).

Despite the challenges in studying the relationship between HIF and aging in mammals, there are several reports linking HIF to age-related phenotypes and pathways in mammalian systems. These reports are promising, considering that much of the initial data on HIF in mammals was based on its negative (from a health perspective) roles in VHL disease and cancer, where HIF activity is known to increase cancer cell survival (G. L. Semenza, 2009). There is growing recognition, however, that HIF activity is important for health span in young and old mammals, and various studies have linked HIF-1α activity with positive health effects. As mentioned earlier, elevated HIF-1α has been associated with enhanced longevity and improved brain function in long-lived MCLK1 heterozygous mutant mice (D. Wang et al., 2010; Zheng et al., 2010). Another study showed that HIF-1α activity improves the inotropic responses of aged cardiac myocytes, suggesting an age-protective effect (Tan, Marín-García, Damle, & Weiss, 2010). HIF-1α is also implicated in the survival of epidermal cells (Rezvani et al., 2011), pancreatic β cells (Choi, Cai, Schroer, Wang, & Woo, 2011), bone-marrow cells (Rey, Luo, Shimoda, & Semenza, 2011), neural stem cells (Roitbak, Surviladze, & Cunningham, 2011), hematopoietic stem cells (Takubo et al., 2010), and in the maintenance of functional telomerase in embryonic stem cells (Davy & Allsopp, 2011). In contrast, HIF-1α disruption in adipocytes is reported to improve insulin sensitivity in mice on a high-fat diet (C. Jiang et al., 2011), and HIF-1α protein levels often increase with age, possibly because of increased hypoxia or oxidative stress, but this increase is alleviated by DR (Kang et al., 2005; H. J. Kim et al., 2002).

HIF function appears to be particularly critical for healthy aging in the mammalian brain. Many age-related diseases—including diseases such as Alzheimer's disease, Parkinson's disease, and diabetes—involve hypoxic conditions that can worsen the disease. Studies examining amyloid beta accumulation in Alzheimer's disease suggest that increased HIF-1α tends to be protective in disease-free states, but that increased HIF-1α levels are also a sign of advanced disease progression (Ogunshola & Antoniou, 2009). This seemingly contradictory data may stem from HIF-1α's role as a stress response protein, in that its upregulation can be either protective or reactive in nature, and the context of measurement is important (Ogunshola & Antoniou, 2009). Several studies in the brain suggest that HIF can function protectively and is necessary for stem cell maintenance (Mannello, Medda, & Tonti, 2011), angiogenesis (Benderro & Lamanna, 2011; Rabie, Kunze, & Marti, 2011; X. Zhang et al., 2011), and protection from prion protein (Jeong et al., 2012).

INTERACTIONS BETWEEN OXYGEN, THE HYPOXIC RESPONSE, AND KNOWN LONGEVITY PATHWAYS

Dietary Restriction

DR, which can be defined as a reduction in nutrient availability in the absence of malnutrition, is the most widely studied intervention to decrease the rate of aging and extend healthy longevity (reviewed in Masoro, 2005). However, although DR is generally effective in organisms ranging from yeast to primates (Colman et al., 2009; Kennedy, Steffen, & Kaeberlein, 2007), there is seemingly no universally accepted effect of DR on oxygen consumption, metabolic rate, or ROS production (Sohal & Orr, 2012). This lack of consensus may arise, in part, from the fact that the experimental methods used to implement a DR state vary quite dramatically in different organisms, and even sometimes within the same organism; or this may reflect a more fundamental lack of conservation in the relationship between nutrient availability and oxygen utilization across divergent species.

In the budding yeast *Saccharomyces cerevisiae*, DR is generally accomplished by reducing glucose availability in the culture medium from 2.0% to 0.5% or lower (M. Kaeberlein, Kirkland, Fields, & Kennedy, 2004; Lin, Defossez, & Guarente, 2000). Budding yeast are a facultative anaerobe that generate ATP primarily through alcoholic anaerobic fermentation when glucose is abundant; however, yeast will switch to respiratory metabolism under glucose-limited conditions such as DR. Thus, DR in yeast results in a substantial increase in mitochondrial biogenesis, respiration, and oxygen consumption (Barros, Bandy, Tahara, & Kowaltowski, 2004; Lin et al., 2002). This increase in oxygen utilization was initially proposed to play a causal role in replicative lifespan extension from DR (Lin et al., 2002), where replicative lifespan is defined as the number of daughter cells produced by a mother cell prior to irreversible cell cycle arrest (reviewed in Longo, Shadel, Kaeberlein, & Kennedy, 2012). Subsequent studies have demonstrated that the effects of DR on respiration are separable from the effects on replicative lifespan because the lifespan of yeast lacking mitochondrial DNA (rho0) can still be extended by DR (M. Kaeberlein, Hu, et al., 2005). DR can also extend chronological lifespan (Murakami, Burtner, Kennedy, & Kaeberlein, 2008; D. L. Smith, McClure, Matecic, & Smith, 2007), which is defined as the length of time a yeast cell can survive in a quiescent stationary phase (Longo et al., 2012). In this case, lifespan extension clearly requires functional mitochondria, which are necessary for proper entry into stationary phase; however, the mechanism by which increased oxygen consumption promotes chronological longevity appears to result primarily from reduced acidification of the culture medium (Burtner, Murakami, Kennedy, & Kaeberlein, 2009; Murakami, Wall, Basisty, & Kaeberlein, 2011). This occurs because acetic acid is produced as a by-product of metabolism of ethanol produced from glucose fermentation; when yeast are cultured under DR conditions, very little ethanol is produced and the culture medium does not become acidic over the course of the chronological aging experiment.

In *C. elegans*, the standard laboratory diet is a lawn of *E. coli* bacteria, and there are numerous protocols for extending lifespan by restricting food availability. Published DR protocols vary in the substrate (liquid vs. solid agar), the amount of bacteria provided (10^8 cells per mL to none), and the timing and frequency of restriction (continuous vs. intermittent; Greer & Brunet, 2009; Mair & Dillin, 2008). The most severe form of DR in *C. elegans* is referred to as bacterial deprivation (BD), where the bacterial food is completely removed, which extends lifespan by approximately 50% (T. L. Kaeberlein et al., 2006; G. D. Lee et al., 2006). This extension of lifespan is seen even when BD is started late in post-reproductive adulthood and argues against a developmental or reproductive effect of DR in lifespan determination (E. D. Smith et al., 2008; Sutphin & Kaeberlein, 2008). The effect of BD and other forms of DR on metabolic rate has been controversial: during acute BD, within 24 hr, the metabolic output of the worm drops to less than 25% of baseline levels as determined by CO_2 output and normalized to worm size (Van Voorhies, 2002); however, when measured by microcalorimetry and fluorescent superoxide probes, and normalized to total worm protein, the metabolic rate of DR worms has been reported as not statistically different or higher than fed controls (Houthoofd et al., 2002a, 2002b). A similar lack of consensus exists regarding the effect of reduced insulin/IGF-1-like signaling on metabolic rate. Temperature sensitive *daf-2* alleles, which contain partial loss of function mutations in the *C. elegans* insulin/IGF-like receptor, result in worms that live twice as long as controls (Kenyon et al., 1993; Kimura, Tissenbaum, Liu, & Ruvkun, 1997; Larsen, Albert, & Riddle, 1995). Van Voorheis reported that long-lived *daf-2* worms have a metabolic rate roughly half that of wild type (Van Voorhies & Ward, 1999), suggesting that in terms of "physiological lifespan," *daf-2* animals are unchanged from wild type. In contrast, the Vanfleteren group concluded that although *daf-2* worms showed a lower rate of oxygen consumption on a per worm basis, when normalized to total protein levels, *daf-2* worms showed a rate of oxygen consumption roughly the same or slightly higher than wild type, owing to lower protein density in the *daf-2* animals. They also showed that protein density fluctuated with age and concluded that, based on allometric scaling of the data, *daf-2* animals have metabolic rates identical to wild type (Braeckman, Houthoofd, & Vanfleteren, 2002). These types of analyses are further complicated by the fact that nearly 90% of worm metabolic activity in adult worms is directed to reproduction, which is often altered in long-lived mutants and which ceases altogether under BD. It is our opinion that this controversy remains unsettled, and that the assumption that total protein level on a per animal basis does not vary between strains or conditions (e.g., fully fed vs. BD) is not valid. Thus, the effect of BD and other forms of DR on metabolic rate and oxygen consumption in *C. elegans* remains unclear.

Fortunately, fruit flies are large enough to be weighed easily, and the effects of DR on oxygen consumption in *Drosophila* and other insects seem more straightforward. Like *C. elegans*, however, numerous different DR protocols are used within the fruit fly community to modulate longevity, and there is little consensus regarding methodology (Grandison, Wong, Bass, Partridge, & Piper, 2009; Ja et al., 2009; Skorupa, Dervisefendic, Zwiener, & Pletcher, 2008; Tatar, 2011). The relationship between metabolic rate and DR in flies has not been studied extensively; however, the Partridge group tested directly the influence of DR on oxygen consumption and found that in DR regimes that extend lifespan, there was no significant change in metabolic rate (Hulbert et al., 2004).

In mice and rats, the situation is again controversial, despite the methodology for DR being more consistent. Studies of effects of DR on oxygen consumption and metabolic rate have reported these parameters to be increased, decreased, and unchanged (Ferguson, Sohal, Forster, & Sohal, 2007; Hunt et al., 2006; Ramsey & Hagopian, 2006; Selman et al., 2005). On the surface, this lack of consensus regarding the relationship between DR and metabolic rate is somewhat surprising. The natural assumption would be that as nutrient intake declines for a mammal, metabolic rate should also decline, and indeed this appears to be the case at the whole body level. This analysis is complicated, however, by the fact that animals on DR are smaller than fed controls; and upon normalization for whole body mass, organ mass, or body composition, the relationship is less clear. This lack of consensus also extends to whether DR induces mitochondrial biogenesis or changes in mitochondrial function at the tissue or cellular level in mice and rats (Gouspillou & Hepple, 2013; Hancock, Han, Higashida, Kim, & Holloszy, 2011), which is clearly related to oxygen consumption and metabolic rate. Current studies appear to suggest that DR enhances or maintains mitochondrial function during aging without a large increase in mitochondrial density or translation of mitochondrial proteins (Hempenstall, Page, Wallen, & Selman, 2012; Lanza et al., 2012; B. F. Miller, Robinson, Bruss, Hellerstein, & Hamilton, 2012); although, this may be highly dependent on the tissue type, DR protocol, strain background, and other experimental factors. The limited data from controlled human studies appears to consistently indicate that short-term DR results in a reduction in resting metabolic rate in both obese and nonobese individuals (Johannsen et al., 2012; Martin et al., 2007; Redman et al., 2009), although whether this is also true for total energy expenditure after adjusting for changes in body weight and composition is currently unclear.

mTOR

The mechanistic target of rapamycin (mTOR) is a nutrient responsive kinase that has been shown to play a conserved role in modulating growth, stress resistance, and longevity (reviewed in Johnson, Rabinovitch, & Kaeberlein, 2013; Sharp, 2011; Stanfel, Shamieh, Kaeberlein, & Kennedy, 2009). Inhibition of mTOR through genetic manipulations or with the drug rapamycin has been shown to extend lifespan in yeast (M. Kaeberlein, Powers, et al., 2005; Powers, Kaeberlein, Caldwell, Kennedy, & Fields, 2006), worms (Jia, Chen, & Riddle, 2004; Vellai et al., 2003), fruit flies (Bjedov et al., 2010; Kapahi et al., 2004), and mice (Harrison et al., 2009; R. A. Miller et al., 2011). Inhibition by mTOR is also thought to underlie many of the important physiological changes associated with DR, including induction of autophagy, regulation of protein synthesis, and altered mitochondrial respiration (M. Kaeberlein, 2010; Kapahi et al., 2010). As described earlier, the interactions between DR and oxygen consumption are complex and still poorly understood. Genetic evidence has suggested an equally complex interaction between DR/mTOR and HIF transcription factors in nematodes and mammals.

Based on a study in *C. elegans*, it has been proposed that lifespan extension from DR results in part through inhibition of HIF-1 (D. Chen et al., 2009). The authors show that worms deleted for *hif-1* have no additional lifespan extension from DR, whereas activation of HIF-1 by mutation of *egl-9* did not increase lifespan. They interpret these data to mean that under their conditions,

DR modulates lifespan by decreasing HIF-1 activity. This study is supported in part by two studies in mammals that show DR prevents increased HIF-1α activity in the brain and liver, and that suggest the lack of HIF-1α activity is caused by a decrease in ROS (Kang et al., 2005; H. J. Kim et al., 2002).

In mammals, there is a large body of work supporting a direct link between mTOR signaling and hypoxic signaling. HIF-1α is reported to be a substrate of mTOR in certain cell types, where TOR prevents oxygen-dependent degradation of HIF-1α and thus activates HIF-1α (Demidenko & Blagosklonny, 2011; Harada et al., 2009; Hudson et al., 2002). Most of this work focuses on cancer cells, where HIF-1α activation promotes tumorigenesis, and may explain why rapamycin inhibits cancer cell growth. The implication is that when tumors reach a size where hypoxia is inevitable, increased levels of mTOR activity stabilize HIF-1α allowing the tumor to continue to grow. In noncancer cells, there are considerably less data available, but the relationship between HIF-1α and mTOR appears similar. For example, mTOR activates HIF-1α in neutrophils to control trap formation (McInturff et al., 2012), in neurons to prevent apoptosis (H. Chen et al., 2012), and in pancreatic β cells to mediate the positive effects of incretin on cell survival (Van de Velde, Hogan, & Montminy, 2011). The general relevance of mTOR regulation of HIF-1α and vice versa in vivo remains to be determined, but the link between mTOR and HIF-1α may be useful in differentiating the positive and negative effects of HIF-1α in mammals.

Sirtuins and HIF Proteins

Sirtuins are a family of NAD-dependent protein deacetylases implicated in aging in various species, including yeast, worms, fruit flies, and mice (reviewed in Finkel, Deng, & Mostoslavsky, 2009; Houtkooper, Pirinen, & Auwerx, 2012). Overexpression of yeast SIR2 was first shown to increase replicative lifespan (M. Kaeberlein, McVey, & Guarente, 1999), and subsequent studies reported similar effects from overexpression of SIR2 orthologs in worms (Tissenbaum & Guarente, 2001) and flies (Rogina & Helfand, 2004). Activation of the mammalian SIR2 ortholog, SIRT1, has not been found to increase lifespan but has been linked to multiple age-related diseases (Finkel et al., 2009). Another Sirtuin, SIRT6, has been suggested to play a more direct role in mouse aging because knockout results in genomic instability and accelerated aging phenotypes (Mostoslavsky et al., 2006, p. 6) and overexpression extends lifespan in male mice (Kanfi et al., 2012). In 2009, Dioum et al. reported that SIRT1 binds and deacetylates HIF-2α to promote HIF activation in response to hypoxia. The authors suggest that HIF-2α is more responsive to subtle changes in oxygen than HIF-1α, and that SIRT1 is necessary for its activation and "fine-tuning" of the hypoxic response. Another study (Zhong et al., 2010) suggests that HIF-1α is regulated by SIRT6 through deacetylation of histones near HIF-1α target genes that deactivates their promoters. They provide evidence that the extreme hypoglycemia of SIRT6 knockout mice results from cellular glucose uptake caused in large part by HIF-1α activation. Another report contends that a mitochondrial Sirtuin, SIRT3, deactivates HIF-1α and that this deactivation in cancer cells is crucial to preventing growth (Haigis, Deng, Finley, Kim, & Gius, 2012). Together, these reports suggest that HIF and Sirtuins have a complex relationship that may involve specific modification of the hypoxic response.

CONCLUSIONS

In this review, we have focused on how environmental alterations in oxygen affect aging, how the hypoxic response pathway influences the aging process, how hypoxic responses change during aging, how the hypoxic response affects diseases associated with aging, and how the hypoxia-signaling pathway interacts with other pathways known to influence aging. The supply of oxygen along with other dietary nutrients and temperature are key environmental modulators of the aging process in many animals. Although it is generally accepted that altering oxygen concentration alters the production of ROS and that ROS plays some role in the aging process, the molecular mechanisms through which ROS influences aging remains unclear. Since the discovery of in vivo ROS production, the study of ROS in biology has focused primarily on their damaging effects. However, the last decade has seen an explosion in the field of ROS or redox signaling (reviewed in Forman, Maiorino, & Ursini, 2010). It has even been suggested that more subtle disruptions in the redox balance of aged cells, resulting from long-term oxidative stress, prevents normal redox signaling and leads to the pathogenic effects we call aging (Sohal & Orr, 2012). This hypothesis has been termed the "redox stress hypothesis." In this regard the paradoxical effects of hypoxia and hyperoxia and HIF activation or HIF inhibition may begin to make sense. Because both hyperoxia and hypoxia can generate ROS and if ROS, like hydrogen peroxide, function primarily as signaling molecules, it is not surprising that—depending on the developmental stage, the degree of activation, and the cellular context—these signals could have vastly different effects. It is also not surprising that the hypoxic response coevolved to coordinate with other nutritional response pathways like mTOR and the Sirtuins to allow the organism to survive adversity. The nonlinear effects of oxygen concentration on aging are also reminiscent of the effects of mitochondrial inhibition on lifespan. Moderate inhibition of mitochondrial function leads to longevity but more severe inhibition is highly detrimental (Rea, Ventura, & Johnson, 2007). This inverted U-shaped dose response curve typically describes a hormetic effect (Calabrese &

Baldwin, 2001), and it has been suggested that ROS-induced hormetic effects in the mitochondria underlay lifespan extension in worms (Schulz et al., 2007). Certainly, FOXO/DAF-16 activation in response to hypoxic stress supports this model, as does the suppression of lifespan extension in mitochondrial mutants by antioxidants (Leiser et al., 2013; Yang & Hekimi, 2010).

Does this apply to higher animals? Mammalian physiology has evolved homeostatic mechanisms to provide the organism with a constant supply of oxygen despite environmental fluctuations. These mechanisms provide some resistance to hypoxic exposure, but at the tissue and cellular level, hypoxia is a challenge to which mammalian cells must adequately respond or die. Even at the organismal level, there is some evidence that limiting environmental oxygen may have benefits in mammals (Sung et al., 2011; Weinberg et al., 1987). The conserved and crucial role of the HIF pathway in higher animals suggests that many of the insights gained in invertebrate model systems may lead to an increased understanding of the pathways that influence human aging and possibly afford new therapies to intervene in the treatment of age-related disease.

REFERENCES

Ackerman, D., & Gems, D. (2012). Insulin/IGF-1 and hypoxia signaling act in concert to regulate iron homeostasis in caenorhabditis elegans. *PLoS Genetics*, 8(3), e1002498. http://dx.doi.org/10.1371/journal.pgen.1002498

Austad, S. N., & Fischer, K. E. (1991). Mammalian aging, metabolism, and ecology: Evidence from the bats and marsupials. *Journal of Gerontology*, 46(2), B47–B53.

Barros, M. H., Bandy, B., Tahara, E. B., & Kowaltowski, A. J. (2004). Higher respiratory activity decreases mitochondrial reactive oxygen release and increases life span in Saccharomyces cerevisiae. *The Journal of Biological Chemistry*, 279(48), 49883–49888. http://dx.doi.org/10.1074/jbc.M408918200

Bellier, A., Chen, C.-S., Kao, C.-Y., Cinar, H. N., & Aroian, R. V. (2009). Hypoxia and the hypoxic response pathway protect against pore-forming toxins in C. elegans. *PLoS Pathogens*, 5(12), e1000689. http://dx.doi.org/10.1371/journal.ppat.1000689

Benderro, G. F., & Lamanna, J. C. (2011). Hypoxia-induced angiogenesis is delayed in aging mouse brain. *Brain Research*, 1389, 50–60. http://dx.doi.org/10.1016/j.brainres.2011.03.016

Benita, Y., Kikuchi, H., Smith, A. D., Zhang, M. Q., Chung, D. C., & Xavier, R. J. (2009). An integrative genomics approach identifies Hypoxia Inducible Factor-1 (HIF-1)-target genes that form the core response to hypoxia. *Nucleic Acids Research*, 37(14), 4587–4602. http://dx.doi.org/10.1093/nar/gkp425

Bishop, T., Lau, K. W., Epstein, A. C. R., Kim, S. K., Jiang, M., O'Rourke, D., . . . Ratcliffe, P. J. (2004). Genetic analysis of pathways regulated by the von Hippel-Lindau tumor suppressor in Caenorhabditis elegans. *PLoS Biology*, 2(10), e289. http://dx.doi.org/10.1371/journal.pbio.0020289

Bjedov, I., Toivonen, J. M., Kerr, F., Slack, C., Jacobson, J., Foley, A., & Partridge, L. (2010). Mechanisms of life span extension by rapamycin in the fruit fly Drosophila melanogaster. *Cell Metabolism*, *11*(1), 35–46. http://dx.doi.org/10.1016/j.cmet.2009.11.010

Bolli, R., & Marbán, E. (1999). Molecular and cellular mechanisms of myocardial stunning. *Physiological Reviews*, *79*(2), 609–634.

Braeckman, B. P., Houthoofd, K., & Vanfleteren, J. R. (2002). Assessing metabolic activity in aging Caenorhabditis elegans: Concepts and controversies. *Aging Cell*, *1*(2), 82–88. http://dx.doi.org/10.1046/j.1474-9728.2002.00021.x

Burtner, C. R., Murakami, C. J., Kennedy, B. K., & Kaeberlein, M. (2009). A molecular mechanism of chronological aging in yeast. *Cell Cycle (Georgetown, Tex.)*, *8*(8), 1256–1270.

Calabrese, E. J., & Baldwin, L. A. (2001). The frequency of U-shaped dose responses in the toxicological literature. *Toxicological Sciences*, *62*(2), 330–338. http://dx.doi.org/10.1093/toxsci/62.2.330

Chang, A. J., Chronis, N., Karow, D. S., Marletta, M. A., & Bargmann, C. I. (2006). A distributed chemosensory circuit for oxygen preference in C. elegans. *PLoS Biology*, *4*(9), e274. http://dx.doi.org/10.1371/journal.pbio.0040274

Chen, D., Thomas, E. L., & Kapahi, P. (2009). HIF-1 modulates dietary restriction-mediated lifespan extension via IRE-1 in Caenorhabditis elegans. *PLoS Genetics*, *5*(5), e1000486. http://dx.doi.org/10.1371/journal.pgen.1000486

Chen, H., Xiong, T., Qu, Y., Zhao, F., Ferriero, D., & Mu, D. (2012). mTOR activates hypoxia-inducible factor-1α and inhibits neuronal apoptosis in the developing rat brain during the early phase after hypoxia-ischemia. *Neuroscience Letters*, *507*(2), 118–123. http://dx.doi.org/10.1016/j.neulet.2011.11.058

Choi, D., Cai, E. P., Schroer, S. A., Wang, L., & Woo, M. (2011). Vhl is required for normal pancreatic β cell function and the maintenance of β cell mass with age in mice. *Laboratory Investigation*, *91*(4), 527–538. http://dx.doi.org/10.1038/labinvest.2010.207

Colman, R. J., Anderson, R. M., Johnson, S. C., Kastman, E. K., Kosmatka, K. J., Beasley, T. M., . . . Weindruch, R. (2009). Caloric restriction delays disease onset and mortality in rhesus monkeys. *Science (New York, N.Y.)*, *325*(5937), 201–204. http://dx.doi.org/10.1126/science.1173635

Conti, B. (2008). Considerations on temperature, longevity and aging. *Cellular and Molecular Life Sciences: CMLS*, *65*(11), 1626–1630. http://dx.doi.org/10.1007/s00018-008-7536-1

Danovaro, R., Dell'Anno, A., Pusceddu, A., Gambi, C., Heiner, I., & Kristensen, R. M. (2010). The first metazoa living in permanently anoxic conditions. *BMC Biology*, *8*(1), 30. http://dx.doi.org/10.1186/1741-7007-8-30

Darr, D., & Fridovich, I. (1995). Adaptation to oxidative stress in young, but not in mature or old, Caenorhabditis elegans. *Free Radical Biology and Medicine*, *18*(2), 195–201. http://dx.doi.org/10.1016/0891-5849(94)00118-4

Davy, P., & Allsopp, R. (2011). Hypoxia: Are stem cells in it for the long run? *Cell Cycle (Georgetown, Tex.)*, *10*(2), 206–211.

Dawson, T. L., Gores, G. J., Nieminen, A. L., Herman, B., & Lemasters, J. J. (1993). Mitochondria as a source of reactive oxygen species during reductive stress in rat hepatocytes. *The American Journal of Physiology*, *264*(4, Pt. 1), C961–967.

Debonneuil, E. H., Quillard, J., & Baulieu, E.-E. (2006). Hypoxia and dehydroepiandrosterone in old age: A mouse survival study. *Respiratory Research*, *7*, 144. http://dx.doi.org/10.1186/1465-9921-7-144

Demidenko, Z. N., & Blagosklonny, M. V. (2011). The purpose of the HIF-1/PHD feedback loop: To limit mTOR-induced HIF-1α. *Cell Cycle (Georgetown, Tex.)*, *10*(10), 1557–1562.

Dhalla, N. S., Elmoselhi, A. B., Hata, T., & Makino, N. (2000). Status of myocardial antioxidants in ischemia–reperfusion injury. *Cardiovascular Research*, *47*(3), 446–456. http://dx.doi.org/10.1016/S0008-6363(00)00078-X

Dioum, E. M., Chen, R., Alexander, M. S., Zhang, Q., Hogg, R. T., Gerard, R. D., & Garcia, J. A. (2009). Regulation of hypoxia-inducible Factor 2α signaling by the stress-responsive deacetylase sirtuin 1. *Science*, *324*(5932), 1289–1293. http://dx.doi.org/10.1126/science.1169956

Fehrer, C., Brunauer, R., Laschober, G., Unterluggauer, H., Reitinger, S., Kloss, F., . . . Lepperdinger, G. (2007). Reduced oxygen tension attenuates differentiation capacity of human mesenchymal stem cells and prolongs their lifespan. *Aging Cell*, *6*(6), 745–757. http://dx.doi.org/10.1111/j.1474-9726.2007.00336.x

Ferguson, M., Sohal, B. H., Forster, M. J., & Sohal, R. S. (2007). Effect of long-term caloric restriction on oxygen consumption and body temperature in two different strains of mice. *Mechanisms of Ageing and Development*, *128*(10), 539–545. http://dx.doi.org/10.1016/j.mad.2007.07.005

Finkel, T., Deng, C.-X., & Mostoslavsky, R. (2009). Recent progress in the biology and physiology of sirtuins. *Nature*, *460*(7255), 587–591. http://dx.doi.org/10.1038/nature08197

Foe, V. E., & Alberts, B. M. (1985). Reversible chromosome condensation induced in Drosophila embryos by anoxia: Visualization of interphase nuclear organization. *The Journal of Cell Biology*, *100*(5), 1623–1636.

Forman, H. J., Maiorino, M., & Ursini, F. (2010). Signaling functions of reactive oxygen species. *Biochemistry*, *49*(5), 835–842. http://dx.doi.org/10.1021/bi9020378

Gharbi, H., Fabretti, F., Bharill, P., Rinschen, M. M., Brinkkötter, S., Frommolt, P., . . . Müller, R.-U. (2013). Loss of the Birt-Hogg-Dubé gene product folliculin induces longevity in a hypoxia-inducible factor-dependent manner. *Aging Cell*, *12*(4), 593–603. http://dx.doi.org/10.1111/acel.12081

Gouspillou, G., & Hepple, R. T. (2013). Facts and controversies in our understanding of how caloric restriction impacts the mitochondrion. *Experimental Gerontology*, *48*(10), 1075–1084. http://dx.doi.org/10.1016/j.exger.2013.03.004

Grandison, R. C., Wong, R., Bass, T. M., Partridge, L., & Piper, M. D. W. (2009). Effect of a standardised dietary restriction protocol on multiple laboratory strains of Drosophila melanogaster. *PloS One*, *4*(1), e4067. http://dx.doi.org/10.1371/journal.pone.0004067

Greer, E. L., & Brunet, A. (2009). Different dietary restriction regimens extend lifespan by both independent and overlapping genetic pathways in C. elegans. *Aging Cell*, *8*(2), 113–127. http://dx.doi.org/10.1111/j.1474-9726.2009.00459.x

Guzy, R. D., Hoyos, B., Robin, E., Chen, H., Liu, L., Mansfield, K. D., . . . Schumacker, P. T. (2005). Mitochondrial complex III is required for hypoxia-induced ROS production and cellular oxygen sensing. *Cell Metabolism*, *1*(6), 401–408. http://dx.doi.org/10.1016/j.cmet.2005.05.001

Hagen, T. (2012). Oxygen versus reactive oxygen in the regulation of HIF-1α: The balance tips. *Biochemistry Research International*, *2012*, 436981. http://dx.doi.org/10.1155/2012/436981

Haigis, M. C., Deng, C.-X., Finley, L. W. S., Kim, H.-S., & Gius, D. (2012). SIRT3 is a mitochondrial tumor suppressor: A scientific tale that connects aberrant cellular ROS, the Warburg effect, and carcinogenesis. *Cancer Research*, *72*(10), 2468–2472. http://dx.doi.org/10.1158/0008-5472.CAN-11-3633

Hancock, C. R., Han, D.-H., Higashida, K., Kim, S. H., & Holloszy, J. O. (2011). Does calorie restriction induce mitochondrial biogenesis? A reevaluation. *FASEB Journal: Official Publication of the Federation of American Societies for Experimental Biology*, *25*(2), 785–791. http://dx.doi.org/10.1096/fj.10-170415

Harada, H., Itasaka, S., Kizaka-Kondoh, S., Shibuya, K., Morinibu, A., Shinomiya, K., & Hiraoka, M. (2009). The Akt/mTOR pathway assures the synthesis of HIF-1alpha protein in a glucose- and reoxygenation-dependent manner in irradiated tumors. *The Journal of Biological Chemistry*, *284*(8), 5332–5342. http://dx.doi.org/10.1074/jbc.M806653200

Harman, D. (1956). Aging: A theory based on free radical and radiation chemistry. *Journal of Gerontology*, *11*(3), 298–300.

Harrison, D. E., Strong, R., Sharp, Z. D., Nelson, J. F., Astle, C. M., Flurkey, K., . . . Miller, R. A. (2009). Rapamycin fed late in life extends lifespan in genetically heterogeneous mice. *Nature*, *460*(7253), 392–395. http://dx.doi.org/10.1038/nature08221

Hempenstall, S., Page, M. M., Wallen, K. R., & Selman, C. (2012). Dietary restriction increases skeletal muscle mitochondrial respiration but not mitochondrial content in C57BL/6 mice. *Mechanisms of Ageing and Development*, *133*(1), 37–45. http://dx.doi.org/10.1016/j.mad.2011.12.002

Hochachka, P. W., & Somero, G. N. (2002). *Biochemical adaptation: Mechanism and process in physiological evolution* (1st ed.). New York, NY: Oxford University Press.

Holland, H. D. (2006). The oxygenation of the atmosphere and oceans. *Philosophical Transactions of the Royal Society B: Biological Sciences*, *361*(1470), 903–915. http://dx.doi.org/10.1098/rstb.2006.1838

Honda, S., Ishii, N., Suzuki, K., & Matsuo, M. (1993). Oxygen-dependent perturbation of life span and aging rate in the nematode. *Journal of Gerontology*, *48*(2), B57–B61.

Honda, Y., & Honda, S. (2001). Life span extensions associated with upregulation of gene expression of antioxidant enzymes in Caenorhabdms elegans; studies of mutation in the AGE-1, PI3 kinase homologue and short-term exposure to hyperoxia. *Journal of the American Aging Association*, *24*(4), 179–186. http://dx.doi.org/10.1007/s11357-001-0019-z

Honda, Y., Tanaka, M., & Honda, S. (2008). Modulation of longevity and diapause by redox regulation mechanisms under the insulin-like signaling control in Caenorhabditis elegans. *Experimental Gerontology*, *43*(6), 520–529. http://dx.doi.org/10.1016/j.exger.2008.02.009

Houthoofd, K., Braeckman, B. P., Lenaerts, I., Brys, K., De Vreese, A., Van Eygen, S., & Vanfleteren, J. R. (2002a). Axenic growth up-regulates mass-specific metabolic rate, stress resistance, and extends life span in Caenorhabditis elegans. *Experimental Gerontology*, *37*(12), 1371–1378. http://dx.doi.org/10.1016/S0531-5565(02)00173-0

Houthoofd, K., Braeckman, B. P., Lenaerts, I., Brys, K., De Vreese, A., Van Eygen, S., & Vanfleteren, J. R. (2002b). No reduction of metabolic rate in food restricted Caenorhabditis elegans. *Experimental Gerontology*, *37*(12), 1359–1369. http://dx.doi.org/10.1016/S0531-5565(02)00172-9

Houtkooper, R. H., Pirinen, E., & Auwerx, J. (2012). Sirtuins as regulators of metabolism and healthspan. *Nature Reviews. Molecular Cell Biology*, *13*(4), 225–238. http://dx.doi.org/10.1038/nrm3293

Hudson, C. C., Liu, M., Chiang, G. G., Otterness, D. M., Loomis, D. C., Kaper, F., . . . Abraham, R. T. (2002). Regulation of hypoxia-inducible factor 1alpha expression and function by the mammalian target of rapamycin. *Molecular and Cellular Biology*, *22*(20), 7004–7014.

Hulbert, A., Clancy, D. J., Mair, W., Braeckman, B. P., Gems, D., & Partridge, L. (2004). Metabolic rate is not reduced by dietary-restriction or by lowered insulin/IGF-1 signalling and is not correlated with individual lifespan in Drosophila melanogaster. *Experimental Gerontology*, *39*(8), 1137–1143. http://dx.doi.org/10.1016/j.exger.2004.04.006

Hunt, N. D., Hyun, D.-H., Allard, J. S., Minor, R. K., Mattson, M. P., Ingram, D. K., & de Cabo, R. (2006). Bioenergetics of aging and calorie restriction. *Ageing Research Reviews*, *5*(2), 125–143. http://dx.doi.org/10.1016/j.arr.2006.03.006

Iyer, N. V., Kotch, L. E., Agani, F., Leung, S. W., Laughner, E., Wenger, R. H., . . . Semenza, G. L. (1998). Cellular and developmental control of O2 homeostasis by hypoxia-inducible factor 1 alpha. *Genes & Development*, *12*(2), 149–162.

Ja, W. W., Carvalho, G. B., Zid, B. M., Mak, E. M., Brummel, T., & Benzer, S. (2009). Water- and nutrient-dependent effects of dietary restriction on Drosophila lifespan. *Proceedings of the National Academy of Sciences of the United States of America*, *106*(44), 18633–18637. http://dx.doi.org/10.1073/pnas.0908016106

Jackson, M. J., Pye, D., & Palomero, J. (2007). The production of reactive oxygen and nitrogen species by skeletal muscle. *Journal of Applied Physiology*, *102*(4), 1664–1670. http://dx.doi.org/10.1152/japplphysiol.01102.2006

Jamieson, D. (1989). Oxygen toxicity and reactive oxygen metabolites in mammals. *Free Radical Biology and Medicine*, 7(1), 87–108. http://dx.doi.org/10.1016/0891-5849(89)90103-2

Jeong, J.-K., Seo, J.-S., Moon, M.-H., Lee, Y.-J., Seol, J.-W., & Park, S.-Y. (2012). Hypoxia-inducible factor-1 alpha regulates prion protein expression to protect against neuron cell damage. *Neurobiology of Aging*, *33*(5), 1006.e1–1006.e10. http://dx.doi.org/10.1016/j.neurobiolaging.2011.09.037

Jia, K., Chen, D., & Riddle, D. L. (2004). The TOR pathway interacts with the insulin signaling pathway to regulate C. elegans larval development, metabolism and life span. *Development (Cambridge, England)*, *131*(16), 3897–3906. http://dx.doi.org/10.1242/dev.01255

Jiang, C., Qu, A., Matsubara, T., Chanturiya, T., Jou, W., Gavrilova, O., . . . Gonzalez, F. J. (2011). Disruption of hypoxia-inducible factor 1 in adipocytes improves insulin sensitivity and decreases adiposity in high-fat diet-fed mice. *Diabetes*, *60*(10), 2484–2495. http://dx.doi.org/10.2337/db11-0174

Jiang, H., Guo, R., & Powell-Coffman, J. A. (2001). The Caenorhabditis elegans hif-1 gene encodes a bHLH-PAS protein that is required for adaptation to hypoxia. *Proceedings of the National Academy of Sciences*, *98*(14), 7916–7921. http://dx.doi.org/10.1073/pnas.141234698

Johannsen, D. L., Knuth, N. D., Huizenga, R., Rood, J. C., Ravussin, E., & Hall, K. D. (2012). Metabolic slowing with massive weight loss despite preservation of fat-free mass. *The Journal of Clinical Endocrinology and Metabolism*, *97*(7), 2489–2496. http://dx.doi.org/10.1210/jc.2012-1444

Johnson, S. C., Rabinovitch, P. S., & Kaeberlein, M. (2013). mTOR is a key modulator of ageing and age-related disease. *Nature*, *493*(7432), 338–345. http://dx.doi.org/10.1038/nature11861

Kaeberlein, M. (2010). Resveratrol and rapamycin: Are they anti-aging drugs? *BioEssays: News and Reviews in Molecular, Cellular and Developmental Biology*, *32*(2), 96–99. http://dx.doi.org/10.1002/bies.200900171

Kaeberlein, M., Hu, D., Kerr, E. O., Tsuchiya, M., Westman, E. A., Dang, N., . . . Kennedy, B. K. (2005). Increased life span due to calorie restriction in respiratory-deficient yeast. *PLoS Genetics*, *1*(5), e69. http://dx.doi.org/10.1371/journal.pgen.0010069

Kaeberlein, M., & Kapahi, P. (2009). The hypoxic response and aging. *Cell Cycle (Georgetown, Tex.)*, *8*(15), 2324.

Kaeberlein, M., Kirkland, K. T., Fields, S., & Kennedy, B. K. (2004). SIR2-independent life span extension by calorie restriction in yeast. *PLoS Biology*, *2*(9), E296. http://dx.doi.org/10.1371/journal.pbio.0020296

Kaeberlein, M., McVey, M., & Guarente, L. (1999). The SIR2/3/4 complex and SIR2 alone promote longevity in Saccharomyces cerevisiae by two different mechanisms. *Genes & Development*, *13*(19), 2570–2580.

Kaeberlein, M., Powers, R. W., III, Steffen, K. K., Westman, E. A., Hu, D., Dang, N., . . . Kennedy, B. K. (2005). Regulation of yeast replicative life span by TOR and Sch9 in response to nutrients. *Science (New York, N.Y.)*, *310*(5751), 1193–1196. http://dx.doi.org/10.1126/science.1115535

Kaeberlein, T. L., Smith, E. D., Tsuchiya, M., Welton, K. L., Thomas, J. H., Fields, S., . . . Kaeberlein, M. (2006). Lifespan extension in Caenorhabditis elegans by complete removal of food. *Aging Cell*, *5*(6), 487–494. http://dx.doi.org/10.1111/j.1474-9726.2006.00238.x

Kaelin, W. G., Jr. (2002). How oxygen makes its presence felt. *Genes & Development*, *16*(12), 1441–1445. http://dx.doi.org/10.1101/gad.1003602

Kanfi, Y., Naiman, S., Amir, G., Peshti, V., Zinman, G., Nahum, L., . . . Cohen, H. Y. (2012). The sirtuin SIRT6 regulates lifespan in male mice. *Nature*, *483*(7388), 218–221. http://dx.doi.org/10.1038/nature10815

Kang, M. J., Kim, H. J., Kim, H. K., Lee, J. Y., Kim, D. H., Jung, K. J., . . . Chung, H. Y. (2005). The effect of age and calorie restriction on HIF-1-responsive genes in aged liver. *Biogerontology*, *6*(1), 27–37. http://dx.doi.org/10.1007/s10522-004-7381-z

Kapahi, P., Chen, D., Rogers, A. N., Katewa, S. D., Li, P. W.-L., Thomas, E. L., & Kockel, L. (2010). With TOR, less is more: A key role for the conserved nutrient-sensing TOR pathway in aging. *Cell Metabolism*, *11*(6), 453–465. http://dx.doi.org/10.1016/j.cmet.2010.05.001

Kapahi, P., Zid, B. M., Harper, T., Koslover, D., Sapin, V., & Benzer, S. (2004). Regulation of lifespan in Drosophila by modulation of genes in the TOR signaling pathway. *Current Biology: CB*, *14*(10), 885–890. http://dx.doi.org/10.1016/j.cub.2004.03.059

Kennedy, B. K., Steffen, K. K., & Kaeberlein, M. (2007). Ruminations on dietary restriction and aging. *Cellular and Molecular Life Sciences: CMLS*, *64*(11), 1323–1328. http://dx.doi.org/10.1007/s00018-007-6470-y

Kenyon, C., Chang, J., Gensch, E., Rudner, A., & Tabtiang, R. (1993). A *C. elegans* mutant that lives twice as long as wild type. *Nature*, *366*(6454), 461–464. http://dx.doi.org/10.1038/366461a0

Kim, H. J., Jung, K. J., Yu, B. P., Cho, C. G., Choi, J. S., & Chung, H. Y. (2002). Modulation of redox-sensitive transcription factors by calorie restriction during aging. *Mechanisms of Ageing and Development*, *123*(12), 1589–1595. http://dx.doi.org/10.1016/S0047-6374(02)00094-5

Kim, W., & Kaelin, W. G., Jr. (2003). The von Hippel-Lindau tumor suppressor protein: New insights into oxygen sensing and cancer. *Current Opinion in Genetics & Development*, *13*(1), 55–60.

Kimura, K. D., Tissenbaum, H. A., Liu, Y., & Ruvkun, G. (1997). daf-2, an insulin receptor-like gene that regulates longevity and diapause in Caenorhabditis elegans. *Science (New York, N.Y.)*, *277*(5328), 942–946.

Kirienko, N. V., Kirienko, D. R., Larkins-Ford, J., Wählby, C., Ruvkun, G., & Ausubel, F. M. (2013). Pseudomonas aeruginosa disrupts Caenorhabditis elegans iron homeostasis, causing a hypoxic response and death. *Cell Host & Microbe*, *13*(4), 406–416. http://dx.doi.org/10.1016/j.chom.2013.03.003

Kirito, K., Hu, Y., & Komatsu, N. (2009). HIF-1 prevents the overproduction of mitochondrial ROS after cytokine stimulation through induction of PDK-1. *Cell Cycle (Georgetown, Tex.)*, *8*(17), 2844–2849.

Koc, A., Gasch, A. P., Rutherford, J. C., Kim, H.-Y., & Gladyshev, V. N. (2004). Methionine sulfoxide reductase regulation of yeast lifespan reveals reactive oxygen species-dependent and -independent components of aging. *Proceedings of the National Academy of Sciences of the United States of America*, *101*(21), 7999–8004. http://dx.doi.org/10.1073/pnas.0307929101

Lanza, I. R., Zabielski, P., Klaus, K. A., Morse, D. M., Heppelmann, C. J., Bergen, H. R., III, . . . Nair, K. S. (2012). Chronic caloric restriction preserves mitochondrial function in senescence without increasing mitochondrial biogenesis. *Cell Metabolism*, *16*(6), 777–788. http://dx.doi.org/10.1016/j.cmet.2012.11.003

Larsen, P. L., Albert, P. S., & Riddle, D. L. (1995). Genes that regulate both development and longevity in Caenorhabditis elegans. *Genetics*, *139*(4), 1567–1583.

Lee, G. D., Wilson, M. A., Zhu, M., Wolkow, C. A., de Cabo, R., Ingram, D. K., & Zou, S. (2006). Dietary deprivation extends lifespan in Caenorhabditis elegans. *Aging Cell*, *5*(6), 515–524. http://dx.doi.org/10.1111/j.1474-9726.2006.00241.x

Lee, S.-J., Hwang, A. B., & Kenyon, C. (2010). Inhibition of respiration extends C. elegans life span via reactive oxygen species that increase HIF-1 activity. *Current Biology: CB*, *20*(23), 2131–2136. http://dx.doi.org/10.1016/j.cub.2010.10.057

Lefer, D. J., & Granger, D. N. (2000). Oxidative stress and cardiac disease. *The American Journal of Medicine*, *109*(4), 315–323. http://dx.doi.org/10.1016/S0002-9343(00)00467-8

Leiser, S. F., Begun, A., & Kaeberlein, M. (2011). HIF-1 modulates longevity and healthspan in a temperature-dependent manner. *Aging Cell*, *10*(2), 318–326. http://dx.doi.org/10.1111/j.1474-9726.2011.00672.x

Leiser, S. F., Fletcher, M., Begun, A., & Kaeberlein, M. (2013). Life-span extension from hypoxia in Caenorhabditis elegans requires both HIF-1 and DAF-16 and is antagonized by SKN-1. *The Journals of Gerontology. Series A, Biological Sciences and Medical Sciences*, *68*(10), 1135–1144. http://dx.doi.org/10.1093/gerona/glt016

Li, M., & Kim, W. Y. (2011). Two sides to every story: the HIF-dependent and HIF-independent functions of pVHL. *Journal of Cellular and Molecular Medicine*, *15*(2), 187–195. http://dx.doi.org/10.1111/j.1582-4934.2010.01238.x

Lin, S. J., Defossez, P. A., & Guarente, L. (2000). Requirement of NAD and SIR2 for life-span extension by calorie restriction in Saccharomyces cerevisiae. *Science (New York, N.Y.)*, *289*(5487), 2126–2128.

Lin, S. J., Kaeberlein, M., Andalis, A. A., Sturtz, L. A., Defossez, P.-A., Culotta, V. C., . . . Guarente, L. (2002). Calorie restriction extends Saccharomyces cerevisiae lifespan by increasing respiration. *Nature*, *418*(6895), 344–348. http://dx.doi.org/10.1038/nature00829

Liu, T., & Cai, D. (2013). Counterbalance between BAG and URX neurons via guanylate cyclases controls lifespan homeostasis in C. elegans. *The EMBO Journal*, *32*(11), 1529–1542. http://dx.doi.org/10.1038/emboj.2013.75

Loh, K. P., Huang, S. H., De Silva, R., Tan, B. K. H., & Zhu, Y. Z. (2006). Oxidative stress: Apoptosis in neuronal injury. *Current Alzheimer Research*, *3*(4), 327–337.

Longo, V. D., Shadel, G. S., Kaeberlein, M., & Kennedy, B. (2012). Replicative and chronological aging in Saccharomyces cerevisiae. *Cell Metabolism*, *16*(1), 18–31. http://dx.doi.org/10.1016/j.cmet.2012.06.002

Mair, W., & Dillin, A. (2008). Aging and survival: The genetics of life span extension by dietary restriction. *Annual Review of Biochemistry*, *77*, 727–754. http://dx.doi.org/10.1146/annurev.biochem.77.061206.171059

Mannello, F., Medda, V., & Tonti, G. A. (2011). Hypoxia and neural stem cells: From invertebrates to brain cancer stem cells. *The International Journal of Developmental Biology*, *55*(6), 569–581. http://dx.doi.org/10.1387/ijdb.103186fm

Mansfield, K. D., Guzy, R. D., Pan, Y., Young, R. M., Cash, T. P., Schumacker, P. T., & Simon, M. C. (2005). Mitochondrial dysfunction resulting from loss of cytochrome c impairs cellular oxygen sensing and hypoxic HIF-alpha activation. *Cell Metabolism*, *1*(6), 393–399. http://dx.doi.org/10.1016/j.cmet.2005.05.003

Martin, C. K., Heilbronn, L. K., de Jonge, L., DeLany, J. P., Volaufova, J., Anton, S. D., . . . Ravussin, E. (2007). Effect of calorie restriction on resting metabolic rate and spontaneous physical activity. *Obesity (Silver Spring, Md.)*, *15*(12), 2964–2973. http://dx.doi.org/10.1038/oby.2007.354

Masoro, E. J. (2005). Overview of caloric restriction and ageing. *Mechanisms of Ageing and Development*, *126*(9), 913–922. http://dx.doi.org/10.1016/j.mad.2005.03.012

McDonough, M. A., Li, V., Flashman, E., Chowdhury, R., Mohr, C., Liénard, B. M. R., . . . Schofield, C. J. (2006). Cellular oxygen sensing: Crystal structure of hypoxia-inducible factor prolyl hydroxylase (PHD2). *Proceedings of the National Academy of Sciences of the United States of America*, *103*(26), 9814–9819. http://dx.doi.org/10.1073/pnas.0601283103

McInturff, A. M., Cody, M. J., Elliott, E. A., Glenn, J. W., Rowley, J. W., Rondina, M. T., & Yost, C. C. (2012). Mammalian target of rapamycin regulates neutrophil extracellular trap formation via induction of hypoxia-inducible factor 1 α. *Blood*, *120*(15), 3118–3125. http://dx.doi.org/10.1182/blood-2012-01-405993

McNeill, L. A., Flashman, E., Buck, M. R. G., Hewitson, K. S., Clifton, I. J., Jeschke, G., . . . Schofield, C. J. (2005). Hypoxia-inducible factor prolyl hydroxylase 2 has a high affinity for ferrous iron and 2-oxoglutarate. *Molecular BioSystems*, *1*(4), 321–324. http://dx.doi.org/10.1039/b511249b

Mehta, R., Steinkraus, K. A., Sutphin, G. L., Ramos, F. J., Shamieh, L. S., Huh, A., . . . Kaeberlein, M. (2009). Proteasomal regulation of the hypoxic response modulates aging in C. elegans. *Science*, *324*(5931), 1196–1198. http://dx.doi.org/10.1126/science.1173507

Mendenhall, A. R., LaRue, B., & Padilla, P. A. (2006). Glyceraldehyde-3-phosphate dehydrogenase mediates anoxia response and survival in Caenorhabditis elegans. *Genetics*, *174*(3), 1173–1187. http://dx.doi.org/10.1534/genetics.106.061390

Miller, B. F., Robinson, M. M., Bruss, M. D., Hellerstein, M., & Hamilton, K. L. (2012). A comprehensive assessment of mitochondrial protein synthesis and cellular proliferation with age and caloric restriction. *Aging Cell*, *11*(1), 150–161. http://dx.doi.org/10.1111/j.1474-9726.2011.00769.x

Miller, R. A., Harrison, D. E., Astle, C. M., Baur, J. A., Boyd, A. R., de Cabo, R., . . . Strong, R. (2011). Rapamycin, but not resveratrol or simvastatin, extends life span of genetically heterogeneous mice. *The Journals of Gerontology. Series A, Biological Sciences and Medical Sciences*, 66(2), 191–201. http://dx.doi.org/10.1093/gerona/glq178

Mockett, R. J., Sohal, R. S., & Orr, W. C. (1999). Overexpression of glutathione reductase extends survival in transgenic Drosophila melanogaster under hyperoxia but not normoxia. *FASEB Journal: Official Publication of the Federation of American Societies for Experimental Biology*, *13*(13), 1733–1742.

Mostoslavsky, R., Chua, K. F., Lombard, D. B., Pang, W. W., Fischer, M. R., Gellon, L., . . . Alt, F. W. (2006). Genomic instability and aging-like phenotype in the absence of mammalian SIRT6. *Cell*, *124*(2), 315–329. http://dx.doi.org/10.1016/j.cell.2005.11.044

Müller, R.-U., Fabretti, F., Zank, S., Burst, V., Benzing, T., & Schermer, B. (2009). The von Hippel Lindau tumor suppressor limits longevity. *Journal of the American Society of Nephrology: JASN*, *20*(12), 2513–2517. http://dx.doi.org/10.1681/ASN.2009050497

Murakami, C. J., Burtner, C. R., Kennedy, B. K., & Kaeberlein, M. (2008). A method for high-throughput quantitative analysis of yeast chronological life span. *The Journals of Gerontology. Series A, Biological Sciences and Medical Sciences*, *63*(2), 113–121.

Murakami, C. J., Wall, V., Basisty, N., & Kaeberlein, M. (2011). Composition and acidification of the culture medium influences chronological aging similarly in vineyard and laboratory yeast. *PloS One*, *6*(9), e24530. http://dx.doi.org/10.1371/journal.pone.0024530

Ogunshola, O. O., & Antoniou, X. (2009). Contribution of hypoxia to Alzheimer's disease: Is HIF-1alpha a mediator of neurodegeneration? *Cellular and Molecular Life Sciences: CMLS*, *66*(22), 3555–3563. http://dx.doi.org/10.1007/s00018-009-0141-0

Packer, L., & Fuehr, K. (1977). Low oxygen concentration extends the lifespan of cultured human diploid cells. *Nature*, *267*(5610), 423–425.

Pearl, R. (1928). *The rate of living: Being an account of some experimental studies on the biology of life duration*. New York, NY: A.A. Knopf.

Powers, R. W., III, Kaeberlein, M., Caldwell, S. D., Kennedy, B. K., & Fields, S. (2006). Extension of chronological life span in yeast by decreased TOR pathway signaling. *Genes & Development*, *20*(2), 174–184. http://dx.doi.org/10.1101/gad.1381406

Putker, M., Madl, T., Vos, H. R., de Ruiter, H., Visscher, M., van den Berg, M. C. W., . . . Dansen, T. B. (2013). Redox-dependent control of FOXO/DAF-16 by transportin-1. *Molecular Cell*, *49*(4), 730–742. http://dx.doi.org/10.1016/j.molcel.2012.12.014

Rabie, T., Kunze, R., & Marti, H. H. (2011). Impaired hypoxic response in senescent mouse brain. *International Journal of Developmental Neuroscience: The Official Journal of the International Society for Developmental Neuroscience*, *29*(6), 655–661. http://dx.doi.org/10.1016/j.ijdevneu.2011.06.003

Ramsey, J. J., & Hagopian, K. (2006). Energy expenditure and restriction of energy intake: Could energy restriction alter energy expenditure in companion animals? *The Journal of Nutrition*, *136*(7 Suppl.), 1958S–1966S.

Rascón, B., & Harrison, J. F. (2010). Lifespan and oxidative stress show a non-linear response to atmospheric oxygen in Drosophila. *The Journal of Experimental Biology*, *213*(Pt. 20), 3441–3448. http://dx.doi.org/10.1242/jeb.044867

Rea, S. L., Ventura, N., & Johnson, T. E. (2007). Relationship between mitochondrial electron transport chain dysfunction, development, and life extension in Caenorhabditis elegans. *PLoS Biology*, *5*(10), e259. http://dx.doi.org/10.1371/journal.pbio.0050259

Redman, L. M., Heilbronn, L. K., Martin, C. K., de Jonge, L., Williamson, D. A., Delany, J. P., . . . Pennington CALERIE Team. (2009). Metabolic and behavioral compensations in response to caloric restriction: Implications for the maintenance of weight loss. *PloS One*, *4*(2), e4377. http://dx.doi.org/10.1371/journal.pone.0004377

Rey, S., Luo, W., Shimoda, L. A., & Semenza, G. L. (2011). Metabolic reprogramming by HIF-1 promotes the survival of bone marrow–derived angiogenic cells in ischemic tissue. *Blood*, *117*(18), 4988–4998. http://dx.doi.org/10.1182/blood-2010-11-321190

Rezvani, H. R., Ali, N., Nissen, L. J., Harfouche, G., de Verneuil, H., Taïeb, A., & Mazurier, F. (2011). HIF-1α in epidermis: Oxygen sensing, cutaneous angiogenesis, cancer, and non-cancer disorders. *Journal of Investigative Dermatology*, *131*(9), 1793–1805. http://dx.doi.org/10.1038/jid.2011.141

Rogina, B., & Helfand, S. L. (2004). SIR2 mediates longevity in the fly through a pathway related to calorie restriction. *Proceedings of the National Academy of Sciences of the United States of America*, *101*(45), 15998–16003. http://dx.doi.org/10.1073/pnas.0404184101

Roitbak, T., Surviladze, Z., & Cunningham, L. A. (2011). Continuous expression of HIF-1α in neural stem/progenitor cells. *Cellular and Molecular Neurobiology*, *31*(1), 119–133. http://dx.doi.org/10.1007/s10571-010-9561-5

Schofield, C. J., & Ratcliffe, P. J. (2004). Oxygen sensing by HIF hydroxylases. *Nature Reviews. Molecular Cell Biology*, *5*(5), 343–354. http://dx.doi.org/10.1038/nrm1366

Schulz, T. J., Zarse, K., Voigt, A., Urban, N., Birringer, M., & Ristow, M. (2007). Glucose restriction extends Caenorhabditis elegans life span by inducing mitochondrial respiration and increasing oxidative stress. *Cell Metabolism*, *6*(4), 280–293. http://dx.doi.org/10.1016/j.cmet.2007.08.011

Scott, B. A., Avidan, M. S., & Crowder, C. M. (2002). Regulation of hypoxic death in C. elegans by the insulin/IGF receptor homolog DAF-2. *Science (New York, N.Y.)*, *296*(5577), 2388–2391. http://dx.doi.org/10.1126/science.1072302

Selman, C., Phillips, T., Staib, J. L., Duncan, J. S., Leeuwenburgh, C., & Speakman, J. R. (2005). Energy expenditure of calorically restricted rats is higher than predicted from their altered body composition. *Mechanisms of Ageing and Development*, *126*(6–7), 783–793. http://dx.doi.org/10.1016/j.mad.2005.02.004

Semenza, G. (2002). Signal transduction to hypoxia-inducible factor 1. *Biochemical Pharmacology*, *64*(5–6), 993–998.

Semenza, G. L. (2009). Regulation of vascularization by hypoxia-inducible factor 1. *Annals of the New York Academy of Sciences*, *1177*, 2–8. http://dx.doi.org/10.1111/j.1749-6632.2009.05032.x

Severinghaus, J. W. (2002). Priestley, the furious free thinker of the enlightenment, and Scheele, the taciturn apothecary of Uppsala. *Acta Anaesthesiologica Scandinavica*, *46*(1), 2–9. http://dx.doi.org/10.1046/j.0001-5172.2001.00351.x

Shao, Z., Zhang, Y., & Powell-Coffman, J. A. (2009). Two distinct roles for EGL-9 in the regulation of HIF-1-mediated gene expression in Caenorhabditis elegans. *Genetics*, *183*(3), 821–829. http://dx.doi.org/10.1534/genetics.109.107284

Sharp, Z. D. (2011). Aging and TOR: Interwoven in the fabric of life. *Cellular and Molecular Life Sciences: CMLS*, *68*(4), 587–597. http://dx.doi.org/10.1007/s00018-010-0542-0

Shen, C., Nettleton, D., Jiang, M., Kim, S. K., & Powell-Coffman, J. A. (2005). Roles of the HIF-1 hypoxia-inducible factor during hypoxia response in Caenorhabditis elegans. *The Journal of Biological Chemistry*, *280*(21), 20580–20588. http://dx.doi.org/10.1074/jbc.M501894200

Shen, C., & Powell-Coffman, J. A. (2003). Genetic analysis of hypoxia signaling and response in C elegans. *Annals of the New York Academy of Sciences*, *995*, 191–199.

Shen, C., Shao, Z., & Powell-Coffman, J. A. (2006). The Caenorhabditis elegans rhy-1 gene inhibits HIF-1 hypoxia-inducible factor activity in a negative feedback loop that does not include vhl-1. *Genetics*, *174*(3), 1205–1214. http://dx.doi.org/10.1534/genetics.106.063594

Skorupa, D. A., Dervisefendic, A., Zwiener, J., & Pletcher, S. D. (2008). Dietary composition specifies consumption, obesity, and lifespan in Drosophila melanogaster. *Aging Cell*, *7*(4), 478–490. http://dx.doi.org/10.1111/j.1474-9726.2008.00400.x

Smith, D. L., Jr, McClure, J. M., Matecic, M., & Smith, J. S. (2007). Calorie restriction extends the chronological lifespan of Saccharomyces cerevisiae independently of the Sirtuins. *Aging Cell*, *6*(5), 649–662. http://dx.doi.org/10.1111/j.1474-9726.2007.00326.x

Smith, E. D., Kaeberlein, T. L., Lydum, B. T., Sager, J., Welton, K. L., Kennedy, B. K., & Kaeberlein, M. (2008). Age- and calorie-independent life span extension from dietary restriction by bacterial deprivation in Caenorhabditis elegans. *BMC Developmental Biology*, *8*, 49. http://dx.doi.org/10.1186/1471-213X-8-49

Sohal, R. S., Agarwal, S., Dubey, A., & Orr, W. C. (1993). Protein oxidative damage is associated with life expectancy of houseflies. *Proceedings of the National Academy of Sciences of the United States of America*, *90*(15), 7255–7259.

Sohal, R. S., & Orr, W. C. (2012). The redox stress hypothesis of aging. *Free Radical Biology & Medicine*, *52*(3), 539–555. http://dx.doi.org/10.1016/j.freeradbiomed.2011.10.445

Speakman, J. R. (2005). Body size, energy metabolism and lifespan. *Journal of Experimental Biology*, *208*(Pt. 9), 1717–1730. http://dx.doi.org/10.1242/jeb.01556

Stanfel, M. N., Shamieh, L. S., Kaeberlein, M., & Kennedy, B. K. (2009). The TOR pathway comes of age. *Biochimica et Biophysica Acta, 1790*(10), 1067–1074. http://dx.doi.org/10.1016/j.bbagen.2009.06.007

Sung, H. J., Ma, W., Starost, M. F., Lago, C. U., Lim, P. K., Sack, M. N., . . . Hwang, P. M. (2011). Ambient oxygen promotes tumorigenesis. *PLoS One*, *6*(5), e19785. http://dx.doi.org/10.1371/journal.pone.0019785

Sutphin, G. L., & Kaeberlein, M. (2008). Dietary restriction by bacterial deprivation increases life span in wild-derived nematodes. *Experimental Gerontology*, *43*(3), 130–135. http://dx.doi.org/10.1016/j.exger.2007.10.019

Takubo, K., Goda, N., Yamada, W., Iriuchishima, H., Ikeda, E., Kubota, Y., . . . Suda, T. (2010). Regulation of the HIF-1α level is essential for hematopoietic stem cells. *Cell Stem Cell*, *7*(3), 391–402. http://dx.doi.org/10.1016/j.stem.2010.06.020

Tan, T., Marín-García, J., Damle, S., & Weiss, H. R. (2010). Hypoxia-inducible factor-1 improves inotropic responses of cardiac myocytes in ageing heart without affecting mitochondrial activity. *Experimental Physiology*, *95*(6), 712–722. http://dx.doi.org/10.1113/expphysiol.2009.051649

Tatar, M. (2011). The plate half-full: Status of research on the mechanisms of dietary restriction in Drosophila melanogaster. *Experimental Gerontology*, *46*(5), 363–368. http://dx.doi.org/10.1016/j.exger.2010.12.002

Tissenbaum, H. A., & Guarente, L. (2001). Increased dosage of a sir-2 gene extends lifespan in Caenorhabditis elegans. *Nature*, *410*(6825), 227–230. http://dx.doi.org/10.1038/35065638

Tormos, K. V., & Chandel, N. S. (2010). Inter-connection between mitochondria and HIFs. *Journal of Cellular and Molecular Medicine*, *14*(4), 795–804. http://dx.doi.org/10.1111/j.1582-4934.2010.01031.x

Turrens, J. F. (2003). Mitochondrial formation of reactive oxygen species. *The Journal of Physiology*, *552*(2), 335–344. http://dx.doi.org/10.1113/jphysiol.2003.049478

Underwood, E. A. (1944). Lavoisier and the History of Respiration. *Proceedings of the Royal Society of Medicine*, *37*(6), 247–262.

Van de Velde, S., Hogan, M. F., & Montminy, M. (2011). mTOR links incretin signaling to HIF induction in pancreatic beta cells. *Proceedings of the National Academy of Sciences of the United States of America*, *108*(41), 16876–16882. http://dx.doi.org/10.1073/pnas.1114228108

Van Voorhies, W. A. (2002). The influence of metabolic rate on longevity in the nematode Caenorhabditis elegans. *Aging Cell*, *1*(2), 91–101. http://dx.doi.org/10.1046/j.1474-9728.2002.00022.x

Van Voorhies, W. A. (2004). Live fast—live long? A commentary on a recent paper by Speakman et al. *Aging Cell*, *3*(5), 327–330. http://dx.doi.org/10.1111/j.1474-9728.2004.00113.x

Van Voorhies, W. A. (2009). Metabolic function in Drosophila melanogaster in response to hypoxia and pure oxygen. *The Journal of Experimental Biology*, *212*(19), 3132–3141. http://dx.doi.org/10.1242/jeb.031179

Van Voorhies, W. A., & Ward, S. (1999). Genetic and environmental conditions that increase longevity in Caenorhabditis elegans decrease metabolic rate. *Proceedings of the National Academy of Sciences of the United States of America*, *96*(20), 11399–11403.

Van Voorhies, W. A., & Ward, S. (2000). Broad oxygen tolerance in the nematode Caenorhabditis elegans. *The Journal of Experimental Biology*, *203*(Pt. 16), 2467–2478.

Vellai, T., Takacs-Vellai, K., Zhang, Y., Kovacs, A. L., Orosz, L., & Müller, F. (2003). Genetics: Influence of TOR kinase on lifespan in C. elegans. *Nature*, *426*(6967), 620. http://dx.doi.org/10.1038/426620a

Vigne, P., & Frelin, C. (2006). A low protein diet increases the hypoxic tolerance in Drosophila. *PLoS One*, *1*(1), e56. http://dx.doi.org/10.1371/journal.pone.0000056

Waalen, J., & Buxbaum, J. N. (2011). Is older colder or colder older? The association of age with body temperature in 18,630 individuals. *The Journals of Gerontology. Series A, Biological Sciences and Medical Sciences*, *66*(5), 487–492. http://dx.doi.org/10.1093/gerona/glr001

Wang, D., Malo, D., & Hekimi, S. (2010). Elevated mitochondrial reactive oxygen species generation affects the immune response via hypoxia-inducible factor-1alpha in long-lived Mclk1+/- mouse mutants. *Journal of Immunology (Baltimore, Md.: 1950)*, *184*(2), 582–590. http://dx.doi.org/10.4049/jimmunol.0902352

Wang, G. L., Jiang, B. H., Rue, E. A., & Semenza, G. L. (1995). Hypoxia-inducible factor 1 is a basic-helix-loop-helix-PAS heterodimer regulated by cellular O2 tension. *Proceedings of the National Academy of Sciences of the United States of America*, *92*(12), 5510–5514.

Weinberg, C. R., Brown, K. G., & Hoel, D. G. (1987). Altitude, radiation, and mortality from cancer and heart disease. *Radiation Research*, *112*(2), 381–390.

Westerterp-Plantenga, M. S., van Marken Lichtenbelt, W. D., Strobbe, H., & Schrauwen, P. (2002). Energy metabolism in humans at a lowered ambient temperature. *European Journal of Clinical Nutrition*, *56*(4), 288–296. http://dx.doi.org/10.1038/sj.ejcn.1601308

Wikström, M., Krab, K., & Saraste, M. (1981). *Cytochrome oxidase: A synthesis*. New York, NY: Academic Press.

Yang, W., & Hekimi, S. (2010). A mitochondrial superoxide signal triggers increased longevity in Caenorhabditis elegans. *PLoS Biology*, *8*(12), e1000556. http://dx.doi.org/10.1371/journal.pbio.1000556

Yee Koh, M., Spivak-Kroizman, T. R., & Powis, G. (2008). HIF-1 regulation: Not so easy come, easy go. *Trends in Biochemical Sciences*, *33*(11), 526–534. http://dx.doi.org/10.1016/j.tibs.2008.08.002

Zhang, X., Sarkar, K., Rey, S., Sebastian, R., Andrikopoulou, E., Marti, G. P., . . . Harmon, J. W. (2011). Aging impairs the mobilization and homing of bone marrow-derived angiogenic cells to burn wounds. *Journal of Molecular Medicine (Berlin, Germany)*, *89*(10), 985–995. http://dx.doi.org/10.1007/s00109-011-0754-2

Zhang, Y., Shao, Z., Zhai, Z., Shen, C., & Powell-Coffman, J. A. (2009). The HIF-1 hypoxia-inducible factor modulates lifespan in C. elegans. *PLoS One*, *4*(7), e6348. http://dx.doi.org/10.1371/journal.pone.0006348

Zheng, H., Lapointe, J., & Hekimi, S. (2010). Lifelong protection from global cerebral ischemia and reperfusion in long-lived Mclk1(+/)(-) mutants. *Experimental Neurology*, *223*(2), 557–565. http://dx.doi.org/10.1016/j.expneurol.2010.02.002

Zhong, L., D'Urso, A., Toiber, D., Sebastian, C., Henry, R. E., Vadysirisack, D. D., . . . Mostoslavsky, R. (2010). The histone deacetylase Sirt6 regulates glucose homeostasis via Hif1alpha. *Cell*, *140*(2), 280–293. http://dx.doi.org/10.1016/j.cell.2009.12.041

Zimmer, M., Gray, J. M., Pokala, N., Chang, A. J., Karow, D. S., Marletta, M. A., . . . Bargmann, C. I. (2009). Neurons detect increases and decreases in oxygen levels using distinct guanylate cyclases. *Neuron*, *61*(6), 865–879. http://dx.doi.org/10.1016/j.neuron.2009.02.013

CHAPTER 4

Aging, Disease, and Longevity in Mice

David B. Lombard and Richard A. Miller

ABSTRACT

There is now substantial evidence, in some cases compelling and in others fairly preliminary, that mouse lifespan can be extended by 3 dietary interventions (Miller et al. 2005; Sun, Sadighi Akha, Miller, & Harper, 2009; Weindruch & Sohal, 1997), by mutations in numerous genes (Ladiges et al., 2009), and by multiple drugs including rapamycin (Harrison et al., 2009). There are also provocative reports of genetic or nongenetic interventions that seem to convey health benefits to mice without clear improvement in lifespan. These new methods for postponing ill health and/or death provide valuable tools for asking questions, at the level of cell biology and organismic physiology, about the factors that control the rate of aging in mammals and the pathways that link aging to diseases and to death. This research area may also someday be seen as an early step toward the development of preventive medicines that postpone a wide range of human maladies by retarding the common factor, aging, that underlies them.

This chapter will present a status report and murocentric point of view on a series of closely related questions. Do interventions (a term we will use, throughout, to lump mutations, diets, and drugs) that extend lifespan always do so by an effect on aging (summarized in Figure 4.1)? Do interventions that extend lifespan always postpone multiple diseases of aging? What models are available to explore the links between delayed aging and retardation of specific diseases? What criteria can be used to test a claim that a particular intervention has modulated aging,

http://dx.doi.org/10.1891/0198-8794.34.93

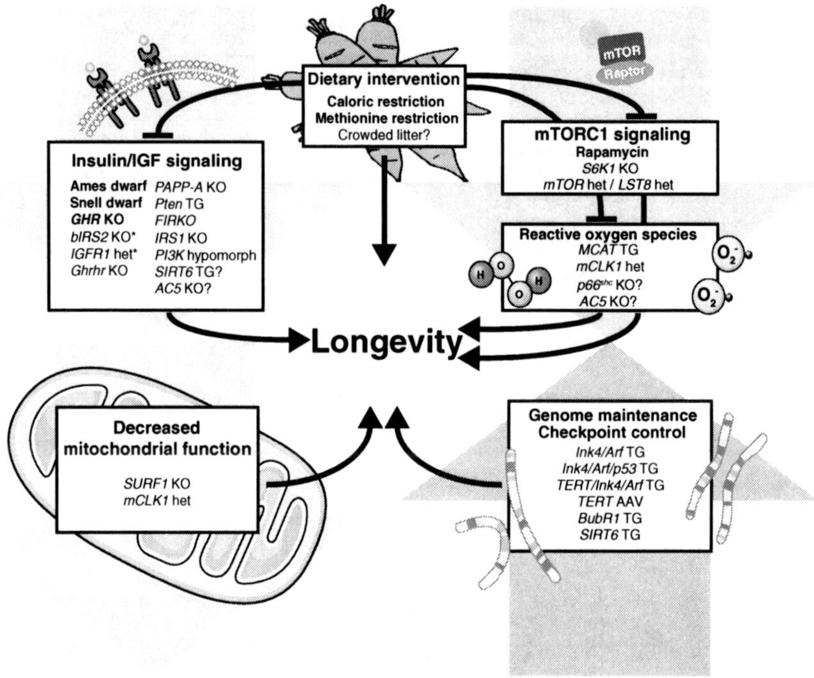

FIGURE 4.1 Summary of longevity-promoting interventions discussed in this chapter. Reductions in insulin/IGF1-like-signaling, mTORC1 signaling, and/or ROS-related damage may all contribute to the beneficial effects of CR. Interventions whose effects have been reproduced in multiple laboratories are designated in bold. Conversely, those for which contradictory results have been reported by different groups are designated with an asterisk. A question mark indicates uncertainty about the relevant molecular pathway. KO = knockout; TG = transgenic; het = heterozygote. Some graphics in this figure were obtained and modified from Servier Medical Art from Servier (http://www.servier.com/Powerpoint-image-bank).

or delayed specific diseases through an effect on aging? Our goal here is not to present an exhaustive review of all published papers relevant to each of these questions but to use selected studies to illustrate how these questions have been, or could be, addressed.

EVALUATION OF SURVIVAL DATA

Many allegations that a diet, drug, or mutation may slow aging start from a demonstration of increased lifespan, so it may be useful to consider the kinds of evidence available from such survival studies. Traditionally, such reports include data on mean, median, and maximal longevity as well as an integrated statistical test of mortality risk, typically the log-rank test based on the Kaplan-Meier model. Although each of these indices has some merit, none is perfectly suited to answering questions about whether a given intervention has slowed the aging process. Increases in mean and median longevity may reflect protection solely against early life hazards. An intervention that increases mean or median survival but has no effect on maximal survival suggests that the intervention may have two effects—lower mortality at early ages accompanied by higher mortality risks in older age groups—a paired effect whose relevance to aging biology may be difficult to untangle.

Estimates of maximal lifespan based on the observed age at death of the longest lived individual are notoriously flawed: they are very dependent on sample size, nonrobust in replication studies, and do not permit statistical comparisons between treated and control groups (Moorad, Promislow, Flesness, & Miller, 2012). A common approach is to do a *t* test to compare mean survival of animals of mice that live longer than 90% (or some other arbitrary large percentage) of the entire group, but this approach is statistically invalid (Wang, Li, Redden, Weindruch, & Allison, 2004). Wang and Allison have proposed and validated an alternate method, in which the proportions of surviving animals are compared (e.g., using the Fisher Exact Test) at the age at which 90% of the mice have died in the pooled, joint distribution, and this method is recommended as superior to the more traditional approaches. In practice, any conclusions about effects of interventions on "maximal" longevity require relatively large numbers of animals to achieve statistical power. For example, a comparison of treated and control groups in which each group initially has 30 mice can produce a significant result using the Wang/Allison method (at $p = .05$, using the 90th percentile) only if 6 mice in the treated group are still alive at the time of the death of the last surviving control mouse. Table 4.1 shows an excerpt of a set of power analyses with various group sizes, to guide in the design (and critical evaluation) of protocols intended to determine if an intervention extends maximal lifespan, or survival to the 90th percentile.

Design and interpretation of longevity experiments is complicated by several points too often ignored by researchers and reviewers alike. If, as is strongly recommended, the protocol includes both males and females, the analytical procedure will either need to consider each sex independently (at higher cost in dollars, or with dramatic loss in statistical power), or else pool across sex with stratification for sex, an approach that could miss effects that are sex specific. If the plan includes simultaneous evaluation of multiple mutant alleles, or multiple drugs, or uses a range of control groups, some adjustment may be needed to control Type I error that might be inflated in a series of multiple comparisons.

TABLE 4.1
Power Analysis for Survival Experiments

Days[a]	Mice[b]	Log-Rank[c]	Max LS[d]
50 (6%)	60	0.34	0.12
50 (6%)	75	0.39	0.23
50 (6%)	90	0.43	0.22
50 (6%)	105	0.50	0.32
50 (6%)	120	0.55	0.34
100 (12%)	60	0.85	0.50
100 (12%)	75	0.93	0.71
100 (12%)	90	0.95	0.74
100 (12%)	105	0.97	0.85
100 (12%)	120	0.99	0.88
110 (13%)	60	0.91	0.59
110 (13%)	75	0.96	0.81
110 (13%)	90	0.98	0.81
110 (13%)	105	0.99	0.92
110 (13%)	120	1.00	0.96
125 (15%)	60	0.95	0.68
125 (15%)	75	0.98	0.88
125 (15%)	90	0.99	0.90
125 (15%)	105	1.00	0.96
125 (15%)	120	1.00	0.98

Note. This table was calculated by Andrzej Galecki, Shu Chen, and Lili Deng using 1,000 simulations for mouse survival data with the following assumptions: mean lifespan of controls 825 days, and survival curves based on those of untreated mice of the UM-HET3 stock (Miller et al., 1999), pooled across genders, housed at the University of Michigan, and evaluated using $\alpha = .05$ for a two-sided comparison. (a) Days = difference (increase or decrease) between experimental group and control group. (b) Number of mice in each group, assuming equal numbers of control and experimental mice. (c) Power to detect this difference using the log-rank test. (d) Power to detect an effect using the Wang/Allison test (Wang et al., 2004), using a two-sided Fisher exact calculation at the age where 90% of the mice in the joint survival distribution had died. For example, in an experiment where a drug causes an increase (or decrease) of 100 days (12% greater than control median), using 60 mice in each group will detect this difference by log-rank test 85% of the time and will show an effect on maximum lifespan 50% of the time.

An alternate approach, adopted by the National Institute on Aging (NIA) Interventions Testing Program (ITP; Miller et al., 2007; Nadon et al., 2008), is to report unadjusted significance tests and a list of the interventions tested in each set of comparisons and to acknowledge the likelihood that some findings of beneficial effect may represent chance events.

Survival distributions can also be compared using parametric methods, most often using the Gompertz model, or equivalent transformations (Finch, Pike, & Witten, 1990). These approaches make the oversimplified assumption that the life table can be adequately represented by two parameters, one reflecting an initial or baseline mortality risk and the other reflecting the age-dependent rate of increase in mortality risk. This line of argument poses many problems: (a) poor statistical power; (b) poor theoretical justification for relating Gompertz parameters to important biological processes; and (c) data that fail to meet the assumption that the logarithm of the risk of mortality increases linearly over the entire lifespan. In practice, with data sets consisting of a few score or few hundred individuals, minor variations in the age at death of the first animals to die can have a dramatic effect on estimates of both Gompertz parameters, without any real connection with the biology of aging.

Evaluation of survival data sets can help to provide an idea of their likely robustness, and of their potential relevance to the underlying question of whether the intervention slows aging. Readers should approach such reports with several questions in mind as follows:

1. Is the control group unusually short-lived, either with respect to previous reports using the same stock or with respect to other stocks used in aging research? There are cases, among them the Ames dwarf model, in which major discoveries have emerged from a mutant that increases lifespan with respect to a short-lived control group (Brown-Borg, Borg, Meliska, & Bartke, 1996), but reports using short-lived control groups, particularly of stocks that show longer lifespan in other vivaria, raise questions about whether poor husbandry conditions may have affected the survival data in ways that are difficult to interpret and replicate.
2. Does the report include information about the cause of death? If most of the mice have died of an infectious cause, for example, or of a lesion (such as fatty liver disease [Pearson, Baur, et al., 2008] or lung tumors [Kanfi et al., 2012]) that is uncommon as a cause of death in mice, this may raise questions about whether the intervention is likely to be of benefit in other strains and other circumstances.
3. Did the investigators take pains to demonstrate that their colony is specific pathogen free, as for example by the use of quarterly evaluation of sentinel

mice for antiviral antibodies and parasites? These issues have been discussed in depth elsewhere (Ladiges et al., 2009). Other housing parameters, such as ambient temperature, can profoundly influence phenotypes of mouse mutants, potentially including lifespan (Bartke & Westbrook, 2012).

4. Perhaps the most important criterion, and one that is particularly hard to document in most initial reports, is that of replication: to what extent is the benefit seen in multiple laboratories and in multiple mouse strains? Publication bias—the preference of investigators and editors for reports of "positive findings" over findings that an intervention does not have an effect—inevitably tilts the published literature toward papers whose results, although honest and accurate, are unrepresentative and which cannot be replicated in follow-up studies. There are now multiple reports, for example, of longevity extension in independent cohorts of pituitary dwarf mutants (Bartke, Coschigano, et al., 2001; Brown-Borg et al., 1996; Flurkey, Papaconstantinou, Miller, & Harrison, 2001; Panici et al., 2010; Vergara, Smith-Wheelock, Harper, Sigler, & Miller, 2004), and in mice lacking growth hormone (GH) receptor (GHR; Bartke, 2002; Bonkowski et al., 2009; Coschigano et al., 2003), representing work on several background stocks and in more than a single laboratory. It thus seems a safe conclusion that maximum longevity can be increased by interference with GH-dependent processes. In other cases, however, influential initial reports have proven difficult to replicate. A report of substantial longevity increase in females hemizygous for the IGF1 receptor (Holzenberger et al., 2003) has been called into question by a subsequent study, in another laboratory, in which husbandry conditions led to much longer lifespan of control animals (Bokov et al., 2011). Similarly, a disparity in outcome between two tests of brain-specific insulin receptor deletions may well reflect the use of a diet relatively high in fat content in the laboratory in which a significant lifespan benefit was noted (Taguchi, Wartschow, & White, 2007), compared to the use of a lower fat diet used by colleagues studying the same stock of mice (Selman et al., 2008; Selman, Lingard, Gems, Partridge, & Withers, 2008). In the NIA Interventions Testing Program, unexplained but consistent differences in lifespan of male control mice among the three test sites complicate interpretations of longevity benefits of the anti-inflammatory drug aspirin and an antioxidant, nordihydroguaiaretic acid (NDGA), each of which was shown (Strong et al., 2008) to produce larger lifespan effects at the sites with the shortest lived male controls.

Replication of initial reports, although expensive and generally time consuming, provides a critical bulwark against the distortions of publication bias. Researchers, reviewers, and editors favor papers reporting benefits of drugs or diets over reports that fail to find an effect; and funding agencies assign low priority to expensive replication studies, leading inevitably to a literature contaminated by misleading reports: honest reports of experimental findings whose conclusions would, if tested, prove to be nonrepresentative. Ioannidis has presented a quantitative argument to show why most published research reports are false (Ioannidis, 2005b), and tabulated examples (Ioannidis, 2005a) of initial reports whose conclusions were later refuted, or dramatically mitigated, by subsequent attempts at replication. The risks of basing conclusions on single reports, based on *p* value thresholds alone, should inspire a healthy dose of caution to readers of isolated reports of longevity effects in modest sized groups of mice. Reports of intervention effects based on studies of a single genotype, whether inbred or F1 hybrid, should also be taken with a mixture of interest and skepticism until confirmed on a wider range of genetic backgrounds, preferably from a segregating cross or, better, on a set of F1 hybrids generated from a foundation stock through diallel matings (Chesler et al., 2008; Churchill, Gatti, Munger, & Svenson, 2012; Institute of Laboratory Animal Resources [U.S.] Committee on Animal Models for Research on Aging, 1981; Miller, Burke, & Nadon, 1999; Miller & Nadon, 2000; Threadgill & Churchill, 2012). Nonetheless, reports of single gene mutants that extend mouse lifespan, in one or both sexes, have been accumulating at a steady pace since 1996 (see Figure 4.2); many of these may prove robust, and the growing mutant collection will continue to pose new ideas about the cellular and systemic factors that delay aging, along with tools to test these ideas.

Reports that a particular intervention apparently does not lead to a lifespan effect must also be carefully evaluated to decide how likely the results are to be robust. There are several studies in which an intervention has not only led to an increase in early life deaths but also to a significant increase in maximal lifespan, complicating interpretation. In a study of the effects of caloric restriction (CR) in wild-derived compared to laboratory-derived mice, for example, early deaths in the restricted wild-derived group contributed to the lack of a significant effect on overall survival evaluated by the log-rank test, convincing the authors that wild mice do not show a lifespan benefit from a CR diet (Harper, Leathers, & Austad, 2006). The life table data, however, show that the CR diet, applied to the wild-derived mice, increased maximal longevity, diminished tumor risk, and led to a significant change in the Gompertz slope parameter, suggesting that the authors' conclusion may have been too pessimistic. Similarly, early life deaths in mice placed on a diet low in methionine produced a survival curve in which mean and median lifespan were unaffected by the diet, despite a significant beneficial effect on maximal longevity (Miller et al. 2005). The effects of background genes may also lead to results that require careful interpretation. In one example, a study of genetic effects on CR effect, using a set of recombinant inbred stocks, showed

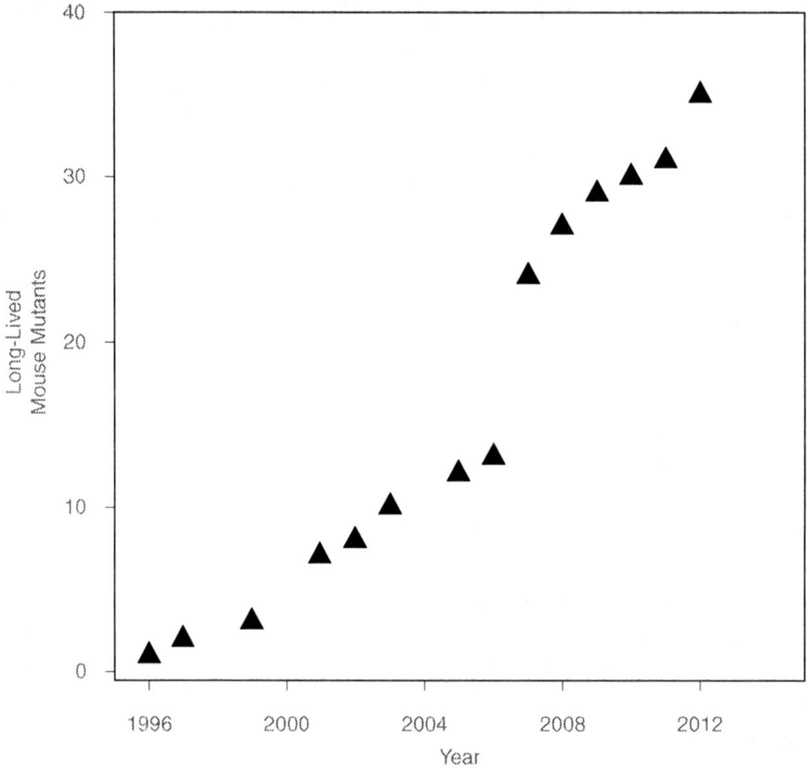

FIGURE 4.2 Cumulative count of mouse genetic loci for which a published report claims mutation can increase lifespan beyond that of control mice, either in a single sex or in both sexes. Data accumulated largely by William Swindell.

that many of the stocks were shorter lived on the CR diet than when fed ad lib, suggesting to the authors that the beneficial effects of CR were highly dependent on genetic background (Liao, Rikke, Johnson, Diaz, & Nelson, 2010). Although there are examples of laboratory mouse stocks for which CR diets do not increase lifespan, it is uncommon to see actual reduction of lifespan below control levels in response to a CR protocol (Weindruch & Walford, 1988), raising the possibility that the set of stocks used by Liao et al. (2010) may harbor background genes, uncommon in other laboratory mice, that lead to ill health on CR diets.

BUILDING A CASE THAT AN INTERVENTION SLOWS AGING

Evidence that an intervention extends lifespan—and preferably maximum lifespan—is usually the first step in testing the idea that the intervention is affecting the underlying aging rate. The framework idea here is that the rate of aging influences a wide range of late-life processes in parallel; thus postponement or deceleration of aging ought to slow accumulation of age-related changes in multiple cells, tissues, and organ systems, including those that can lead to death and those that do not. In some cases, the case is cut and dried: large dog breeds, for example, are not only shorter lived than (most) small breeds of dogs but also show increased age-adjusted rates of neurological, skeletal, cardiac, and neoplastic diseases (Bonnett, Egenvall, Hedhammar, & Olson, 2005; Egenvall, Bonnett, Olson, & Hedhammar, 2000a, 2000b). The long history of work on CR has gradually built a comprehensive case that most aspects of aging, from effects on cataracts (Wolf, Li, Pendergrass, Schmeider, & Turturro, 2000), autoimmune diseases (Fernandes, Friend, Yunis, & Good, 1978), muscle damage (Aspnes et al., 1997), immune defenses (see Table 4.12 in Weindruch & Walford, 1988), learning and memory (Ingram, Weindruch, Spangler, Freeman, & Walford, 1987), myocardial tolerance to ischemia/reperfusion injury (Edwards et al., 2010), reproductive aging (Nelson, Karelus, Bergman, & Felicio, 1995), and a host of late-life lethal diseases are all postponed (Weindruch & Walford, 1988). CR rats can remain physically active and vigorous at very old ages: given access to an exercise wheel, the average 34-month-old CR rat voluntarily runs 4,000 meters/day at an age where fewer than 10% of controls are still alive (McCarter et al., 1997).

It is, however, easy to imagine situations in which an intervention increases mean and maximum lifespan by blocking a disease, or class of diseases, without modulating aging itself. In a mouse stock where most deaths are caused by hemophilia, for example, transgenic restoration of the gene for the missing clotting factor would increase lifespan dramatically, even though it is unlikely that differences in clotting factor levels are the principal regulator of aging. Less trivial examples are easy to find in the recent literature, including the demonstration that lifespan of klotho-deficient mice can be restored by provision of food without vitamin D (Lanske & Razzaque, 2007; Razzaque & Lanske, 2006), or that mice crippled by short telomeres can benefit by elevation of telomerase (Jaskelioff et al., 2011). The relevance of such observations to aging depends on an assessment of the evidence, from other sources, that aging is affected by vitamin D levels or by telomere length in mice. The latter issue is discussed further below.

Evidence is gradually developing that mutant mice with deficits in GH and/or IGF1 signals do indeed age more slowly than control mice. Snell dwarf mice, for example, show delay in many indices of aging, including joint pathology (Silberberg, 1972), collagen cross-linking in tendon (Flurkey et al., 2001), accumulation of memory T cells (Flurkey et al., 2001), cataract formation (Vergara et al., 2004), and kidney pathology (Vergara et al., 2004). Ames dwarf and GHR-knockout (KO) mice retain cognitive function, assessed by tests of learning and memory, better than aging controls (Kinney, Coschigano, Kopchick, Steger, & Bartke, 2001; Kinney, Meliska, Steger, & Bartke, 2001), perhaps because of retention of cell replenishment and local GH/IGF1 production within the brain (Pearson, Baur, et al., 2008). Bone marrow stem cell numbers also seem to be retained in aging GHR-KO mice (Ratajczak et al., 2011), and cataract formation is also delayed (Wolf et al., 2005). Neoplastic diseases also develop more slowly in Ames, Snell, and GHR-KO mice (Ikeno, Bronson, Hubbard, Lee, & Bartke, 2003; Ikeno et al., 2009; Vergara et al., 2004). Similarly, pregnancy-associated plasma protein A (PAPP-A) KO mice also showed later development of neoplastic disease, and slower accumulation of pathological changes in heart, brain, kidney, and immune organs (discussed further below; Conover, Bale, et al., 2010). These observations represent the beginning of an argument that mutants which extend lifespan through alterations in GH and IGF1 slow down the process of aging, and that the lifespan effect is the result of a more general delay or deceleration of a wide range of age-related changes. Such an inference is by no means trivial: the first compelling report of a single gene mutation that extended lifespan in *Caenorhabditis elegans* (Kenyon, Chang, Gensch, Rudner, & Tabtiang, 1993) was preceded by a comprehensive theoretical analysis (Partridge & Barton, 1993) proving that no such gene could exist, and followed by an essay showing that no such mutation could exist in species other than *C. elegans* (Partridge & Harvey, 1993).

The realization that extended lifespan per se is merely suggestive of an effect on aging has led to an admirable trend toward including data on multiple age-sensitive traits in initial reports of putative antiaging interventions (see below). For example, evidence that rapamycin retards age-associated changes in multiple tissues, including some that do not contribute to mortality risk (Wilkinson et al., 2012), has suggested that this drug may be working on some fundamental aspect of the aging process, consistent with longevity effects of mechanistic target of rapamycin (mTOR) inhibition in invertebrate species (Kapahi et al., 2004; Vellai et al., 2003). Reports that rapamycin can slow effects of aging on bone marrow stem cell turnover and humoral immune response to influenza (Chen, Liu, Liu, & Zheng, 2009), retard biochemical and behavioral endpoints in a mouse model of Alzheimer's disease (Caccamo, Majumder, Richardson, Strong, & Oddo, 2010), suppress age-associated obesity (Yang et al., 2012), and improve outcomes in a mouse model of bacterial pneumonia (Hinojosa et al., 2012) are consistent with an antiaging effect. Nonetheless, the hypothesis that rapamycin-mediated longevity in mice reflects primarily a direct effect of this drug on cancer cell biology is still quite plausible (Neff et al., 2013), and additional evidence on rapamycin effects on age-sensitive endpoints is badly needed. Reports that an intervention slows a wide range of age-dependent effects without a benefit to lifespan (Pearson, Baur, et al., 2008; Gonzalez-Suarez, Geserick, Flores, & Blasco, 2005; Herranz et al., 2010) also require careful evaluation; in principle, these may represent an authentic retardation of aging accompanied by some unidentified side effect(s) that limit lifespan.

MOUSE LONGEVITY MODELS

Early, Transient CR Extends Mouse Longevity

We will not review here the extensive studies showing that diminishing food availability in adult mice and rats leads, in nearly all strains tested, to an increase in mean and maximal lifespan, with relative preservation of youthful characteristics in multiple cells, tissues, and organ systems (Flurkey, Astle, & Harrison, 2010; Lipman, Dallal, & Bronson, 1999; Masoro, 2005; Sohal, & Weindruch, 1996; Weindruch & Walford, 1988). The relative effects of modulation of various macronutrients (Iwasaki et al., 1988), of the timing of food availability (Masoro, Shimokawa, Higami, McMahan, & Yu, 1995), and on the effects of CR diets started in middle age (Spindler, 2005; Weindruch & Walford, 1982), as well as on the physiological and biochemical pathways that could mediate benefit of CR, have all been extensively explored without producing, yet, any clear consensus on how CR slows aging. Reductions in insulin/IGF1-like signaling (IIS), mTORC1 signaling, and reactive oxygen species (ROS)-related macromolecular damage, as well as increased AMP-activated protein kinase (AMPK) signaling, altered sirtuin function, and potentially other pathways may contribute to the effects of CR diets on longevity and preservation of health.

Most previous studies of CR in rodents have involved chronic (typically lifelong) food restriction, started in adult life and continued until death. In contrast, Sun and colleagues (2009) recently demonstrated that an expansion of the litter size in mice, effectively imposing a brief period of CR during the preweaning period only, resulted in a significant increase in longevity. These "crowded litter" (CL) mice show reduced size and serum IGF1 levels at the time of weaning, and remain smaller than controls even at 2 years of age. Thus, early food limitation in the CL model imposes durable alterations in physiology that are associated with longevity years later.

Male CL mice, tested at 12 months of age, show increases in certain of the hepatic mRNAs encoding xenobiotic metabolizing enzymes, showing that at least some of the effects of transient early food limitation survive long into adult life (Steinbaugh, Sun, Bartke, & Miller, 2012). The set of mRNAs elevated in the liver of male CL mice is similar to that elevated in adult male CR mice and in GHR-KO, growth hormone releasing hormone (*Ghrhr*)-mutant and Snell dwarf adults, consistent with the idea that disruption of male-specific GH pulse patterns (Waxman & Holloway, 2009) may be a stable feature of the CL mice, shared by CR and some long-lived mutants. Additional studies are needed to document the effects of the transient CL intervention on hormonal patterns, stress resistance, age-associated physiological changes, and late-life diseases. Early life exposure to limited nutrition may induce, in the CL mice, epigenetic alterations in one or more cell types at loci that modulate aging and/or age-associated disease. Identification of these loci would be of general relevance to aging biology. Alternatively or in addition, the CL intervention may promote an altered developmental program that fosters longevity, perhaps by developmental effects on central nervous system (CNS) circuits that control responses to frustration and the psychological stress of transient hunger.

Inhibition of mTORC1 Signaling Extends Mouse Lifespan

The observations that genetic or pharmacologic inhibition of mTOR extends lifespan in yeast (Powers, Kaeberlein, Caldwell, Kennedy, & Fields, 2006), worms (Jia, Chen, & Riddle, 2004; Vellai et al., 2003), and flies (Kapahi et al., 2004) prompted experiments to see if the mTOR inhibitor rapamycin could extend lifespan in mice. Reports from the ITP group showed that rapamycin extends mean and maximum lifespan in genetically heterogeneous mice when started either at 9 or at 20 months of age (Harrison et al., 2009; Miller et al., 2011). Rapamycin also lengthens lifespan when given orally throughout adult life to C57BL/6 male mice (Neff et al., 2013), or from 19 months of age in a separate colony of C57BL/6 mice (Y. Zhang et al., 2013), or for a mere 6 weeks to aged C57BL/6 mice (Chen et al., 2009), or when given by periodic subcutaneous injection to females rendered short-lived and cancer-prone by a HER-2/neu transgene (Anisimov et al., 2010), or to females of the inbred 129/Sv stock (Anisimov et al., 2011). In the ITP studies, beneficial effects were seen at each of the three test sites, in both sexes, and in each of three independent replicate studies, suggesting that the effects are robust. In the published data, median lifespan was increased by 10% in males and by 18% in females (Miller et al., 2011), but experiments using a higher rapamycin dose led to an increase in median lifespan of 23% in males and 26% in females (Miller et al., in press). The proportional benefit was higher in female mice than in male mice in each of the independent replicate studies, although whether this represents differences in blood levels of rapamycin, or sex-specific responses in some aspect of mTOR pathophysiology is still unclear.

It is not yet clear whether the increased lifespan in rapamycin-treated mice reflects a direct effect of this drug on cancer cells, an effect on aging per se (including perhaps age-associated loss of protective anticancer immune responses), or a combination of anticancer and antiaging effects. Necropsies of the genetically heterogeneous mice used by the ITP group show that cancer is responsible for the death of more than 80% of the animals, including both control and rapamycin-treated cohorts, suggesting that direct effects on cancer cell growth might well extend both median and maximal lifespan. The observation that administration of rapamycin at 20 months is as effective as initiation at 9 months (Miller et al., 2011) also argues against delayed aging as the main mode for lifespan extension, suggesting that the key rapamycin-sensitive changes do not occur in mice younger than 20 months. On the other hand, a detailed necropsy evaluation (Wilkinson et al., 2012) showed that mice exposed to rapamycin from 9 to 22 months of age had delayed development of many age-sensitive lesions—including changes in heart, liver, adrenal glands, endometrium, and tendon—with suggestive trends for delayed change in ovaries, thyroid, and lung, suggesting that the drug did indeed retard age-related changes in many organs. In contrast, a more recent, very comprehensive analysis of the effects of rapamycin on multiple systems (Neff et al., 2013) has found many age-associated traits that are not altered by rapamycin, and others in which a rapamycin effect is seen even in young animals. These authors interpret their findings as evidence that rapamycin does not lead to a broad and general deceleration of aging in mice, and that its effects on lifespan principally represent direct effects on neoplasia, although it is worth noting that their work focused on a single inbred stock (C57BL/6), and used only male mice, which are typically less responsive to the lifespan benefits of rapamycin. An accompanying commentary (Richardson, 2013) emphasizes that the beneficial effects of rapamycin, whether caused by improvements in physiological responses throughout life or by retardation of aging change, should prompt further studies of mechanistic target of rapamycin (mTOR) inhibitors as potential preventive medicines in humans.

The role of mTOR in modulation of aging has also been evaluated using genetic tools. Compound heterozygosity of *mTOR* and *lst8* results in a 14% increase in female longevity, with no significant effect on male lifespan (Lamming et al., 2012). Both male and female compound heterozygotes showed reduced S6K1 phosphorylation, indicative of reduced mTORC1 function. By contrast, mTORC2 signaling appeared intact in these animals. Little characterization of aging phenotypes was performed in these strains. Similarly, deletion of the gene encoding the downstream mTORC1 effector *S6K1* is associated with a female-specific 19% increase in lifespan (Selman et al., 2009). Aged *S6K1*-KO mice showed some protection from age-associated pathologies: osteopenia, changes in lymphocyte subsets, and insulin resistance. In addition, old mutant mice manifested improved rotarod performance and activity levels relative to controls. Unfortunately, these parameters were not assessed in young animals for comparison, so it is unclear formally whether S6K1-deficient animals really show attenuation of age-associated decline, or rather whether these phenotypes differ between mutants and controls even at young ages. Surprisingly, *S6K1*-KO animals did not show a difference in the prevalence of macroscopic tumors relative to controls. This result is seemingly at odds with the results from studies using rapamycin, which potently delays cancer onset and/or slows its progression (Harrison et al., 2009; Miller et al., 2011; Neff et al., 2013; Y. Zhang et al., 2013). Curiously, the incidence of macroscopic tumors was only 8% in the *S6K1*-KO studies in both controls and mutants (Selman et al., 2009), whereas a much higher incidence of neoplasia is reported in most strains of mice at the time of death (Anisimov, 2009; Ikeno et al., 2009; Miller & Chrisp, 2002; Miller et al., 2011; Y. Zhang et al., 2013). Further studies are warranted to assess fully the effects of S6K1 deficiency on cancer in mice.

Many Mouse Strains With Reduced Activity of GH and/or IGF1 Show Extended Longevity

The report of lifespan extension by mutations of daf-2 in *C. elegans* (Kenyon et al., 1993) was accompanied by a commentary (Partridge & Harvey, 1993) explaining that single-gene mutations would not be able to extend lifespan in mammals; *C. elegans*, with its alternative dauer stage in larval development, was said to be an exception to the general rule that aging was too complex to be susceptible to deceleration by individual allelic variants (Partridge & Harvey, 1993). In this context, the 1996 report (Brown-Borg et al., 1996) of dramatically extended maximal longevity in male and female mice homozygous for the Ames dwarf mutation (df/df, an allele of *Prop1*), was particularly momentous. This one-page report established three major themes that remain central drivers for modern biogerontology. First, it effectively refuted the pessimistic notion that aging was a mere grab bag of unrelated deleterious events that happened to occur late in life, helping to establish the more productive idea of aging as a unifying process, with effects on many physiological endpoints but potentially malleable in its own right. Second, it focused attention on endocrine pathways, and in particular those related to GH and IGF1, as regulators of aging and multiple forms of age-associated disease. Lastly, the growing realization that hormones related to GH and insulin regulated the timing of aging in invertebrates as well as in mammals (Tatar, Bartke, & Antebi, 2003) served as the impetus for renewed and reciprocal interactions between researchers working in mammalian and invertebrate aging, prompting integrated exploitation of the genetic and logistic advantages of work in nonmammalian organisms to guide work on rodents as surrogates for mammals like us.

The Bartke report was soon followed by evidence for extended lifespan in the closely related Snell dwarf mutant (Flurkey et al., 2001), in which disrupted embryogenesis of the pituitary led to the same trio of endocrine defects (reduced GH, prolactin, and the thyroid stimulating hormone [TSH]) responsible for the Ames dwarf phenotype. Observations suggesting that Snell and Ames dwarf mice show delayed aging in multiple cell and tissue types has been reviewed earlier. The importance of the GH/IGF1 pathway was highlighted by the report (Coschigano, Clemmons, Bellush, & Kopchick, 2000) of extended longevity in mice lacking the GH receptor (GHR-KO, the "Laron dwarf" mice). Mice in which secretion of GH is impaired by mutations in Ghrhr are also long-lived (Flurkey et al., 2001). It is still uncertain whether the antiaging effects in these three varieties of mice reflect diminished GH signals, or diminished IGF1 action. A report of extended lifespan in mice with reduced levels of the IGF1 receptor (Holzenberger et al., 2003) suggested that disruption of IGF1 signals, rather than changes in GH stimulation per se, was the key element of the endocrine picture leading to lifespan benefits in this set of mice, but a subsequent report, using a colony with superior survival of control mice, found much smaller effects of IGF1 receptor mutations (Bokov et al., 2011). The improved lifespan of mice lacking PAPP-A, a protease that cleaves IGF1 binding proteins, also hints that IGF1 signals, in some unidentified set of responder cells and tissues, may be responsible for slower aging in mice with alterations in GH or IGF1 (Conover & Bale, 2007; Conover, Bale, et al., 2010). It is also possible that the factors contributing to lifespan benefit in this set of mice may vary somewhat among models: Ames dwarf mice, for example, respond to CR diets with further improvements in lifespan (Bartke, Wright, et al., 2001), whereas GHR-KO mice seem not to do so (Bonkowski et al., 2009). More detailed discussion of the effects of altered GH, IGF1, and insulin levels in mouse lifespan can be found in other recent reviews (Bartke, 2011; Ladiges et al., 2009).

It is not yet clear whether the health benefits of low GH and/or IGF1 signals reflect early life developmental effects, endocrine support for disease processes that occur only in late life, or a combination of early and later influences. There is some evidence that early life exposure to GH or IGF1 may have long-lasting effects, molding the risks or speed of disease much later in life. For example, transient exposure to GH in Ames dwarf mice starting at 2 weeks of age reduces longevity to that of WT controls (Panici et al., 2010). Interestingly, GH treatment of Snell dwarf mice starting at 4 weeks does not have any such effect (Vergara et al., 2004), suggesting that the window of opportunity for GH-dependent effects on the pace of aging may indeed be quite transient. Work with the CL model described earlier is consistent with the idea that GH and IGF1 levels present in young animals may play important role in determining an organism's eventual longevity. However, hepatic deletion of the *IGF1* gene in young adult animals also provokes a modest increase in lifespan (Svensson et al., 2011), suggesting that postdevelopmental activities of IGF1 also affect longevity.

It is important to make a clear distinction between factors that modulate the systemic levels of GH and IGF1, and those that affect local levels of these hormones in specific cell types and tissue beds. In Ames dwarf mice, for example, levels of GH and IGF1 produced locally within the hippocampus seem normal in young adults, and then remain at youthful levels at ages at which control mice show decreases (Sun, Al-Regaiey, Masternak, Wang, & Bartke, 2005), suggesting that low serum levels of GH/IGF1 may lead to compensatory overproduction of these proteins in specific tissues. Exploitation of mouse stocks in which GH receptor is ablated in single tissues (List et al., 2013), and in which GH/IGF1 signals can be modulated experimentally at specific ages, will help to further define the cellular basis for preservation of health in mice with disrupted endocrine circuits.

Several other genetic models with reduced insulin or IGF1 function have been reported to show increased longevity. Increased lifespan is generally more pronounced in female than male mutants. These models include adipose-specific insulin receptor (*IR*) KOs (FIRKO mice; Bluher, Kahn, & Kahn, 2003), liver-specific adult *IGF1* KOs (Svensson et al., 2011), *Pten* transgenics (Ortega-Molina et al., 2012), *PI3K* hypomorphs (Foukas et al., 2013), *IRS1* KOs (Selman, Lingard, Choudhury, et al., 2008), and mice lacking the PAPP-A protease (Conover & Bale, 2007), discussed further elsewhere in this chapter. As noted earlier, longevity claims regarding mice heterozygous for *IGFR1* mutations are currently controversial (Bokov et al., 2011; Holzenberger et al., 2003), as are those regarding mice lacking IRS2 in the brain (Selman, Lingard, Choudhury, et al., 2008; Selman, Lingard, Gems, et al., 2008; Taguchi et al., 2007). The effects of these genetic manipulations on aspects of age-associated disease have been explored in varied depth (Ladiges et al., 2009).

PAPP-A may represent an especially attractive target for eventual antiaging therapies. PAPP-A is an extracellular Metzincin family protease that cleaves IGF binding proteins (primarily IGFBP4) to regulate local IGF1 bioavailability (reviewed in Conover, 2012). The fact that PAPP-A is an extracellular protease implies that putative small molecule PAPP-A inhibitors need not cross the cell membrane to be effective, potentially minimizing side effects. PAPP-A deficiency is associated with increased median and maximal longevity (Conover & Bale, 2007; Conover, Bale, et al., 2010). Thirty percent of *PAPP-A* KO animals died with no pathological evidence of lethal lesions, whereas only 6% of wild-type (WT) controls did so. The onset of fatal neoplastic disease was delayed in *PAPP-A* KOs, and age-associated degenerative changes in the heart, kidney, brain, immune system, and gonads occurred less frequently in mutants than controls (Conover, Bale, et al., 2010; Vallejo et al., 2009). Although WT mice do not normally develop atherosclerosis, PAPP-A deficiency is protective against this condition in susceptible genetic backgrounds under atherogenic dietary conditions (Boldt et al., 2013; Conover,

Mason, et al., 2010; Harrington, Simari, & Conover, 2007). Thus, PAPP-A deficiency seems to have broad positive effects on age-associated pathologies. Further efforts to elucidate more fully the effects of PAPP-A deficiency during aging are warranted. For example, it will be of great interest to test whether *PAPP-A* KO animals are protected from age-associated memory deficits, renal impairment, cardiac dysfunction, and other clinically relevant effects of mouse aging. Development of a conditional KO *PAPP-A* allele—permitting tissue- and temporal-specific gene deletion—will allow detailed characterization of where and when PAPP-A activity is most important in regulating health and lifespan. Very recently, such an allele has been described (Conover, Bale, & Powell, 2013).

Checkpoint Controls and Longevity

Genetic and epigenetic damage accumulation has long been thought to contribute to the degenerative effects of aging (Lopez-Otin, Blasco, Partridge, Serrano, & Kroemer, 2013). Unrepaired DNA lesions can lead to deleterious consequences such as cellular senescence and tissue dysfunction, cell death, or neoplastic transformation. Therefore, cells have evolved an elaborate network of DNA damage sensors, repair proteins, and cell cycle checkpoint control mechanisms. p53 and the proteins encoded by the *Ink4/Arf* locus ($p16^{Ink4a}$, $p19^{Arf}$, and $p15^{Ink4b}$, collectively termed Ink4/Arf herein) are checkpoint factors that play major tumor suppressor roles in mammals (Matheu, Maraver, & Serrano, 2008). Potential roles for these proteins in regulating aging have been the subject of active investigation. Mice expressing truncated *p53* alleles show evidence of early life pathology that has been interpreted as a form of accelerated aging (Maier et al., 2004; Tyner, 2002). Moreover, $p16^{Ink4a}$ limits stem cell proliferation and tissue renewal in the CNS, pancreatic β-cells, and hematopoietic system during aging (Sharpless & DePinho, 2007). These results imply that DNA damage checkpoints may contribute to phenotypes of aging.

However, other studies have shown that p53 and Ink4/Arf actually play important roles in preserving health in mice, in the context of both neoplastic and non-neoplastic pathologies. Mice with transgenes encoding Ink4/Arf alone, or p53 and Ink4/Arf, expressed from their endogenous promoters, showed protection from a wide variety of neoplasms and increased median (although not maximal) longevity (Matheu et al., 2009; Matheu et al., 2007). Transgenic animals showed reduced DNA damage levels and improved late-life health: reduced cancer incidence, superior neuromuscular performance, and more rapid hair regrowth.

Interestingly, *p53* transgenesis on its own did not increase lifespan, although it was even more effective than *Ink4/Arf* in suppressing neoplasia. One possible explanation for this discrepancy is that these proteins promote longevity through mechanisms at least in part unrelated to tumor surveillance. This would be unexpected, given the high rate of spontaneous lethal tumors observed, in most laboratories, in the strain of mice (C57BL/6) used in this study (Anisimov, 2009). Another possible interpretation is that *Ink4/Arf* and *p53/Ink4/Arf* trangenesis not only increase median lifespan through improved tumor suppression but also exert some other negative effects very late in life that prevent extension of maximal longevity. This seems plausible: an increase in median longevity without change in maximum lifespan implies increased rates of mortality at older ages. Yet another possibility is that factors independent of Ink4/Arf and p53—for example, telomere attrition—may play roles in limiting very late-life longevity in mice, a possibility we discuss below (Garcia-Cao et al., 2006).

Increased Telomerase Dosage Extends Murine Lifespan

The repetitive terminal ends of chromosomes—the telomeres—have been the focus of much attention in aging biology. Ordinarily, telomeres are protected by a multisubunit protein complex termed *shelterin* (reviewed in Donate, & Blasco, 2011). Because of the inability of DNA polymerase to copy linear chromosomes to their very distal tips, telomeres erode during each cell division in many cell types, eventually reaching a critical length threshold, leading to telomere deprotection and induction of a DNA damage response. Telomere dysfunction also provokes metabolic dysfunction via reductions in PGC-1α and β levels (Sahin et al., 2011).

To avoid this occurrence, critical cell types such as germ and stem cells express the enzyme telomerase (telomerase reverse transcriptase [TERT]) that stabilizes telomere lengths. Several observations have suggested links between telomere shortening and the diseases of aging, in mouse and humans (Donate & Blasco, 2011). In human cells, telomere length is typically limiting for replicative capacity. Telomeres shorten with age in many human and mouse tissues, and many age-related pathologies in humans are marked by the presence of cells with shortened telomeres (reviewed in Blasco, 2005). Moreover, mouse strains lacking telomerase activity show progressively reduced lifespan over successive generations and develop defects in proliferative tissues and degenerative phenotypes. Similar defects are observed in patients with genetic defects in telomerase. Although laboratory mice have much longer telomeres than humans, it has been shown that telomeres also erode in this organism with age, both in differentiated tissues and in stem cell pools (Flores et al., 2008; Vera, Bernardes de Jesus, Foronda, Flores, & Blasco, 2012). In addition, mouse telomeres shorten with age much faster than do those of humans (Vera et al., 2012). Collectively, these findings raise the question of whether improved telomere maintenance might affect healthy aging.

Addressing this question is complicated by the fact that telomere shortening is an important tumor suppressor mechanism in mammals (Donate & Blasco, 2011). Indeed, increased telomerase activity from birth predisposes animals to neoplasia, potentially obscuring beneficial effects of this intervention on aging per se (Gonzalez-Suarez et al., 2005). Telomerase transgenics do show improved renal function and germline maintenance with age (Gonzalez-Suarez et al., 2005).

To circumvent this cancer predisposition, mice with increased telomerase activity in multiple epithelial compartments were bred to *p53* and *Ink4/Arf* transgenics (Tomas-Loba et al., 2008). Triply transgenic mice (*Tert;p53;Ink4/Arf*) showed large increases in median lifespan as well as the average age of the oldest mice, with improved maintenance of epithelial integrity, and lower levels of DNA damage. Intriguingly, these animals showed other improvements as well, seemingly unrelated to epithelial function, including improved neuromuscular coordination and glucose tolerance. The authors speculate that these effects may result from better maintenance of serum IGF1 levels with age in the transgenic mice versus controls. More recently, studies have been performed in which aged WT mice have been reconstituted with telomerase via viral infection, leading to increased median and maximal lifespan along with improved health in old age: better maintenance of bone density, insulin sensitivity, and rotarod performance in aged animals (Bernardes de Jesus et al., 2012). Altogether, these data argue for an important role for telomere attrition in limiting lifespan in mice.

Longevity Associated With Mitochondrial Defects

Progressive impairment of mitochondrial function is a feature of mammalian aging (Lopez-Otin et al., 2013). Surprisingly, specific genetic lesions that impair mitochondrial oxidative function are associated with longevity in mice. SURF1 is an assembly factor for mitochondrial cytochrome *c* oxidase. In humans, mutations in the *SURF1* gene lead to severe mitochondrial defects and fatal encephalomyelopathy. By contrast, mutation of this gene in mice leads to a remarkably mild phenotype, along with a 21% increase in median lifespan (Dell'agnello et al., 2007). The mechanistic basis for this longevity is currently unclear, although recent work indicates that SURF1 deficiency leads to several metabolic benefits: increased fat metabolism, improved insulin sensitivity, and elevated mitochondrial biogenesis (Deepa et al., 2013). Murine SURF1 deficiency may lead to the recently described phenomenon of "mitonuclear protein imbalance," a stoichiometric imbalance between mitochondrially and nuclearly encoded mitochondrial proteins that activates a mitochondrial unfolded protein response to promote longevity in an evolutionarily conserved manner (Houtkooper et al., 2013). It will be of significant interest to elucidate fully the spectrum of age-associated pathologies affected by SURF1 deficiency. Longevity has also been observed in mice heterozygous for *MCLK1*, a gene encoding a protein required for ubiquinone biosynthesis, a molecule playing roles in mitochondrial respiration and numerous other physiologic processes (Liu et al., 2005). In invertebrates, specific mitochondrial defects present early in development can extend lifespan in a tissue-non-autonomous manner (Durieux, Wolff, & Dillin, 2011): longevity of mouse *SURF1* KOs and *MCLK1* heterozygotes may reflect a conserved biological phenomenon.

Uncertainties Regarding Longevity of the p66^{shc} Mutant

p66^{shc} is a multifunctional adaptor protein with roles in inhibiting growth factor signaling, promoting stress-induced apoptosis, and elevating cellular ROS levels (reviewed in Natalicchio, Tortosa, Perrini, Laviola, & Giorgino, 2011). The median lifespan of p66^{shc}-deficient mice was initially reported to be 28% greater than controls (Migliaccio et al., 1999). Little information is available regarding pathologies in aging *p66*^{shc} KO mice. Initial mechanistic models regarding the basis for the longevity of this mutant focused on the role of p66^{shc} in increasing cellular ROS levels (Migliaccio et al., 1999). However, a recently generated independent line of p66^{shc}-deficient animals shows key molecular differences with the original strain (Tomilov et al., 2011). This study potentially implicates increased expression of *p46*^{shc}, a gene product expressed from the same locus as *p66*^{shc}, in the longevity of the originally described *p66*^{shc} KO. Increased *p46*^{shc} expression in turn leads to reduced insulin signaling in adipose tissue, with concomitant reduction in overall adiposity, similar to that occurring in the long-lived FIRKO mutant (Bluher et al., 2003).

BubR1 Links Improved Maintenance of Euploidy With Increased Longevity

BubR1 is a mitotic checkpoint protein, helping to ensure that daughter cells receive an appropriate chromosomal complement during each cell division to promote maintenance of euploidy. Hypomorphic mutations in *BubR1* lead to degenerative phenotypes (Baker et al., 2004). Strikingly, high-level overexpression of BubR1 extended longevity of mice, and conferred protection against both spontaneous and experimentally induced neoplasia (Baker et al., 2012). These effects were more pronounced in male than in female mice. BubR1 also promoted several aspects of health unrelated to cancer resistance. Overexpressors showed increased cardiac stress resistance, improved exercise tolerance, and reduced renal fibrosis in old age. Other aspects of age-related decline, such as osteopenia and cataract formation, were not affected by BubR1 overexpression. Mechanistically, BubR1 overexpression antagonized the accumulation of aneuploid cells normally observed in mice during aging. These studies suggest that improved maintenance of euploidy can enhance healthy aging and even increase longevity. It will be of interest to assess other aspects of physiology in a longitudinal manner in BubR1 overexpressors as they age, particularly neurologic function and other aspects of health not directly related to cell proliferation.

Adenylyl Cyclase 5 Deficiency Promotes Cardiac Stress Resistance and Longevity

Members of the adenylyl cyclase (AC) protein family catalyze conversion of ATP into cyclic AMP to activate downstream protein kinase A (PKA) signaling and other pathways. Unexpectedly, deletion of the *AC5* gene in the mouse produced a 32% increase in median lifespan extension in both males and females, along with protection from cardiomyopathy and bone loss (Yan et al., 2007). *AC5* mutants may show reduced incidence of lymphoma as well, although this has not been rigorously quantitated. Like the Ames, Snell, and GHR-KO mutations (Salmon et al., 2005), AC5 deficiency is associated with increased cellular stress resistance, potentially contributing to the increased longevity of these mutant mice. *AC5* KOs also possess reduced GH levels, perhaps leading to reduced IGF1 signaling. Although they eat more than littermate controls, AC5-deficient mice weigh less and show reduced adiposity (Yan et al., 2012), effects that could also contribute to their extended lifespan. AC5 is highly expressed not only in myocardium but also in the brain, in particular in regions regulating motor control (reviewed in Chester & Watts, 2007). Consequently, *AC5* mutants show various neurologic phenotypes, such as motor defects resembling a Parkinson's disease (Iwamoto et al., 2003). The relationship between these effects and the longevity, if any, remains to be established. Tissue- and temporal-specific *AC5* KOs would be very helpful in separating effects of this protein in the CNS from those in myocardium and other tissues.

MODELS WITH IMPROVED HEALTHSPAN BUT NOT LIFESPAN

In contrast to the models discussed earlier, there are situations where genetic or pharmacologic interventions improve aspects of healthy aging in rodents, without concomitantly increasing lifespan per se. This may occur if interventions exert mixed effects, for example, enhancing health in young animals but exerting deleterious effects later in life. Alternatively, such outcomes can occur if an intervention modulates age-dependent disorders that are not the principal causes of mortality in that strain. For example, if most animals on a particular strain background die of cancer, an intervention that improves metabolic fitness exclusively may have little or no effect on lifespan, although it might have major benefits in the context of particular stressors (e.g., high fat feeding). Interventions that fall into this category could represent disease-specific therapies rather than measures modulating the aging process itself. Similarly, tissue-specific interventions may ameliorate the effects of aging in a particular organ system without affecting overall longevity.

Reactive Oxygen Species: Complex Relationships With Aging and Age-Associated Disease

The idea that reactive oxygen species (ROS), generated primarily as byproducts of mitochondrial metabolism, might cause progressive damage to cellular macromolecules, eventually contributing to the degenerative changes of aging (Harman, 1972), has long been influential in aging biology, although a long history of failed predictions has made it clear that the original suggestion was at best oversimplified (Perez, Bokov, et al., 2009; Perez, Van Remmen, et al., 2009). To test the "oxidative damage" hypothesis, numerous mouse models with altered levels of antioxidant enzymes have been generated (reviewed in Hamilton, Walsh, & Van Remmen, 2012). Mice with defects in antioxidative defense systems show a wide spectrum of phenotypes. These range in severity from prenatal lethality to an increased incidence of neoplasia; to very subtle, tissue-specific defects that can only be elicited on directed testing; and to no apparent phenotype. In the case of one antioxidant gene, *Gpx4* (phospholipid hydroperoxide glutathione peroxidase) heterozygosity actually seems to improve health during aging, by reducing age-associated glomerulonephritis and lymphoma, associated with a slight but significant increase in mean lifespan (Ran et al., 2007). These phenotypes were ascribed to a greater sensitivity to apoptosis induction in *Gpx4* heterozygous cells. This effect might potentially allow premalignant cells to be culled before becoming full-blown cancers, reducing the incidence of observable neoplasias.

Conversely, overexpression of single antioxidant enzymes does not, as a rule, extend lifespan in mouse models, although in some cases it enhances resistance to certain age-associated pathologies and specific stressors (e.g., reperfusion injury; Hamilton et al., 2012). Taken as a whole, this set of studies points to important roles for ROS in the pathogenesis of specific disease states rather than as a major control point regulating aging per se. The strongest current evidence that aging can be decelerated by diminished oxidative damage alone involves a mouse strain overexpressing catalase artificially targeted to mitochondria (mitochondria-targeted catalase [MCAT] mice). These animals showed reduced levels of oxidative damage, along with a median 17%–21% lifespan extension (Schriner et al., 2005). In addition, necropsies performed on moribund mice revealed that MCAT transgenics showed relative protection against diverse age-associated pathologies, including cardiac lesions, cataracts, nonhematopoietic malignancies, and inflammation (Schriner et al., 2005; Treuting et al., 2008). Other age-associated diseases, such as glomerulonephritis and hematopoietic malignancies, were not affected by MCAT expression. In future studies, it would be helpful to evaluate this and related mutations on a wider range of background stocks and in other animal colonies, and to assess age-associated parameters in cohorts of MCAT transgenics and controls at defined ages throughout the life cycle, to test the robustness of the effects and to assess more rigorously how MCAT expression may modulate the appearance of age-associated phenotypes. Overall, there is little evidence to support the hypothesis that reduced ROS, by itself, can increase mammalian longevity as a general rule (Hamilton et al., 2012; Perez, Bokov, et al., 2009), although it seems plausible that interventions that do slow aging may act by protecting cells against many forms of injury, oxidative injuries among them (Johnson, Lithgow, & Murakami, 1996; Lithgow & Miller, 2008; Miller, 2009a).

Sirtuins: Complex Relationships With Health and Lifespan

The sirtuins are a conserved family of NAD+-dependent deacetylases that regulate many key biological processes, particularly those involving metabolism. On balance, data from invertebrates indicates that overexpression of sirtuins leads to lifespan extension, although published data remain somewhat controversial (Banerjee et al., 2012; Burnett et al., 2011; Longo & Kennedy, 2006; Rizki et al., 2011; Rogina, Helfand, & Frankel, 2002; Tissenbaum & Guarente, 2001; Viswanathan & Guarente, 2011). Mammals possess seven sirtuins, termed SIRT1–SIRT7. A large literature indicates that several sirtuins—particularly SIRT1, SIRT3, and SIRT6—play roles in suppressing specific age-associated diseases and promoting cellular and organismal homeostasis (reviewed in Hall, Dominy, Lee, & Puigserver, 2013). Most of this work has focused on SIRT1, the closest mammalian homolog of *Saccharomyces cerevisiae* SIR2. SIRT1 deacetylates dozens of cellular transcription factors and other proteins to influence diverse processes including glucose and lipid homeostasis, genomic integrity, inflammation, stress responses, and others. Studies using mice with experimentally altered SIRT1 levels (overexpression and gene KO studies) have revealed roles for this protein in suppressing neurodegeneration, metabolic syndrome, cardiac failure, neoplasia, and other age-associated pathologies.

Given the data on invertebrate sirtuins, there has been particular interest in assessing the impact of global SIRT1 overexpression on longevity and health (Banks et al., 2008; Bordone et al., 2007; Pfluger, Herranz, Velasco-Miguel, Serrano, & Tschop, 2008). In models with an extra copy of the SIRT1 genomic locus, SIRT1 overexpression preserves metabolic homeostasis in response to a high-fat diet challenge (Banks et al., 2008; Pfluger et al., 2008). These transgenics, as they age, show improved glucose sensitivity, better maintenance of bone density, more effective wound healing, and superior tightrope performance compared to controls (Herranz et al., 2010). They also show relative protection from certain neoplasms: spontaneous carcinomas and sarcomas, as well as experimentally induced liver cancer. However, global SIRT1 transgenics do not live longer, potentially because the incidence of lymphoma, a common age-associated malignancy in C57BL/6 mice, was not affected by SIRT1 transgenesis (Herranz et al., 2010). In contrast, a recent study showed that SIRT1 overexpression in the brain specifically did extend longevity in mice, likely through hypothalamic effects (Satoh et al., 2013).

SIRT3 is a mitochondrial matrix protein that deacetylates many protein targets in this organelle (Lombard et al., 2007). Although SIRT3-deficient mice appear normal under basal conditions, studies of SIRT3-deficient mice allowed to age, or exposed to stress conditions, have revealed roles for SIRT3 in modulating many core mitochondrial functions such as ROS management, ATP generation, fatty acid β-oxidation, amino acid catabolism, and ketone body formation (reviewed in Lombard & Zwaans, 2013). As a consequence of these activities, SIRT3 plays major roles in suppressing age-associated pathologies such as mammary cancer, metabolic syndrome, cardiomyopathy, hearing loss, and hematopoietic stem cell decline (Bell, Emerling, Ricoult, & Guarente, 2011; Brown et al., 2013; Finley et al., 2011; Hirschey et al., 2010; Hirschey et al., 2011; Kim et al., 2010; Pillai et al., 2010; Qiu, Brown, Hirschey, Verdin, & Chen, 2010; Shimazu et al., 2010; Someya et al., 2010; Sundaresan, Samant, Pillai, Rajamohan, & Gupta, 2008). With a few exceptions, most of these studies were performed in the context of global SIRT3 loss-of-function. It will be of significant interest to test potential effects of SIRT3 overexpression on age-associated pathologies and longevity. Importantly, a recent study analyzing liver-specific and skeletal muscle-specific *SIRT3* KO mice could not reproduce many of the findings reported using global *SIRT3* KO mice (Fernandez-Marcos et al., 2012). This discrepancy implies that either the phenotypes of SIRT3 deficiency are extremely sensitive to variations in experimental protocol, and/or that SIRT3 plays tissue-non-autonomous roles in regulating mitochondrial functions. In addition, SIRT3 appears to play oncogenic roles in certain human malignancies (Alhazzazi et al., 2011), and an extra copy of SIRT3 along with its flanking genes has been associated with tumor susceptibility in humans (Aury-Landas et al., 2013). Clearly, further studies are needed to assess the effects of SIRT3 on mammalian health and longevity, and elucidate how SIRT3 exerts its influence.

The sirtuin SIRT6 is found mainly in the nucleus, associated with chromatin (Mostoslavsky et al., 2006). SIRT6 acts as a histone deacetylase, functioning as a transcriptional corepressor for key cellular transcription factors: for example, NF-kB, hypoxia-inducible factor (HIF-1α), c-Myc, and c-Jun (reviewed in Zwaans & Lombard, in press). SIRT6 also facilitates maintenance of genome integrity by multiple mechanisms. By means of these activities, SIRT6 promotes diverse aspects of mammalian health: metabolic homeostasis, tumor suppression, and cardiac function. As with several other sirtuins, SIRT6 has a complex relationship with neoplasia: it functions as a tumor suppressor in the contexts of intestinal and hepatocellular cancer (Marquardt et al., 2013; Sebastian et al., 2012), but may play an oncogenic role in breast carcinoma (Khongkow et al., 2013).

A major question in sirtuin biology has been whether any sirtuin proteins can actually extend lifespan in mammals when overexpressed. Kanfi and colleagues showed that SIRT6 overexpression modestly increases the longevity of male mice (median extension of 15% and 9% in two independent transgenic lines, respectively; Kanfi et al., 2012). Male transgenics (but not females) showed lower circulating IGF1 levels, potentially identifying reduced IGF1 as the cause of longevity in these animals. Relative protection against lung cancer may explain some of the male-specific longevity (Lombard & Miller, 2012). In future studies, it will be necessary to perform histopathological analysis in cohorts of SIRT6 transgenics and controls at defined ages to rigorously test whether SIRT6 overexpression might delay the onset or slow the progression of age-associated pathologies.

Proteostasis Promotes Maintenance of Organ Function With Age

A growing body of evidence from invertebrates and mammals implicates age-associated impairment of protein quality control (proteostasis) in the pathobiology of many diseases of aging, and perhaps in limiting longevity itself (reviewed in Hubbard, Valdor, Macian, & Cuervo, 2012; Lopez-Otin et al., 2013). In invertebrates, macroautophagy, a major proteostatic pathway that degrades large cytosolic regions or whole organelles in lysosomes, is crucial for increased lifespan in response to multiple pro-longevity interventions (Gelino & Hansen, 2012). In mammalian liver, macroautophagy function declines with age, an effect rescued by CR (Hubbard et al., 2012). The function of chaperone-mediated autophagy (CMA), a distinct proteostatic pathway whereby single proteins are degraded and recycled in lysosomes, is also reduced with age in mammals (Hubbard et al., 2012). One mechanism of age-associated CMA impairment in mammals involves a reduction in levels of lysosome-associated membrane protein type 2A (LAMP2A; Cuervo & Dice, 2000). Transgenic restoration of LAMP2A protein levels in the livers of aged mice restores CMA in this tissue (C. Zhang & Cuervo, 2008). Remarkably, this rescue leads to a concomitant reduction in levels of oxidatively damaged proteins, along with maintenance of hepatocyte function and reduced cell death. It will be of great interest to test whether enhanced CMA in other mammalian tissues ameliorates other types of age-associated decline, and whether this might extend longevity.

Resveratrol Protects Against Sequelae of High Fat Feeding

Resveratrol is a polyphenol naturally found in plants, and was found to be a SIRT1 activator in an early screen for such activators (Howitz et al., 2003). Subsequently, other putative sirtuin activating compounds (STACs) were identified, structurally unrelated to resveratrol (Milne et al., 2007). It is currently debated whether these compounds activate SIRT1, and if so, whether the action is direct or occurs indirectly via effects on upstream signaling factors such as AMPK (Baur, Ungvari, Minor, Le Couteur, & de Cabo, 2012; Hubbard et al., 2013). Space does not permit an adequate discussion of STAC biology; the reviewer is referred to one of the many dedicated reviews in this area (e.g., Baur et al., 2012). Sirtuins have been proposed as mediators of the organismal response to CR, and as a consequence, resveratrol and other STACs have been evaluated for their effects on health span and lifespan in mice and other aging model systems. Only the data from mammals will be outlined here. Long before it had been implicated as a possible sirtuin activator, older literature suggested various beneficial effects conferred by resveratrol, including cardioprotection and suppression of various experimentally induced cancers (Baur & Sinclair, 2006). More recent studies showed that resveratrol increased survival of mice on a high-fat diet, but not on normal chow (Baur et al., 2006; Miller et al., 2011; Pearson, Baur, et al., 2008; Strong et al., 2013). The principal cause of death in mice on the high-fat diet used in these studies appears to be fat accumulation in the liver, leading to pulmonary congestion and edema (Pearson, Baur, et al., 2008), a cause of death seldom seen in normal aging rodents or people.

Despite the failure of resveratrol to increase lifespan of mice on a normal diet, it did ameliorate various age-associated phenotypes in this context: osteopenia, cataract, and endothelial dysfunction. In multiple organs, resveratrol shifts the gene expression profile toward a more CR-like state (Barger et al., 2008; Pearson, Baur, et al., 2008). Resveratrol has been reported to promote mitochondrial biogenesis and increase aerobic capacity in mice (Lagouge et al., 2006), although contradictory results have recently been described (Higashida et al., 2013). Despite these positive effects, resveratrol did not afford protection against age-associated neoplasia (Pearson, Baur, et al., 2008). Thus, although it is likely that resveratrol offers some protection against a pathogenic diet in mice and perhaps even in humans (Timmers et al., 2011), and may blunt some age-associated phenotypes, it seems unlikely that resveratrol modulates the aging process itself in mammals.

FUTURE AVENUES

The last two decades of work on the biology of aging and longevity have produced remarkable progress, with many new tools, ideas, and provocative findings. Work in rodents and other model organisms has identified conserved pathways, involving GH, IGF1, and mTOR signaling, that modulate health and longevity across species. These studies have firmly established that lifespan is a phenotype highly amenable to genetic and pharmacological manipulation, a notion that was controversial until relatively recently (Partridge & Barton, 1993). The fact that simple dietary, genetic, and pharmacologic interventions can promote healthy aging and increase longevity in rodents strongly suggests that the insights of aging biology may eventually be successfully deployed for the betterment of human health (Butler et al., 2008; Miller, 2002; Miller, 2009b). However, there are many important issues that remain to be addressed.

A major outstanding question in aging research concerns the temporal and tissue requirements for health span and lifespan extension by specific interventions. Work in *C. elegans* has revealed that some pathways that regulate overall organismal longevity act only within restricted time windows and/or in specific tissues (Lapierre & Hansen, 2012). In this regard, it would be surprising if longevity determinants in mammals were not as least as complex as those in *C. elegans*. To date, most studies testing the effects of single-gene mutations on mammalian longevity have used germline KO mice, in which the gene of interest is deleted in all tissues from the time of conception. This approach will completely obscure potential temporal and spatial requirements for genes in regulating organismal longevity. Worse, it may altogether miss factors with mixed effects; for example, putative genes that limit lifespan in some tissues but promote longevity in others, or exert beneficial effects during some periods of life but detrimental effects in others. These issues are important to resolve because eventual antiaging therapies in humans may need to be carefully targeted, both to specific cell types and at specific ages or within specific time frames, to achieve therapeutic benefits without unacceptable side effects. These questions can be addressed using inducible gene KO models or pharmacologic inhibitors to test timing requirements; and tissue-specific KOs to assess spatial requirements. Unfortunately, performing such studies in rodents in a comprehensive fashion represents a major expense.

Current data already suggest that pathways playing major roles in regulating longevity in mammals differ from one another in timing and tissue requirements. For example, the mTOR inhibitor rapamycin yields equivalent increases in lifespan when administered at either 9 months (early middle age) of age or 20 months of age (old age; Harrison et al., 2009; Miller et al., 2011). This result suggests that the critical pro-aging pathways targeted by rapamycin may exert their deleterious effects mostly late in life. Consistent with this model, mTORC1 signaling increases in the POMC hypothalamic neurons with age in mice, contributing to age-associated obesity; these effects are blocked by rapamycin (Yang et al., 2012). Alternatively, rapamycin may retard many aging processes throughout life but delay mortality mostly by inhibiting cancer, a disease primarily of older animals. The tissue requirements for mTOR signaling in the context of longevity in mammals are currently uncharacterized.

In contrast, as noted earlier, GH treatment of Ames dwarf mice for a brief (6-week) period starting one week prior to weaning deprives them of cellular stress resistance and longevity (Panici et al., 2010), suggesting that GH may exert effects, very early in postnatal life, which regulate longevity through pathways not accessible at later ages. Tissue-specific gene deletion studies suggest roles for IIS in CNS and adipose tissue in restricting longevity (Bluher et al., 2003; Taguchi et al., 2007). Further tissue- and temporal-specific gene ablation experiments studies will no doubt refine the current picture of the requirements for hormonal action in regulating mammalian longevity.

Another outstanding issue concerns potential genetic overlap among pathways regulating mammalian lifespan, a question that can be addressed experimentally using compound mutants. In *C. elegans*, the ease of genetic manipulation, coupled with the availability of a genetic model for CR (the *eat-2* mutant), has facilitated a fairly comprehensive epistatic analysis of longevity (e.g., Greer, & Brunet, 2009). Because new genes that regulate lifespan are identified in this organism, their relationships with well-established pathways can be rapidly elucidated to provide useful functional insights. In contrast, very few epistasis studies have been performed in mammals in the context of longevity because in part of the formidable expenditures involved in breeding and aging compound mutant mice and appropriate controls. Construction of compound mutants that combine alleles that slow aging along with alleles that mimic important human diseases—such as Alzheimer's disease, diabetes, or atherosclerosis—may help delineate the basis for age-dependent increases in disease risk and suggest strategies to protect against these and other common afflictions.

A related question concerns mechanistic overlap of genetically defined longevity pathways with CR. In mammals, most of the published work in this regard has assessed the impact of CR on longevity in different strains of dwarf mice. The results of these studies were decidedly mixed; the long lifespan of the Ames dwarf was further extended by CR, but in contrast GH receptor KO mice did not show increased longevity in response to CR (Bartke, Wright, et al., 2001; Bonkowski et al., 2009; Bonkowski, Rocha, Masternak, Al Regaiey, & Bartke, 2006). A third case involved macrophage inhibitory factor (MIF), a proinflammatory cytokine and a component of the innate immune system (Fingerle-Rowson & Bucala, 2001). *MIF* KO mice are long-lived, and CR diets further extend the lifespan of

MIF KO mice, but the effects are not additive, and CR-treated MIF-KO mice do not live any longer than CR-treated control mice (Harper, Wilkinson, & Miller, 2010). FOXO1 and NRF2 are both reported to be required for the tumor suppressive effects of CR, but not the longevity effect of the CR diet (Pearson, Lewis, et al., 2008; Yamaza et al., 2010), although the latter report is complicated by the short lifespan of NRF2-deficient mice compared to controls. Obtaining a deep understanding of relationships between pro-longevity interventions in mammals will require similar studies for many mutants.

Studies in yeast, worms, and flies have frequently initially identified pathways regulating longevity that are subsequently discovered to behave similarly in vertebrates. As examples, IIS, mTOR signaling, and sirtuins were all found to regulate lifespan in invertebrates long before similar conclusions were reached in rodent models. Further insights into determinants of mammalian longevity will no doubt continue to rely heavily on work in simpler organisms. For example, a large body of evidence from *C. elegans* and *Drosophila* shows that, somewhat counter-intuitively, reductions in mitochondrial respiratory function can actually extend lifespan, at least in part by provoking a compensatory stress response (Durieux et al., 2011). As noted earlier, emerging evidence in mouse models suggests that certain mitochondrial defects in mammals can similarly induce longevity (Dell'agnello et al., 2007; Houtkooper et al., 2013). In flies and worms, the perception of food, as opposed to its actual ingestion, exerts a powerful negative influence on lifespan (Linford, Kuo, Chan, & Pletcher, 2011). Roles for sensory perception in modulating mammalian longevity have not been explored, but data from invertebrate animals suggest that such studies might be fruitful.

LONGEVITY WITHOUT GOOD HEALTH: TITHONIAN PARANOIA

Tricky Zeus: asked by Eos to make her lover Tithonus immortal, he complied, but sadistically failed to provide antiaging interventions, thus condemning Tithonus to wither slowly in his lover's arms, "a white-hair'd shadow roaming like a dream the ever-silent spaces of the East," envious "of happy men that have the power to die" (Tennyson, 1859). This paranoid fantasy, common to the deliberations of both Miss Alabama 1994 (http://www.gather.com/viewArticle.action?articleId=281474976768893) and the President's Council on Bioethics (Kass, 2003, p. 352), often enters into discussions of the merits and postulated risks of interventions that might be used to slow aging in people, and thus deserves to be discussed in the context of this review.

We wish to offer four responses to the idea that (future) interventions that might slow aging would make people stay sick and unhappy for a long time.

First, as reviewed earlier, there is now substantial and accumulating evidence that interventions which slow aging—such as restricted diets, well-tested single gene mutations, and perhaps some drugs like rapamycin—do not create rodents that cling to life, demented and disease-ridden, bodies all aching and wracked with pain. Extension of lifespan, not too surprisingly, seems to result from postponement of multiple forms of lethal illness, and is typically accompanied in these experimental situations with postponement of other age-dependent diseases and disabilities which, if left unchecked, would be unpleasant although not lethal.

This is not to say that all interventions that extend lifespan render mice perfectly healthy and resistant to all forms of injury. Rapamycin, for example, seems to increase cataracts in mice (Wilkinson et al., 2012); impairs testosterone production in mice, rats, and humans (Huyghe et al., 2007; Rovira et al., 2012; Wilkinson et al., 2012); and leads to impaired glucose tolerance (Lamming et al., 2013). Rodents on CR diets, although resistant to heat stress (Heydari, Wu, Takahashi, Strong, & Richardson, 1993), are vulnerable to certain infectious agents (Gardner, 2005) and show impaired wound healing (Reed et al., 1996) possibly because each of these challenges calls upon energy stores that are not available to the exceptionally lean CR animals. Pituitary dwarf mice, although resistant to many effects of aging, are physically weaker than controls and show impaired fertility; they would presumably not do well in a natural setting in competition with nonmutant mice. The value of these experimental systems is not that they create animals superior to controls in every measure of physical and mental fitness but rather that they seem to retard, in parallel, many or perhaps even most forms of debility that accompany old age in mammals. They thus provide invaluable tools for learning more about the pathways that coordinate and synchronize the consequences of aging, whether the intervention has any potential for clinical use. It is quite unlikely that homozygous deletion of the *Pit1* (Snell dwarf) gene from newborn babies will prove helpful as preventive medicine, but possible that a detailed understanding of how altered patterns of pituitary hormones stave off multiple aspects of aging could contribute to the development of useful antiaging pharmaceuticals.

Secondly, it is possible that work on drugs that slow aging will serve as the first step in a multistage refinement process toward agents that have a favorable ratio of benefits to side effects. Changes in chemical structure, in targeting vehicle, in dosage schedule, and in cofactors that blunt harmful effects may result in preventive agents that do indeed delay or decelerate, in parallel, multiple aspects of aging without unacceptable toxicity. Such studies will be facilitated by improved insights into the factors that time aging (as distinct from the specific diseases whose risks increase as a consequence of aging), but are still likely to require extensive commitment of resources, and patience, through a series of trial and error studies using expensive endpoints. Development of surrogate endpoints, which predict to some extent the outcome of direct tests for antiaging effects, will also be hard to validate but could potentially pay off if they improve the success rate of tests using whole, aging animals. Such surrogate endpoints could include evaluation in convenient invertebrate models, or tests for effects on cellular stress resistance or gene expression patterns, but in any case will be helpful only to the extent that they can be proven to have both sensitivity and selectivity as predictors of effect in mice.

The third argument involves pointing out that it is clearly possible to develop new stocks of dogs (Bonnett et al., 2005), and probably horses (Brosnahan & Paradis, 2003), and opossums (Austad, 1993), that live longer and age more slowly than their immediate ancestors, and to create such new strains without sacrificing physical fitness and resistance to environmental hazards. The number of changes (in these instances selected genetic changes) needed to delay aging while retaining vigor is not yet known, nor is it clear whether the same physiological systems are involved in the evolution, by natural or artificial selection, of long-lived strains and species. Comparative biology thus makes a strong case that aging can indeed be retarded without loss of vigor, although providing valuable but lamentably understudied systems for learning more about which cells or hormones or pathways can be altered to good effect.

Lastly, we should point out that agents which merely prolong the period of late-life debility—leading (hypothetically) to years or decades of dementia, immobility, and pain—are not likely to be accepted by patients or physicians. Even if such agents could be produced (and there is as yet no evidence that they can), a vengeful Zeus would be required to incorporate them into the health care system. It is, we feel, time to put away the Tithonus fantasy as an impediment to public (and scientific) acceptance of the remarkable promise of research into the biology of aging and paths to its postponement.

ACKNOWLEDGMENTS

Work in the Lombard laboratory is supported by NIH (R01GM101171 and R21CA177925) and the Ellison Medical Foundation (AG-NS-0583-09). Work in the Miller laboratory is supported by grants from NIH (including AG013283 and AG024824), and by the Ellison Medical Foundation. The authors would like to thank Andrzej Galecki, Shu Chen, and Lili Deng for the analyses shown in Table 4.1; Billy Giblin for preparation of Figure 4.1; and William Swindell for much of the information shown in Figure 4.2. The authors confirm that they have no conflicts of interest regarding this Chapter.

REFERENCES

Alhazzazi, T. Y., Kamarajan, P., Joo, N., Huang, J. Y., Verdin, E., D'Silva, N. J., & Kapila, Y. L. (2011). Sirtuin-3 (SIRT3), a novel potential therapeutic target for oral cancer. *Cancer*, *117*(8), 1670–1678.

Anisimov, V. N. (2009). Carcinogenesis and aging 20 years after: Escaping horizon. *Mechanisms of Ageing and Development*, *130*(1–2), 105–121.

Anisimov, V. N., Zabezhinski, M. A., Popovich, I. G., Piskunova, T. S., Semenchenko, A. V., Tyndyk, M. L., . . . Blagosklonny, M. V. (2010). Rapamycin extends maximal lifespan in cancer-prone mice. *The American Journal of Pathology*, *176*(5), 2092–2097.

Anisimov, V. N., Zabezhinski, M. A., Popovich, I. G., Piskunova, T. S., Semenchenko, A. V., Tyndyk, M. L., . . . Blagosklonny, M. V. (2011). Rapamycin increases lifespan and inhibits spontaneous tumorigenesis in inbred female mice. *Cell Cycle*, *10*(24), 4230–4236.

Aspnes, L. E., Lee, C. M., Weindruch, R., Chung, S. S., Roecker, E. B., & Aiken, J. M. (1997). Caloric restriction reduces fiber loss and mitochondrial abnormalities in aged rat muscle. *FASEB Journal: Official Publication of the Federation of American Societies for Experimental Biology*, *11*(7), 573–581.

Aury-Landas, J., Bougeard, G., Castel, H., Hernandez-Vargas, H., Drouet, A., Latouche, J. B., . . . Flaman, J. M. (2013). Germline copy number variation of genes involved in chromatin remodelling in families suggestive of Li-Fraumeni syndrome with brain tumours. *European Journal of Human Genetics: EJHG*, *21*(12), 1369–1376.

Austad, S. N. (1993). Retarded senescence in an insular population of Virginia opossums (Didelphis virginiana). *Journal of Zoology*, *229*, 695–708.

Baker, D. J., Dawlaty, M. M., Wijshake, T., Jeganathan, K. B., Malureanu, L., van Ree, J. H., . . . van Deursen, J. M. (2012). Increased expression of BubR1 protects against aneuploidy and cancer and extends healthy lifespan. *Nature Cell Biology*, *15*(1), 96–102.

Baker, D. J., Jeganathan, K. B., Cameron, J. D., Thompson, M., Juneja, S., Kopecka, A., . . . van Deursen, J. M. (2004). BubR1 insufficiency causes early onset of aging-associated phenotypes and infertility in mice. *Nature Genetics*, *36*(7), 744–749.

Banerjee, K. K., Ayyub, C., Ali, S. Z., Mandot, V., Prasad, N. G., & Kolthur-Seetharam, U. (2012). dSir2 in the Adult Fat Body, but not in muscles, regulates life span in a diet-dependent manner. *Cell Reports*, *2*(6), 1485–1491.

Banks, A. S., Kon, N., Knight, C., Matsumoto, M., Gutierrez-Juarez, R., Rossetti, L., . . . Accili, D. (2008). SIRT1 gain of function increases energy efficiency and prevents diabetes in mice. *Cell Metabolism*, *8*(4), 333–341.

Barger, J. L., Kayo, T., Vann, J. M., Arias, E. B., Wang, J., Hacker, T. A., . . . Prolla, T. A. (2008). A low dose of dietary resveratrol partially mimics caloric restriction and retards aging parameters in mice. *PLoS One*, *3*(6), e2264.

Bartke, A. (2002). Insulin-like growth factor 1 and mammalian aging. *Science of Aging Knowledge Environment: SAGE KE*, *2002*(16), vp4.

Bartke, A. (2011). Growth hormone, insulin and aging: The benefits of endocrine defects. *Experimental Gerontology*, *46*(2–3), 108–111.

Bartke, A., Coschigano, K., Kopchick, J., Chandrashekar, V., Mattison, J., Kinney, B., & Hauck, S. (2001). Genes that prolong life: Relationships of growth hormone and growth to aging and life span. *The Journals of Gerontology. Series A, Biological Sciences and Medical Sciences*, 56, B340–B349.

Bartke, A., & Westbrook, R. (2012). Metabolic characteristics of long-lived mice. *Frontiers in Genetics*, 3, 288.

Bartke, A., Wright, J. C., Mattison, J. A., Ingram, D. K., Miller, R. A., & Roth, G. S. (2001). Extending the lifespan of long-lived mice. *Nature*, *414*(6862), 412.

Baur, J. A., Pearson, K. J., Price, N. L., Jamieson, H. A., Lerin, C., Kalra, A., . . . Sinclair, D. A. (2006). Resveratrol improves health and survival of mice on a high-calorie diet. *Nature*, *444*(7117), 337–342.

Baur, J. A., & Sinclair, D. A. (2006). Therapeutic potential of resveratrol: The in vivo evidence. *Nature Reviews. Drug Discovery*, 5(6), 493–506.

Baur, J. A., Ungvari, Z., Minor, R. K., Le Couteur, D. G., & de Cabo, R. (2012). Are sirtuins viable targets for improving healthspan and lifespan? *Nature Reviews. Drug Discovery*, *11*(16), 443–461.

Bell, E. L., Emerling, B. M., Ricoult, S. J., & Guarente, L. (2011). SIRT3 suppresses hypoxia inducible factor 1 alpha and tumor growth by inhibiting mitochondrial ROS production. *Oncogene*, *30*(26), 2986–2996.

Bernardes de Jesus, B., Vera, E., Schneeberger, K., Tejera, A. M., Ayuso, E., Bosch, F., & Blasco, M. A. (2012). Telomerase gene therapy in adult and old mice delays aging and increases longevity without increasing cancer. *EMBO Molecular Medicine*, 4, 691–704.

Blasco, M. A. (2005). Telomeres and human disease: Ageing, cancer and beyond. *Nature Reviews Genetics*, 6(8), 611–622.

Bluher, M., Kahn, B. B., & Kahn, C. R. (2003). Extended longevity in mice lacking the insulin receptor in adipose tissue. *Science*, *299*(5606), 572–574.

Bokov, A. F., Garg, N., Ikeno, Y., Thakur, S., Musi, N., DeFronzo, R. A., . . . Richardson, A. (2011). Does reduced IGF-1R signaling in Igf1r+/− mice alter aging? *PLoS One*, 6(11), e26891.

Boldt, H. B., Bale, L. K., Resch, Z. T., Oxvig, C., Overgaard, M. T., & Conover, C. A. (2013). Effects of mutated pregnancy-associated plasma protein-a on atherosclerotic lesion development in mice. *Endocrinology*, *154*, 246–252.

Bonkowski, M. S., Dominici, F. P., Arum, O., Rocha, J. S., Al Regaiey, K. A., Westbrook, R., . . . Bartke, A. (2009). Disruption of growth hormone receptor prevents calorie restriction from improving insulin action and longevity. *PLoS One*, 4(2), e4567.

Bonkowski, M. S., Rocha, J. S., Masternak, M. M., Al Regaiey, K. A., & Bartke, A. (2006). Targeted disruption of growth hormone receptor interferes with the beneficial actions of calorie restriction. *Proceedings of the National Academy of Sciences of the United States of America*, *103*(20), 7901–7905.

Bonnett, B. N., Egenvall, A., Hedhammar, A., & Olson, P. (2005). Mortality in over 350,000 insured Swedish dogs from 1995–2000: I. Breed-, gender-, age- and cause-specific rates. *Acta Veterinaria Scandinavica*, *46*(3), 105–120.

Bordone, L., Cohen, D., Robinson, A., Motta, M. C., van Veen, E., Czopik, A., . . . Gu, W., Guarente, L. (2007). SIRT1 transgenic mice show phenotypes resembling calorie restriction. *Aging Cell*, *6*(6), 759–767.

Brosnahan, M. M., & Paradis, M. R. (2003). Demographic and clinical characteristics of geriatric horses: 467 cases (1989–1999). *Journal of the American Veterinary Medical Association*, *223*(1), 93–98.

Brown, K., Xie, S., Qiu, X., Mohrin, M., Shin, J., Liu, Y., . . . Chen, D. (2013). SIRT3 reverses aging-associated degeneration. *Cell Reports*, *3*(2), 319–327.

Brown-Borg, H. M., Borg, K. E., Meliska, C. J., & Bartke, A. (1996). Dwarf mice and the ageing process. *Nature*, *384*, 33.

Burnett, C., Valentini, S., Cabreiro, F., Goss, M., Somogyvari, M., Piper, M. D., . . . Gems, D. (2011). Absence of effects of SIR2 overexpression on lifespan in C. elegans and Drosophila. *Nature*, *477*(7365), 482–485.

Butler, R. N., Miller, R. A., Perry, D., Carnes, B. A., Williams, T. F., Cassel, C., . . . Olshansky, S. J. (2008). New model of health promotion and disease prevention for the 21st century. *British Medical Journal*, *337*, a399.

Caccamo, A., Majumder, S., Richardson, A., Strong, R., & Oddo, S. (2010). Molecular interplay between mammalian target of rapamycin (mTOR), amyloid-beta, and Tau: Effects on cognitive impairments. *The Journal of Biological Chemistry*, *285*(17), 13107–13120.

Chen, C., Liu, Y., Liu, Y., & Zheng, P. (2009). mTOR regulation and therapeutic rejuvenation of aging hematopoietic stem cells. *Science Signaling*, *2*, ra75.

Chesler, E. J., Miller, D. R., Branstetter, L. R., Galloway, L. D., Jackson, B. L., Philip, V. M., . . . Manly, K. F. (2008). The Collaborative Cross at Oak Ridge National Laboratory: Developing a powerful resource for systems genetics. *Mammalian Genome*, *19*(6), 382–389.

Chester, J. A., & Watts, V. J. (2007). Adenylyl cyclase 5: A new clue in the search for the "fountain of youth?" *Science's STKE: Signal Transduction Knowledge Environment*, *2007*(413), pe64.

Churchill, G. A., Gatti, D. M., Munger, S. C., & Svenson, K. L. (2012). The diversity outbred mouse population. *Mammalian Genome*, *23*(9–10), 713–718.

Conover, C. A. (2012). Key questions and answers about pregnancy-associated plasma protein-A. *Trends in Endocrinology and Metabolism: TEM*, *23*(5), 242–249.

Conover, C. A., & Bale, L. K. (2007). Loss of pregnancy-associated plasma protein A extends lifespan in mice. *Aging Cell*, *6*(5), 727–729.

Conover, C. A., Bale, L. K., Mader, J. R., Mason, M. A., Keenan, K. P., & Marler, R. J. (2010). Longevity and age-related pathology of mice deficient in pregnancy-associated plasma protein-A. *The Journals of Gerontology. Series A, Biological Sciences and Medical Sciences*, *65*(6), 590–599.

Conover, C. A., Bale, L. K., & Powell, D. R. (2013). Inducible knock out of pregnancy-associated plasma protein-a gene expression in the adult mouse: Effect on vascular injury response. *Endocrinology*, *154*(8), 2734–2738.

Conover, C. A., Mason, M. A., Bale, L. K., Harrington, S. C., Nyegaard, M., Oxvig, C., & Overgaard, M. T. (2010). Transgenic overexpression of pregnancy-associated plasma protein-A in murine arterial smooth muscle accelerates atherosclerotic lesion development. *American Journal of Physiology. Heart and Circulatory Physiology, 299*, H284–H291.

Coschigano, K. T., Clemmons, D., Bellush, L. L., & Kopchick, J. J. (2000). Assessment of growth parameters and life span of GHR/BP gene-disrupted mice. *Endocrinology, 141*, 2608–2613.

Coschigano, K. T., Holland, A. N., Riders, M. E., List, E. O., Flyvbjerg, A., & Kopchick, J. J. (2003). Deletion, but not antagonism, of the mouse growth hormone receptor results in severely decreased body weights, insulin, and insulin-like growth factor I levels and increased life span. *Endocrinology, 144*(9), 3799–3810.

Cuervo, A. M., & Dice, J. F. (2000). Age-related decline in chaperone-mediated autophagy. *The Journal of Biological Chemistry, 275*, 31505–31513.

Deepa, S. S., Pulliam, D., Hill, S., Shi, Y., Walsh, M. E., Salmon, A., . . . Van Remmen, H. (2013). Improved insulin sensitivity associated with reduced mitochondrial complex IV assembly and activity. *FASEB Journal: Official Publication of the Federation of American Societies for Experimental Biology, 27*(4), 1371–1380.

Dell'agnello, C., Leo, S., Agostino, A., Szabadkai, G., Tiveron, C., Zulian, A., . . . Zeviani, M. (2007). Increased longevity and refractoriness to Ca(2+)-dependent neurodegeneration in Surf1 knockout mice. *Human Molecular Genetics, 16*(4), 431–444.

Donate, L. E., & Blasco, M. A. (2011). Telomeres in cancer and ageing. *Philosophical Transactions of the Royal Society of London. Series B, Biological Sciences, 366*(1561), 76–84.

Durieux, J., Wolff, S., & Dillin, A. (2011). The cell-non-autonomous nature of electron transport chain-mediated longevity. *Cell, 144*(1), 79–91.

Edwards, A. G., Donato, A. J., Lesniewski, L. A., Gioscia, R. A., Seals, D. R., & Moore, R. L. (2010). Life-long caloric restriction elicits pronounced protection of the aged myocardium: A role for AMPK. *Mechanisms of Ageing and Development, 131*(11–12), 739–742.

Egenvall, A., Bonnett, B. N., Olson, P., & Hedhammar, A. (2000a). Gender, age, breed and distribution of morbidity and mortality in insured dogs in Sweden during 1995 and 1996. *The Veterinary Record, 146*(18), 519–525.

Egenvall, A., Bonnett, B. N., Olson, P., & Hedhammar, A. (2000b). Gender, age, and breed pattern of diagnoses for veterinary care in insured dogs in Sweden during 1996. *The Veterinary Record, 146*, 551–557.

Fernandes, G., Friend, P., Yunis, E. J., & Good, R. A. (1978). Influence of dietary restriction on immunologic function and renal disease in (NZB x NZW) F1 mice. *Proceedings of the National Academy of Sciences of the United States of America, 75*, 1500–1504.

Fernandez-Marcos, P. J., Jeninga, E. H., Canto, C., Harach, T., de Boer, V. C., Andreux, P., . . . Auwerx, J. (2012). Muscle or liver-specific SIRT3 deficiency induces hyperacetylation of mitochondrial proteins without affecting global metabolic homeostasis. *Scientific Reports, 2*, 425.

Finch, C. E., Pike, M. C., & Witten, M. (1990). Slow mortality rate accelerations during aging in some animals approximate that of humans. *Science, 249*(4971), 902–905.

Fingerle-Rowson, G. R., & Bucala, R. (2001). Neuroendocrine properties of macrophage migration inhibitory factor (MIF). *Immunology and Cell Biology, 79*(4), 368–375.

Finley, L. W., Carracedo, A., Lee, J., Souza, A., Egia, A., Zhang, J., . . . Haigis, M. C. (2011). SIRT3 opposes reprogramming of cancer cell metabolism through HIF1alpha destabilization. *Cancer Cell*, *19*(3), 416–428.

Flores, I., Canela, A., Vera, E., Tejera, A., Cotsarelis, G., & Blasco, M. A. (2008). The longest telomeres: A general signature of adult stem cell compartments. *Genes & Development*, 22(5), 654–667.

Flurkey, K., Astle, C. M., & Harrison, D. E. (2010). Life extension by diet restriction and N-acetyl-L-cysteine in genetically heterogeneous mice. *The Journals of Gerontology. Series A, Biological Sciences and Medical Sciences*, *65*(12), 1275–1284.

Flurkey, K., Papaconstantinou, J., Miller, R. A., & Harrison, D. E. (2001). Lifespan extension and delayed immune and collagen aging in mutant mice with defects in growth hormone production. *Proceedings of the National Academy of Sciences of the United States of America*, *98*(12), 6736–6741.

Foukas, L. C., Bilanges, B., Bettedi, L., Pearce, W., Ali, K., Sancho, S., . . . Vanhaesebroeck, B. (2013). Long-term p110alpha PI3K inactivation exerts a beneficial effect on metabolism. *EMBO Molecular Medicine*, *5*(4), 563–571.

Garcia-Cao, I., Garcia-Cao, M., Tomas-Loba, A., Martin-Caballero, J., Flores, J. M., Klatt, P., . . . Serrano, M. (2006). Increased p53 activity does not accelerate telomere-driven ageing. *EMBO Reports*, *7*(5), 546–552.

Gardner, E. M. (2005). Caloric restriction decreases survival of aged mice in response to primary influenza infection. *The Journals of Gerontology. Series A, Biological Sciences and Medical Sciences*, *60*(5), 688–694.

Gelino, S., & Hansen, M. (2012). Autophagy—An emerging anti-aging mechanism? *Journal of Clinical & Experimental Pathology*, (Suppl. 4).

Gonzalez-Suarez, E., Geserick, C., Flores, J. M., & Blasco, M. A. (2005). Antagonistic effects of telomerase on cancer and aging in K5-mTert transgenic mice. *Oncogene*, *24*(13), 2256–2270.

Greer, E. L., & Brunet, A. (2009). Different dietary restriction regimens extend lifespan by both independent and overlapping genetic pathways in C. elegans. *Aging Cell*, *8*(2), 113–127.

Hall, J. A., Dominy, J. E., Lee, Y., & Puigserver, P. (2013). The sirtuin family's role in aging and age-associated pathologies. *The Journal of Clinical Investigation*, *123*(3), 973–979.

Hamilton, R. T., Walsh, M. E., & Van Remmen, H. (2012). Mouse models of oxidative stress indicate a role for modulating healthy aging. *Journal of Clinical & Experimental Pathology*, (Suppl. 4).

Harman, D. (1972). The biologic clock: The mitochondria? *Journal of the American Geriatrics Society*, *20*(4), 145–147.

Harper, J. M., Leathers, C. W., & Austad, S. N. (2006). Does caloric restriction extend life in wild mice? *Aging Cell*, *5*(6), 441–449.

Harper, J. M., Wilkinson, J. E., & Miller, R. A. (2010). Macrophage migration inhibitory factor-knockout mice are long lived and respond to caloric restriction. *FASEB Journal: Official Publication of the Federation of American Societies for Experimental Biology*, *24*(7), 2436–2442.

Harrington, S. C., Simari, R. D., & Conover, C. A. (2007). Genetic deletion of pregnancy-associated plasma protein-A is associated with resistance to atherosclerotic lesion development in apolipoprotein E-deficient mice challenged with a high-fat diet. *Circulation Research*, *100*, 1696–1702.

Harrison, D. E., Strong, R., Sharp, Z. D., Nelson, J. F., Astle, C. M., Flurkey, K., . . . Miller, R. A. (2009). Rapamycin fed late in life extends lifespan in genetically heterogeneous mice. *Nature*, *460*(7253), 392–395.

Herranz, D., Munoz-Martin, M., Canamero, M., Mulero, F., Martinez-Pastor, B., Fernandez-Capetillo, O., & Serrano, M. (2010). SIRT1 improves healthy ageing and protects from metabolic syndrome-associated cancer. *Nature Communications*, *1*, 3.

Heydari, A. R., Wu, B., Takahashi, R., Strong, R., & Richardson, A. (1993). Expression of heat shock protein 70 is altered by age and diet at the level of transcription. *Molecular and Cellular Biology*, *13*(5), 2909–2918.

Higashida, K., Kim, S. H., Jung, S. R., Asaka, M., Holloszy, J. O., & Han, D. H. (2013). Effects of Resveratrol and SIRT1 on PGC-1alpha Activity and Mitochondrial Biogenesis: A Reevaluation. *PLoS Biology*, *11*(7), e1001603.

Hinojosa, C. A., Mgbemena, V., Van Roekel, S., Austad, S. N., Miller, R. A., & Bose, S., & Orihuela, C. J. (2012). Enteric-delivered rapamycin enhances resistance of aged mice to pneumococcal pneumonia through reduced cellular senescence. *Experimental Gerontology*, *47*, 958–965.

Hirschey, M. D., Shimazu, T., Goetzman, E., Jing, E., Schwer, B., Lombard, D. B., . . . Verdin, E. (2010). SIRT3 regulates mitochondrial fatty-acid oxidation by reversible enzyme deacetylation. *Nature*, *464*(7285), 121–125.

Hirschey, M. D., Shimazu, T., Jing, E., Grueter, C. A., Collins, A. M., Aouizerat, B., . . . Verdin, E. (2011). SIRT3 deficiency and mitochondrial protein hyperacetylation accelerate the development of the metabolic syndrome. *Molecular Cell*, *44*, 177–190.

Holzenberger, M., Dupont, J., Ducos, B., Leneuve, P., Geloen, A., Even, P. C., . . . Le Bouc, Y. (2003). IGF-1 receptor regulates lifespan and resistance to oxidative stress in mice. *Nature*, *421*(6919), 182–187.

Houtkooper, R. H., Mouchiroud, L., Ryu, D., Moullan, N., Katsyuba, E., Knott, G., . . . Auwerx, J. (2013). Mitonuclear protein imbalance as a conserved longevity mechanism. *Nature*, *497*(7450), 451–457.

Howitz, K. T., Bitterman, K. J., Cohen, H. Y., Lamming, D. W., Lavu, S., Wood, J. G., . . . Sinclair, D. A. (2003). Small molecule activators of sirtuins extend Saccharomyces cerevisiae lifespan. *Nature*, *425*(6954), 191–196.

Hubbard, B. P., Gomes, A. P., Dai, H., Li, J., Case, A. W., Considine, T., . . . Sinclair, D. A. (2013). Evidence for a common mechanism of SIRT1 regulation by allosteric activators. *Science*, *339*(6124), 1216–1219.

Hubbard, V. M., Valdor, R., Macian, F., & Cuervo, A. M. (2012). Selective autophagy in the maintenance of cellular homeostasis in aging organisms. *Biogerontology*, *13*(1), 21–35.

Huyghe, E., Zairi, A., Nohra, J., Kamar, N., Plante, P., & Rostaing, L. (2007). Gonadal impact of target of rapamycin inhibitors (sirolimus and everolimus) in male patients: An overview. *Transplant International: Official Journal of the European Society for Organ Transplantation*, *20*(4), 305–311.

Ikeno, Y., Bronson, R. T., Hubbard, G. B., Lee, S., & Bartke, A. (2003). Delayed occurrence of fatal neoplastic diseases in Ames dwarf mice: Correlation to extended longevity.

The Journals of Gerontology. Series A, Biological Sciences and Medical Sciences, *58*(4), 291–296.

Ikeno, Y., Hubbard, G. B., Lee, S., Cortez, L. A., Lew, C. M., Webb, C. R., . . . Bartke, A. (2009). Reduced incidence and delayed occurrence of fatal neoplastic diseases in growth hormone receptor/binding protein knockout mice. *The Journals of Gerontology. Series A, Biological Sciences and Medical Sciences*, *64*(5), 522–529.

Ingram, D. K., Weindruch, R., Spangler, E. L., Freeman, J. R., & Walford, R. L. (1987). Dietary restriction benefits learning and motor performance of aged mice. *Journal of Gerontology*, *42*, 78–81.

Institute of Laboratory Animal Resources (U.S.) Committee on Animal Models for Research on Aging. (1981). *Mammalian models for research on aging*. Washington, DC: National Academy Press.

Ioannidis, J. P. (2005a). Contradicted and initially stronger effects in highly cited clinical research. *JAMA: The Journal of the American Medical Association*, *294*, 218–228.

Ioannidis, J. P. (2005b). Why most published research findings are false. *PLoS Medicine*, *2*(8), e124.

Iwamoto, T., Okumura, S., Iwatsubo, K., Kawabe, J., Ohtsu, K., Sakai, I., . . . Ishikawa, Y. (2003). Motor dysfunction in type 5 adenylyl cyclase-null mice. *The Journal of Biological Chemistry*, *278*(19), 16936–16940.

Iwasaki, K., Gleiser, C. A., Masoro, E. J., McMahan, C. A., Seo, E. J., & Yu, B. P. (1988). Influence of the restriction of individual dietary components on longevity and age-related disease of Fischer rats: the fat component and the mineral component. *Journal of Gerontology*, *43*(1), B13–B21.

Jaskelioff, M., Muller, F. L., Paik, J. H., Thomas, E., Jiang, S., Adams, A. C., . . . Depinho, R. A. (2011). Telomerase reactivation reverses tissue degeneration in aged telomerase-deficient mice. *Nature*, *469*(7328), 102–106.

Jia, K., Chen, D., & Riddle, D. L. (2004). The TOR pathway interacts with the insulin signaling pathway to regulate C. elegans larval development, metabolism and life span. *Development*, *131*(16), 3897–3906.

Johnson, T. E., Lithgow, G. J., & Murakami, S. (1996). Hypothesis: Interventions that increase the response to stress offer the potential for effective life prolongation and increased health. *The Journals of Gerontology. Series A, Biological Sciences and Medical Sciences*, *51*(6), B392–B395.

Kanfi, Y., Naiman, S., Amir, G., Peshti, V., Zinman, G., Nahum, L., . . . Cohen, H. Y. (2012). The sirtuin SIRT6 regulates lifespan in male mice. *Nature*, *483*(7388), 218–221.

Kapahi, P., Zid, B. M., Harper, T., Koslover, D., Sapin, V., & Benzer, S. (2004). Regulation of lifespan in Drosophila by modulation of genes in the TOR signaling pathway. *Current Biology*, *14*(10), 885–890.

Kass, L. (2003). *Beyond therapy: Biotechnology and the pursuit of happiness*. Wahington, DC: President's Council on Bioethics.

Kenyon, C., Chang, J., Gensch, E., Rudner, A., & Tabtiang, R. (1993). A C. elegans mutant that lives twice as long as wild type. *Nature*, *366*(6454), 461–464.

Khongkow, M., Olmos, Y., Gong, C., Gomes, A. R., Monteiro, L. J., Yague, E., . . . Lam, E. W. (2013). SIRT6 modulates paclitaxel and epirubicin resistance and survival in breast cancer. *Carcinogenesis*, *34*(7), 1476–1486.

Kim, H. S., Patel, K., Muldoon-Jacobs, K., Bisht, K. S., Aykin-Burns, N., Pennington, J. D., . . . Gius, D. (2010). SIRT3 is a mitochondria-localized tumor suppressor required for maintenance of mitochondrial integrity and metabolism during stress. *Cancer Cell*, *17*(1), 41–52.

Kinney, B. A., Coschigano, K. T., Kopchick, J. J., Steger, R. W., & Bartke, A. (2001). Evidence that age-induced decline in memory retention is delayed in growth hormone resistant GH-R-KO (Laron) mice. *Physiology & Behavior*, *72*(5), 653–660.

Kinney, B. A., Meliska, C. J., Steger, R. W., & Bartke, A. (2001). Evidence that Ames dwarf mice age differently from their normal siblings in behavioral and learning and memory parameters. *Hormones & Behavior*, *39*(4), 277–284.

Ladiges, W., Van Remmen, H., Strong, R., Ikeno, Y., Treuting, P., Rabinovitch, P., & Richardson, A. (2009). Lifespan extension in genetically modified mice. *Aging Cell*, *8*(4), 346–352.

Lagouge, M., Argmann, C., Gerhart-Hines, Z., Meziane, H., Lerin, C., Daussin, F., . . . Auwerx, J. (2006). Resveratrol improves mitochondrial function and protects against metabolic disease by activating SIRT1 and PGC-1alpha. *Cell*, *127*(6), 1109–1122.

Lamming, D. W., Ye, L., Astle, C. M., Baur, J. A., Sabatini, D. M., & Harrison, D. E. (2013). Young and old genetically heterogeneous HET3 mice on a rapamycin diet are glucose intolerant but insulin sensitive. *Aging Cell*, *12*(4), 712–718.

Lamming, D. W., Ye, L., Katajisto, P., Goncalves, M. D., Saitoh, M., Stevens, D. M., . . . Baur, J. A. (2012). Rapamycin-induced insulin resistance is mediated by mTORC2 loss and uncoupled from longevity. *Science*, *335*(6076), 1638–1643.

Lanske, B., & Razzaque, M. S. (2007). Premature aging in klotho mutant mice: Cause or consequence? *Ageing Research Reviews*, *6*(1), 73–79.

Lapierre, L. R., & Hansen, M. (2012). Lessons from C. elegans: Signaling pathways for longevity. *Trends in Endocrinology and Metabolism: TEM*, *23*(12), 637–644.

Liao, C. Y., Rikke, B. A., Johnson, T. E., Diaz, V., & Nelson, J. F. (2010). Genetic variation in the murine lifespan response to dietary restriction: From life extension to life shortening. *Aging Cell*, *9*, 92–95.

Linford, N. J., Kuo, T. H., Chan, T. P., & Pletcher, S. D. (2011). Sensory perception and aging in model systems: From the outside in. *Annual Review of Cell and Developmental Biology*, *27*, 759–785.

Lipman, R. D., Dallal, G. E., & Bronson, R. T. (1999). Effects of genotype and diet on age-related lesions in ad libitum fed and calorie-restricted F344, BN, and BNF3F1 rats. *The Journals of Gerontology. Series A, Biological Sciences and Medical Sciences*, *54*, B478–B491.

List, E. O., Berryman, D. E., Funk, K., Gosney, E. S., Jara, A., Kelder, B., . . . Kopchick, J. J. (2013). The role of GH in adipose tissue: Lessons from adipose-specific GH receptor gene-disrupted mice. *Molecular Endocrinology*, *27*(3), 524–535.

Lithgow, G. J., & Miller, R. A. (2008). The determination of aging rate by coordinated resistance to multiple forms of stress. In L. P. Guarente, L. Partridge, & D. Wallace (Eds.), *Molecular biology of aging* (pp. 427–482). Cold Spring Harbor, NY: Cold Spring Harbor Laboratory Press.

Liu, X., Jiang, N., Hughes, B., Bigras, E., Shoubridge, E., & Hekimi, S. (2005). Evolutionary conservation of the clk-1-dependent mechanism of longevity: Loss of mclk1 increases cellular fitness and lifespan in mice. *Genes & Development, 19*(20), 2424–2434.

Lombard, D. B., Alt, F. W., Cheng, H. L., Bunkenborg, J., Streeper, R. S., Mostoslavsky, R., . . . Schwer, B. (2007). Mammalian SIR2 homolog SIRT3 regulates global mitochondrial lysine acetylation. *Molecular and Cellular Biology, 27*(24), 8807–8814.

Lombard, D. B., & Miller, R. A. (2012). Ageing: Sorting out the sirtuins. *Nature, 483*(7388), 166–167.

Lombard, D. B., & Zwaans, B. M. (2013). SIRT3: As simple as it seems? *Gerontology*. Advance online publication.

Longo, V. D., & Kennedy, B. K. (2006). Sirtuins in aging and age-related disease. *Cell, 126*(2), 257–268.

Lopez-Otin, C., Blasco, M. A., Partridge, L., Serrano, M., & Kroemer, G. (2013). The hallmarks of aging. *Cell, 153*(6), 1194–1217.

Maier, B., Gluba, W., Bernier, B., Turner, T., Mohammad, K., Guise, T., . . . Scrable, H. (2004). Modulation of mammalian life span by the short isoform of p53. *Genes & Development, 18*(3), 306–319.

Marquardt, J. U., Fischer, K., Baus, K., Kashyap, A., Ma, S., Krupp, M., . . . Strand, S. (2013). Sirtuin-6-dependent genetic and epigenetic alterations are associated with poor clinical outcome in HCC patients. *Hepatology, 58*(3), 1054–1064.

Masoro, E. J. (2005). Overview of caloric restriction and ageing. *Mechanisms of Ageing and Development, 126*(9), 913–922.

Masoro, E. J., Shimokawa, I., Higami, Y., McMahan, C. A., & Yu, B. P. (1995). Temporal pattern of food intake not a factor in the retardation of aging processes by dietary restriction. *The Journals of Gerontology. Series A, Biological Sciences and Medical Sciences, 50A*(1), B48–B53.

Matheu, A., Maraver, A., Collado, M., Garcia-Cao, I., Canamero, M., Borras, C., . . . Serrano, M. (2009). Anti-aging activity of the Ink4/Arf locus. *Aging Cell, 8*(2), 152–161.

Matheu, A., Maraver, A., Klatt, P., Flores, I., Garcia-Cao, I., Borras, C., . . . Serrano, M. (2007). Delayed ageing through damage protection by the Arf/p53 pathway. *Nature, 448*(7151), 375–379.

Matheu, A., Maraver, A., & Serrano, M. (2008). The Arf/p53 pathway in cancer and aging. *Cancer Research, 68*(15), 6031–6034.

McCarter, R. J. M., Shimokawa, I., Ikeno, Y., Higami, Y., Hubbard, G. B., Yu, B. P., & McMahan, C. A. (1997). Physical activity as a factor in the action of dietary restriction on aging: effects in Fischer 344 rats. *Aging: Clinical and Experimental Research, 9*(1–2), 73–79.

Migliaccio, E., Giorgio, M., Mele, S., Pelicci, G., Reboldi, P., . . . Pelicci, P. G. (1999). The p66shc adaptor protein controls oxidative stress response and life span in mammals. *Nature, 402*, 309–313.

Miller, R. A. (2002). Extending life: Scientific prospects and political obstacles. *The Milbank Quarterly, 80*(1), 155–174.

Miller, R. A. (2009a). Cell stress and aging: New emphasis on multiplex resistance mechanisms. *The Journals of Gerontology. Series A, Biological Sciences and Medical Sciences, 64*(2), 179–182.

Miller, R. A. (2009b). "Dividends" from research on aging—Can biogerontologists, at long last, find something useful to do? *The Journals of Gerontology. Series A, Biological Sciences and Medical Sciences*, *64*(2), 157–160.

Miller, R. A., Buehner, G., Chang, Y., Harper, J. M., Sigler, R., & Smith-Wheelock, M. (2005). Methionine-deficient diet extends mouse lifespan, slows immune and lens aging, alters glucose, T4, IGF-I and insulin levels, and increases hepatocyte MIF levels and stress resistance. *Aging Cell*, *4*(3), 119–125.

Miller, R. A., Burke, D., & Nadon, N. (1999). Announcement: four-way cross mouse stocks: A new, genetically heterogeneous resource for aging research. *The Journals of Gerontology. Series A, Biological Sciences and Medical Sciences*, *54*, B358–B360.

Miller, R. A., & Chrisp, C. (2002). T cell subset patterns that predict resistance to spontaneous lymphoma, mammary adenocarcinoma, and fibrosarcoma in mice. *Journal of Immunology*, *169*(3), 1619–1625.

Miller, R. A., Harrison, D. E., Astle, C. M., Baur, J. A., Boyd, A. R., de Cabo, R., . . . Strong, R. (2011). Rapamycin, but not resveratrol or simvastatin, extends life span of genetically heterogeneous mice. *The Journals of Gerontology. Series A, Biological Sciences and Medical Sciences*, *66*(2), 191–201.

Miller, R. A., Harrison, D. E., Astle, C. M., Floyd, R. A., Flurkey, K., Hensley, K. L., . . . Strong, R. (2007). An Aging Interventions Testing Program: Study design and interim report. *Aging Cell*, *6*(4), 565–575.

Miller, R. A., Harrison, D. E., Astle, C. M., Fernandez, E., Flurkey, K., Han, M., . . . Strong, R. (in press). Rapamycin-mediated lifespan increase in mice is dose and sex-dependent and metabolically distinct from dietary restriction. *Aging Cell*.

Miller, R. A., & Nadon, N. (2000). Principles of animal use for gerontological research. *Journal of Gerontology: Biological Sciences*, *55A*, B117–B123.

Milne, J. C., Lambert, P. D., Schenk, S., Carney, D. P., Smith, J. J., Gagne, D. J., . . . Westphal, C. H. (2007). Small molecule activators of SIRT1 as therapeutics for the treatment of type 2 diabetes. *Nature*, *450*(7170), 712–716.

Moorad, J. A., Promislow, D. E., Flesness, N., & Miller, R. A. (2012). A comparative assessment of univariate longevity measures using zoological animal records. *Aging Cell*, *11*(6), 940–948.

Mostoslavsky, R., Chua, K. F., Lombard, D. B., Pang, W. W., Fischer, M. R., Gellon, L., . . . Alt, F. W. (2006). Genomic instability and aging-like phenotype in the absence of mammalian SIRT6. *Cell*, *124*, 315–329.

Nadon, N. L., Strong, R., Miller, R. A., Nelson, J., Javors, M., Sharp, Z. D., . . . Harrison, D. E. (2008). Design of aging intervention studies: The NIA interventions testing program. *AGE*, *30*(4), 187–199.

Natalicchio, A., Tortosa, F., Perrini, S., Laviola, L., & Giorgino, F. (2011). p66Shc, a multifaceted protein linking Erk signalling, glucose metabolism, and oxidative stress. *Archives of Physiology and Biochemistry*, *117*(3), 116–124.

Neff, F., Flores-Dominguez, D., Ryan, D. P., Horsch, M., Schroder, S., Adler, T., . . . Ehninger, D. (2013). Rapamycin extends murine lifespan but has limited effects on aging. *The Journal of Clinical Investigation*, *123*(8), 3272–3291.

Nelson, J. F., Karelus, K., Bergman, M. D., & Felicio, L. S. (1995). Neuroendocrine involvement in aging: Evidence from studies of reproductive aging and caloric restriction. *Neurobiology of Aging*, *16*(5), 837–843; discussion 855–856.

Ortega-Molina, A., Efeyan, A., Lopez-Guadamillas, E., Munoz-Martin, M., Gomez-Lopez, G., Canamero, M., . . . Serrano, M. (2012). Pten positively regulates brown adipose function, energy expenditure, and longevity. *Cell Metabolism*, *15*(3), 382–394.

Panici, J. A., Harper, J. M., Miller, R. A., Bartke, A., Spong, A., & Masternak, M. M. (2010). Early life growth hormone treatment shortens longevity and decreases cellular stress resistance in long-lived mutant mice. *FASEB Journal: Official Publication of the Federation of American Societies for Experimental Biology*, *24*(12), 5073–5079.

Partridge, L., & Barton, N. H. (1993). Optimality, mutation and the evolution of ageing. *Nature*, *362*(6418), 305–311.

Partridge, L., & Harvey, P. H. (1993). Methusalah among nematodes. *Nature*, *366*(6454), 404–405.

Pearson, K. J., Baur, J. A., Lewis, K. N., Peshkin, L., Price, N. L., Labinskyy, N., . . . de Cabo, R. (2008). Resveratrol delays age-related deterioration and mimics transcriptional aspects of dietary restriction without extending life span. *Cell Metabolism*, *8*(2), 157–168.

Pearson, K. J., Lewis, K. N., Price, N. L., Chang, J. W., Perez, E., Cascajo, M. V., . . . de Cabo, R. (2008). Nrf2 mediates cancer protection but not prolongevity induced by caloric restriction. *Proceedings of the National Academy of Sciences of the United States of America*, *105*(7), 2325–2330.

Perez, V. I., Bokov, A., Van Remmen, H., Mele, J., Ran, Q., Ikeno, Y., & Richardson, A. (2009). Is the oxidative stress theory of aging dead? *Biochimica et Biophysica Acta*, *1790*(10), 1005–1014.

Perez, V. I., Van Remmen, H., Bokov, A., Epstein, C. J., Vijg, J., & Richardson, A. (2009). The overexpression of major antioxidant enzymes does not extend the lifespan of mice. *Aging Cell*, *8*(1), 73–75.

Pfluger, P. T., Herranz, D., Velasco-Miguel, S., Serrano, M., & Tschop, M. H. (2008). SIRT1 protects against high-fat diet-induced metabolic damage. *Proceedings of the National Academy of Sciences of the United States of America*, *105*(28), 9793–9798.

Pillai, V. B., Sundaresan, N. R., Kim, G., Gupta, M., Rajamohan, S. B., Pillai, J. B., . . . Gupta, M. P. (2010). Exogenous NAD blocks cardiac hypertrophic response via activation of the SIRT3-LKB1-AMP-activated kinase pathway. *The Journal of Biological Chemistry*, *285*(5), 3133–3144.

Powers, R. W., III, Kaeberlein, M., Caldwell, S. D., Kennedy, B. K., & Fields, S. (2006). Extension of chronological life span in yeast by decreased TOR pathway signaling. *Genes & Development*, *20*(2), 174–184.

Qiu, X., Brown, K., Hirschey, M. D., Verdin, E., & Chen, D. (2010). Calorie restriction reduces oxidative stress by SIRT3-mediated SOD2 activation. *Cell Metabolism*, *12*(6), 662–667.

Ran, Q., Liang, H., Ikeno, Y., Qi, W., Prolla, T. A., Roberts, L. J., II, & Richardson, A. (2007). Reduction in glutathione peroxidase 4 increases life span through increased sensitivity to apoptosis. *The Journals of Gerontology. Series A, Biological Sciences and Medical Sciences*, *62*(9), 932–942.

Ratajczak, J., Shin, D. M., Wan, W., Liu, R., Masternak, M. M., Piotrowska, K., . . . Ratajczak, M. Z. (2011). Higher number of stem cells in the bone marrow of circulating low Igf-1 level Laron dwarf mice—Novel view on Igf-1, stem cells and aging. *Leukemia, 25*(4), 729–733.

Razzaque, M. S., & Lanske, B. (2006). Hypervitaminosis D and premature aging: lessons learned from Fgf23 and Klotho mutant mice. *Trends in Molecular Medicine, 12*(7), 298–305.

Reed, M. J., Penn, P. E., Li, Y., Birnbaum, R., Vernon, R. B., Johnson, T. S., . . . Wolf, N. S. (1996). Enhanced cell proliferation and biosynthesis mediate improved wound repair in refed, caloric-restricted mice. *Mechanisms of Ageing and Development, 89*(1), 21–43.

Richardson, A. (2013). Rapamycin, anti-aging, and avoiding the fate of Tithonus. *Journal of Clinical Investigation, 123*(8), 3204–3206.

Rizki, G., Iwata, T. N., Li, J., Riedel, C. G., Picard, C. L., Jan, M., & Lee, S. S. (2011). The evolutionarily conserved longevity determinants HCF-1 and SIR-2.1/SIRT1 collaborate to regulate DAF-16/FOXO. *PLoS Genetics, 7*(9), e1002235.

Rogina, B., Helfand, S. L., & Frankel, S. (2002). Longevity regulation by Drosophila Rpd3 deacetylase and caloric restriction. *Science, 298*(5599), 1745.

Rovira, J., Diekmann, F., Ramirez-Bajo, M. J., Bañon-Maneus, E., Moya-Rull, D., & Campistol, J. M. (2012). Sirolimus-associated testicular toxicity: Detrimental but reversible. *Transplantation, 93*(9), 874–879.

Sahin, E., Colla, S., Liesa, M., Moslehi, J., Muller, F. L., Guo, M., . . . DePinho, R. A. (2011). Telomere dysfunction induces metabolic and mitochondrial compromise. *Nature, 470*(7334), 359–365.

Salmon, A. B., Murakami, S., Bartke, A., Kopchick, J., Yasumura, K., & Miller, R. A. (2005). Fibroblast cell lines from young adult mice of long-lived mutant strains are resistant to multiple forms of stress. *American Journal of Physiology. Endocrinology and Metabolism, 289*(1), E23–E29.

Satoh, A., Brace, C. S., Rensing, N., Cliften, P., Wozniak, D. F., Herzog, E. D., . . . Imai, S. (2013). Sirt1 extends life span and delays aging in mice through the regulation of Nk2 homeobox 1 in the DMH and LH. *Cell Metabolism, 18*(3), 416–430.

Schriner, S. E., Linford, N. J., Martin, G. M., Treuting, P., Ogburn, C. E., Emond, M., . . . Rabinovitch, P. S. (2005). Extension of murine life span by overexpression of catalase targeted to mitochondria. *Science, 308*(5730), 1909–1911.

Sebastian, C., Zwaans, B. M., Silberman, D. M., Gymrek, M., Goren, A., Zhong, L., . . . Mostoslavsky, R. (2012). The histone deacetylase SIRT6 is a tumor suppressor that controls cancer metabolism. *Cell, 151*(6), 1185–1199.

Selman, C., Lingard, S., Choudhury, A. I., Batterham, R. L., Claret, M., Clements, M., . . . Withers, D. J. (2008). Evidence for lifespan extension and delayed age-related biomarkers in insulin receptor substrate 1 null mice. *FASEB Journal: Official Publication of the Federation of American Societies for Experimental Biology, 22*(3), 807–818.

Selman, C., Lingard, S., Gems, D., Partridge, L., & Withers, D. J. (2008). Comment on "Brain IRS2 signaling coordinates life span and nutrient homeostasis." *Science, 320*(5879), 1012; author reply 1012.

Selman, C., Tullet, J. M., Wieser, D., Irvine, E., Lingard, S. J., Choudhury, A. I., . . . Gems, D., Withers, D. J. (2009). Ribosomal protein S6 kinase 1 signaling regulates mammalian life span. *Science*, *326*(5949), 140–144.

Sharpless, N. E., & DePinho, R. A. (2007). How stem cells age and why this makes us grow old. *Nature Reviews. Molecular Cell Biology*, *8*(9), 703–713.

Shimazu, T., Hirschey, M. D., Hua, L., Dittenhafer-Reed, K. E., Schwer, B., Lombard, D. B., . . . Verdin, E. (2010). SIRT3 deacetylates mitochondrial 3-hydroxy-3-methylglutaryl CoA synthase 2 and regulates ketone body production. *Cell Metabolism*, *12*(6), 654–661.

Silberberg, R. (1972). Articular aging and osteoarthritis in dwarf mice. *Pathologia et Microbiologia*, *38*(6), 417–430.

Sohal, R. S., & Weindruch, R. (1996). Oxidative stress, caloric restriction, and aging. *Science*, *273*(5271), 59–63.

Someya, S., Yu, W., Hallows, W. C., Xu, J., Vann, J. M., Leeuwenburgh, C., . . . Prolla, T. A. (2010). SIRT3 mediates reduction of oxidative damage and prevention of age-related hearing loss under caloric restriction. *Cell*, *143*(5), 802–812.

Spindler, S. R. (2005). Rapid and reversible induction of the longevity, anticancer and genomic effects of caloric restriction. *Mechanisms of Ageing and Development*, *126*(9), 960–966.

Steinbaugh, M. J., Sun, L. Y., Bartke, A., & Miller, R. A. (2012). Activation of genes involved in xenobiotic metabolism is a shared signature of mouse models with extended lifespan. *American Journal of Physiology. Endocrinology and Metabolism*, *303*(4), E488–E495.

Strong, R., Miller, R. A., Astle, C. M., Baur, J. A., de Cabo, R., Fernandez, E., . . . Harrison, D. E. (2013). Evaluation of resveratrol, green tea extract, curcumin, oxaloacetic acid, and medium-chain triglyceride oil on life span of genetically heterogeneous mice. *The Journals of Gerontology. Series A, Biological Sciences and Medical Sciences*, *68*(1), 6–16.

Strong, R., Miller, R. A., Astle, C. M., Floyd, R. A., Flurkey, K., Hensley, K. L., . . . Harrison, D. E. (2008). Nordihydroguaiaretic acid and aspirin increase lifespan of genetically heterogeneous male mice. *Aging Cell*, *7*(5), 641–650.

Sun, L. Y., Al-Regaiey, K., Masternak, M. M., Wang, J., & Bartke, A. (2005). Local expression of GH and IGF-1 in the hippocampus of GH-deficient long-lived mice. *Neurobiology of Aging*, *26*(6), 929–937.

Sun, L., Sadighi Akha, A. A., Miller, R. A., & Harper, J. M. (2009). Life-span extension in mice by preweaning food restriction and by methionine restriction in middle age. *The Journals of Gerontology. Series A, Biological Sciences and Medical Sciences*, *64*, 711–722.

Sundaresan, N. R., Samant, S. A., Pillai, V. B., Rajamohan, S. B., & Gupta, M. P. (2008). SIRT3 is a stress-responsive deacetylase in cardiomyocytes that protects cells from stress-mediated cell death by deacetylation of Ku70. *Molecular and Cellular Biology*, *28*(20), 6384–6401.

Svensson, J., Sjogren, K., Faldt, J., Andersson, N., Isaksson, O., Jansson, J. O., & Ohlsson, C. (2011). Liver-derived IGF-I regulates mean life span in mice. *PLoS One*, *6*(7), e22640.

Taguchi, A., Wartschow, L. M., & White, M. F. (2007). Brain IRS2 signaling coordinates life span and nutrient homeostasis. *Science*, *317*(5836), 369–372.

Tatar, M., Bartke, A., & Antebi, A. (2003). The endocrine regulation of aging by insulin-like signals. *Science*, *299*(5611), 1346–1351.

Tennyson, A. L. (1859). *Tithonus*. Retrieved from http://www.poetryfoundation.org/poem/174656

Threadgill, D. W., & Churchill, G. A. (2012). Ten years of the Collaborative Cross. *Genetics*, *190*(2), 291–294.

Timmers, S., Konings, E., Bilet, L., Houtkooper, R. H., van de Weijer, T., Goossens, G. H., . . . Schrauwen, P. (2011). Calorie restriction-like effects of 30 days of resveratrol supplementation on energy metabolism and metabolic profile in obese humans. *Cell Metabolism*, *14*(5), 612–622.

Tissenbaum, H. A., & Guarente, L. (2001). Increased dosage of a sir-2 gene extends lifespan in Caenorhabditis elegans. *Nature*, *410*(6825), 227–230.

Tomas-Loba, A., Flores, I., Fernandez-Marcos, P. J., Cayuela, M. L., Maraver, A., Tejera, A., . . . Blasco, M. A. (2008). Telomerase reverse transcriptase delays aging in cancer-resistant mice. *Cell*, *135*(4), 609–622.

Tomilov, A. A., Ramsey, J. J., Hagopian, K., Giorgio, M., Kim, K. M., Lam, A., . . . Cortopassi, G. A. (2011). The Shc locus regulates insulin signaling and adiposity in mammals. *Aging Cell*, *10*(1), 55–65.

Treuting, P. M., Linford, N. J., Knoblaugh, S. E., Emond, M. J., Morton, J. F., Martin, G. M., . . . Ladiges, W. C. (2008). Reduction of age-associated pathology in old mice by overexpression of catalase in mitochondria. *The Journals of Gerontology. Series A, Biological Sciences and Medical Sciences*, *63*(8), 813–822.

Tyner, S. D., Venkatachalam, S., Choi, J., Jones, S., Ghebranious, N., Igelmann, H., . . . Donehower, L. A. (2002). p53 mutant mice that display early ageing-associated phenotypes. *Nature*, *415*(6867), 45–53.

Vallejo, A. N., Michel, J. J., Bale, L. K., Lemster, B. H., Borghesi, L., & Conover, C. A. (2009). Resistance to age-dependent thymic atrophy in long-lived mice that are deficient in pregnancy-associated plasma protein A. *Proceedings of the National Academy of Sciences of the United States of America*, *106*, 11252–11257.

Vellai, T., Takacs-Vellai, K., Zhang, Y., Kovacs, A. L., Orosz, L., & Müller, F. (2003). Genetics: Influence of TOR kinase on lifespan in C. elegans. *Nature*, *426*, 620.

Vera, E., Bernardes de Jesus, B., Foronda, M., Flores, J. M., & Blasco, M. A. (2012). The rate of increase of short telomeres predicts longevity in mammals. *Cell Reports*, *2*(4), 732–737.

Vergara, M., Smith-Wheelock, M., Harper, J. M., Sigler, R., & Miller, R. A. (2004). Hormone-treated snell dwarf mice regain fertility but remain long lived and disease resistant. *The Journals of Gerontology. Series A, Biological Sciences and Medical Sciences*, *59*(12), 1244–1250.

Viswanathan, M., & Guarente, L. (2011). Regulation of Caenorhabditis elegans lifespan by sir-2.1 transgenes. *Nature*, *477*(7365), E1–E2.

Wang, C., Li, Q., Redden, D. T., Weindruch, R., & Allison, D. B. (2004). Statistical methods for testing effects on "maximum lifespan." *Mechanisms of Ageing and Development*, *125*(9), 629–632.

Waxman, D. J., & Holloway, M. G. (2009). Sex differences in the expression of hepatic drug metabolizing enzymes. *Molecular Pharmacology*, *76*(2), 215–228.

Weindruch, R., & Sohal, R. S. (1997). Seminars in medicine of the Beth Israel Deaconess Medical Center. Caloric intake and aging. *The New England Journal of Medicine*, *337*(14), 986–994.

Weindruch, R., & Walford, R. L. (1982). Dietary restriction in mice beginning at 1 year of age: Effect on life span and spontaneous cancer incidence. *Science*, *215*(4538), 1415–1418.

Weindruch, R., & Walford, R. L. (1988). *The retardation of aging and disease by dietary restriction*. Springfield, IL: Charles C. Thomas.

Wilkinson, J. E., Burmeister, L., Brooks, S. V., Chan, C. C., Friedline, S., Harrison, D. E., . . . Miller, R. A. (2012). Rapamycin slows aging in mice. *Aging Cell*, *11*(4), 675–682.

Wolf, N. S., Li, Y., Pendergrass, W., Schmeider, C., & Turturro, A. (2000). Normal mouse and rat strains as models for age-related cataract and the effect of caloric restriction on its development. *Experimental Eye Research*, *70*(5), 683–692.

Wolf, N., Penn, P., Pendergrass, W., Van Remmen, H., Bartke, A., Rabinovitch, P., & Martin, G. M. (2005). Age-related cataract progression in five mouse models for anti-oxidant protection or hormonal influence. *Experimental Eye Research*, *81*(3), 276–285.

Yamaza, H., Komatsu, T., Wakita, S., Kijogi, C., Park, S., Hayashi, H., . . . Shimokawa, I. (2010). FOXO1 is involved in the antineoplastic effect of calorie restriction. *Aging Cell*, *9*(3), 372–382.

Yan, L., Park, J. Y., Dillinger, J. G., De Lorenzo, M. S., Yuan, C., Lai, L., . . . Vatner, S. F. (2012). Common mechanisms for calorie restriction and adenylyl cyclase type 5 knockout models of longevity. *Aging Cell*, *11*(6), 1110–1120.

Yan, L., Vatner, D. E., O'Connor, J. P., Ivessa, A., Ge, H., Chen, W., . . . Vatner, S. F. (2007). Type 5 adenylyl cyclase disruption increases longevity and protects against stress. *Cell*, *130*(2), 247–258.

Yang, S. B., Tien, A. C., Boddupalli, G., Xu, A. W., Jan, Y. N., & Jan, L. Y. (2012). Rapamycin ameliorates age-dependent obesity associated with increased mTOR signaling in hypothalamic POMC neurons. *Neuron*, *75*(3), 425–436.

Zhang, C., & Cuervo, A. M. (2008). Restoration of chaperone-mediated autophagy in aging liver improves cellular maintenance and hepatic function. *Nature Medicine*, *14*(9), 959–965.

Zhang, Y., Bokov, A., Gelfond, J., Soto, V., Ikeno, Y., Hubbard, G., . . . Fischer, K. (2013). Rapamycin Extends Life and Health in C57BL/6 Mice. *The Journals of Gerontology. Series A, Biological Sciences and Medical Sciences*. Advance online publication.

Zwaans, B. M., & Lombard, D. B. (in press). Diverse roles for SIRT6 in mammalian healthspan and longevity. In R. H. Houtkooper (Ed.), *Sirtuins*. New York, NY: Springer.

CHAPTER 5

Primate Models for Human Brain Aging and Neurological Diseases

Caleb Finch and Steve Austad

ABSTRACT

As the longest lived primate species, humans present a remarkable divergence from brain aging processes of their lineage. One way to investigate genetic influences on aging is to make informative comparisons among closely related species. Even though they are nearly identical to chimpanzees and bonobos in nucleotide sequence, humans appear unique in the primate lineages in their vulnerability to neurodegeneration at later ages, although this level of neurodegeneration was not common until the 20th century. The great apes typically have minor neurodegenerative changes of aging relative to the longer lived humans after the age of 70 years or even compared to shorter lived monkeys by the age of 20 years. Surprisingly, an even shorter lived monkey (marmoset) and a prosimian (grey mouse lemur) have extensive earlier deposits of brain amyloid before 10 years, which offer experimental opportunity for interventions into brain aging.

INTRODUCTION

Of all the changes the body undergoes with aging, perhaps the most alarming is our decline in normal cognitive functions during middle-age and, after 60 years, the increasing risk of one or more neurological impairments or chronic diseases, particularly Alzheimer's disease (AD) or Parkinson's disease (PD), which have exponentially increasing incidence. Each condition may be said to intensify underlying aging processes that may not reach clinical grade by life's end.

http://dx.doi.org/10.1891/0198-8794.34.139

The incidence of age-related tremor not only increases from PD but also from the more common "essential" tremor of aging which may involve neurodegeneration in the cerebellum as well as the substantia nigra (Adler, Shill, & Beach, 2011; Louis, 2011). AD and PD are worsened by sporadic strokes.

Later age degenerative conditions may be presaged by modest progressive brain aging changes during middle-age that can be detected in most individuals by age 30 years even when most people appear reasonably healthy, and these processes continue into older ages (Finch, 2009). Changes include slower cognitive processing and increased errors during multitasking. Other mammals show similar trends for changes during middle-age, but with major differences among species as described in our recent review (Finch & Austad, 2012) and discussed below. However, it is remarkable that at ages approaching the limit of recorded lifespan, no aging primate species spontaneously develops severe neurodegeneration with neuron loss comparable to clinical grade AD or PD. Here we further describe the main primate species used as models for laboratory study that are available for future studies of environmental factors in neurological aging.

The genetic influence on aging, its pattern and tempo, may be most cleanly seen in comparisons among species. Therefore, in this volume focused on genetic influences on aging, we concentrate on comparing primate species differences in brain aging. Primates are the most cognitively sophisticated mammals and also our closest relatives, therefore comparing neurodegenerative processes across species, particularly combined with emerging discoveries in comparative primate genomics and transcriptomics, should yield insight into the underlying genetic basis of these degenerative processes.

Chimpanzees and bonobos, our closest relatives, are 99% identical to humans at the nucleotide level (Prüfer et al., 2012). Yet, despite this genetic affinity, they differ dramatically from humans not only in cognitive prowess but also in the manner and degree of neurodegeneration as we discuss below. Surprisingly, patterns of brain aging appear to be more similar to humans in more genetically divergent primate species such as lemurs and Old World monkeys.

Not all aspects of brain aging are genetic in origin, however. Environmental influences on brain aging are strongly documented in human populations. For instance, cognitive status in 90 years and older Danish cohorts born 10 years apart was significantly enhanced in both sexes. In the 1915 cohort, the percentage of probants achieving the maximum score on the mini-mental state exam (MMSE) was almost twofold higher than in the 1905 birth cohort (Christensen et al., 2013). Education level has a specific effect on risk of AD, particularly in developed countries (Sharp & Gatz, 2011), for example in East Boston, the risk was 15% lower per year of additional education (Evans et al., 1997). These associations with education level are consistent with the well-documented and robust influences of socioeconomic status (SES) on the health span and lifespan, in which the "poor" suffer a loss of about 15 years life expectancy from faster aging with earlier and more prevalent disease relative to nonpoor (Crimmins, Kim, Seeman, 2009). For PD, environmental factors are modestly documented and include occupational hazards for exposure to pesticides (Freire & Koifman, 2012; Van Maele-Fabry, Hoet, Vilain, & Laison, 2012) and a possible neuroprotective effect of nicotine (Quik, Perez, & Bordia, 2012). The risk of stroke also has lifestyle and environmental influences in all SES strata, including dietary fat and exercise (Goldstein et al., 2011; Kokubo, 2012).

Effects of SES and environment on outcomes of aging are best understood as lifelong gene-environment interactions, beginning before birth, involving sex and gender, as well as individual gene variations. Because maternal oocytes are completely formed in the maternal grandmother's uterus, there may be prezygotic effects with transgenerational potential (Finch & Loehlin, 1998). Thus far, caloric restriction of macaques is the only long-term manipulation of neurological aging in any nonhuman primate.

OVERVIEW OF MAJOR PRIMATE MODELS FOR AGING

Our synopsis of aging in primates recalls the origins of laboratory studies in the 1920s. Robert Yerkes, a pioneer psychobiologist and ardent eugenicist, established a colony of chimpanzees and other primate species for research on the comparative intelligence of species closely related to humans (Thomas, 2006). Aging studies on primates also soon entered the research arena with the work of the charlatan/scientist Serge Voronoff, who grafted testicles into people from various monkey and ape species including chimpanzees and rhesus macaques in the hopes of slowing or reversing aging processes (Haber, 2004).

Chimpanzees

Of special interest for understanding the evolution of human aging are the chimpanzees (common chimpanzee, *Pan troglodytes* [hereafter called simply the chimpanzee] and the bonobo, *Pan paniscus*), our closest living relatives (see Figure 5.1). The chimpanzee lineage diverged from that of humans 5–7 million years ago and the two chimpanzee species themselves diverged about 1 million years ago (Chatterjee, Ho, Barnes, & Groves, 2009; Fabre, Rodrigues, & Douzery, 2009; Prüfer et al. 2012). At the nucleotide level, both chimpanzee species are greater than 98% identical to humans (Chimpanzee Sequencing & Analysis Consortium, 2005; Prüfer et al., 2012). Both chimpanzee species live in complex

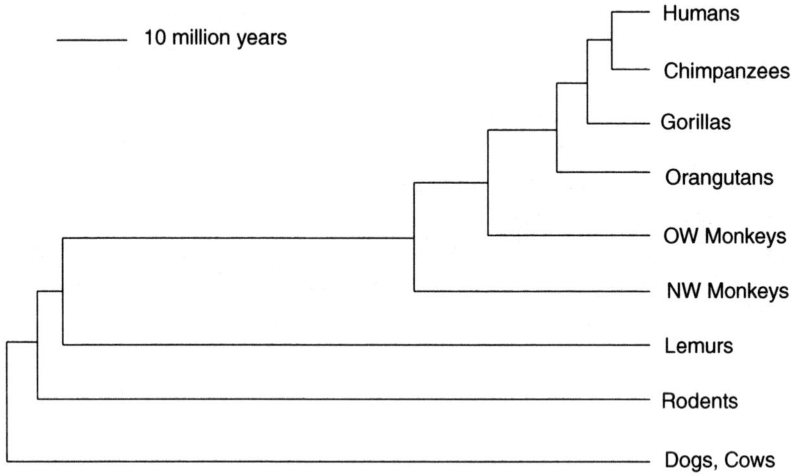

FIGURE 5.1 Phylogeny of primates and humans in relation to other mammals. OW = Old World; NW = New World. Redrawn from Finch & Austad, 2012.

social groups of several dozen to greater than 100 individuals. Body weights in the wild are roughly the same (males: 35–70 kg; females: 25–50 kg), overlapping with some human populations including extant hunter-gatherers (Hill & Hurtado, 1996; Nowak, 1999). Certain aspects of the behavior of the two chimpanzee species differ dramatically. For instance, male chimpanzees use aggression to compete for dominance rank and sex, form alliances with other males, and sometimes use lethal aggression to defend their home range. By contrast, bonobo males are often subordinate to females, do not compete intensely for dominance rank, and lethal aggression between groups has never been observed (Prüfer et al., 2012).

Despite these differences, their reproductive life histories are quite similar, both in the wild and in captivity. First births occur in wild populations of chimpanzees at 10–17 years compared with 9–11 years in captivity (De Lathouwers & Van Elsacker, 2005) and the interval between births averages about 4.5 years in both captive and wild populations. Little information is available on bonobo longevity but it is likely to resemble the chimpanzee. Synthetic life tables constructed from data on multiple captive chimpanzees indicate that life expectancy at birth and at reproductive maturity is about 30 years (Gage, 1998). By contrast, similar analyses from wild populations indicate life expectancies at both birth and at reproductive maturity is about 15 years (Hill et al., 2001). Female chimpanzees live longer than males both in the wild and in captivity (see Figure 5.2). No chimpanzee has been validated to live longer than 60 years, challenging a

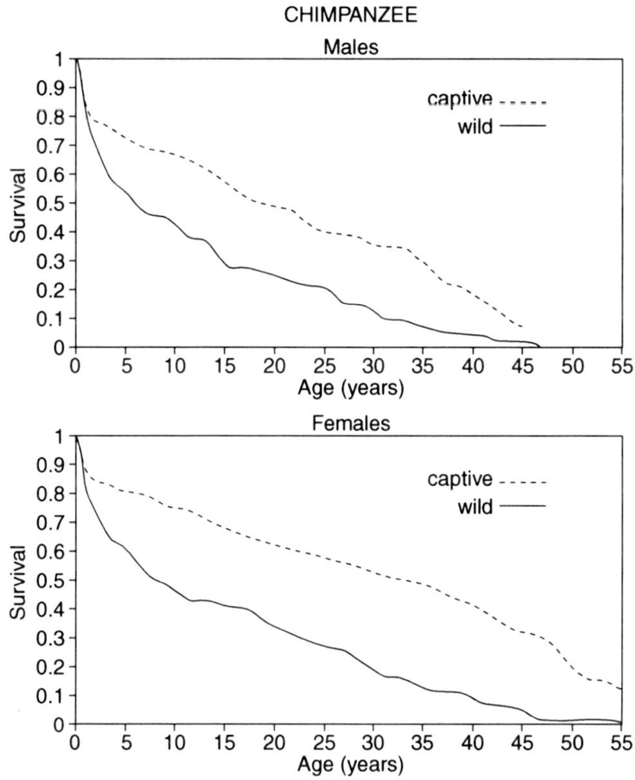

FIGURE 5.2 Survival of chimpanzees in captivity versus wild. Curves for wild populations are synthesized from five different study sites. Captive data were assembled by Gage (1998). Figure redrawn from Hill et al., 2001.

persistent popular myth (R. D. Rosen, 2008). Interestingly, past the age of about 5 years, age-specific mortality rates—particularly of females—in captivity do not appear to substantially differ from females in the wild (Hill et al., 2001), suggesting that the captive husbandry of chimpanzees may not be as advanced as for several other primate species. Another factor supporting this hypothesis of suboptimal husbandry is that the oldest female reported from the wild was still alive at an estimated age of 55 years (Hill et al., 2001), which is not much different than the greatest validated age in captivity—59 years (Weigl, 2005). Orangutans are similarly longevous: the longest wild individual lifespan (a male at least 58 years old; Wich et al., 2004) is virtually identical to the longest lived captive (59 years; Weigl, 2005). The difficult husbandry of captive orangutans is well-documented (Wich et al., 2009).

In recent years, heart disease has been the most common cause of death in aged chimpanzees as it is in humans in many developed countries, although the type of disease differs (Varki et al., 2009). Unlike humans, chimpanzees in current lab populations show cardiac failure caused by diffuse interstitial cardiac fibrosis of unknown cause, distinct from coronary artery atherosclerosis. Nonetheless, classic coronary ischemia was reported from earlier studies (Finch & Stanford, 2004; Appendix Table 1.3), for example, in female of 8 years (Manning, 1943), which may not have used appropriate diets. Neoplasia is also reasonably common in chimpanzees, although it is mostly benign and in females most common in the urogenital tract (Brown et al., 2009).

There are still tremendous gaps in understanding the evolution of human aging compared to that in chimpanzees and bonobos. For instance, the impact of SES on health and longevity may be mimicked in chimpanzees by the effect on longevity of dominance rank (Pusey, Williams, & Goodall, 1997). We anticipate important information on social status and gender interactions on outcomes of aging in chimpanzees. Much can be learned with relatively noninvasively regular physical assessments similar to a human annual physical exam, close behavioral observations, modern imaging, and thorough necropsies. Unfortunately, the recent proposal by the United States Fish and Wildlife Service to declare captive chimpanzees as endangered and the decision by the National Institutes of Health to move all but 50 of its chimpanzees to sanctuaries rather than maintaining them at research institutions (Kaiser, 2013) threatens further research on age-related changes in chimpanzee behavior and cognition. Sanctuaries are not typically organized to conduct even these relatively noninvasive observations and procedures.

Macaques

The workhorse of primate biomedical research has for decades been the rhesus macaque, *Macaca mulatta*. It is one of 20 species of macaques, a widely distributed, diurnal, group-living (group size: 8 to >100), largely terrestrial, largely vegetarian group of Old World monkeys, all of which have arboreal capabilities (Nowak, 1999). Old World monkeys diverged from the human lineage about 25 million years ago (see Figure 5.1; Glazko & Nei, 2003). Several other closely related species of the same subgenus are also used in biomedical research, in particular the smaller cynomolgus macaque (*M. fascicularis*)—known as the crab-eating or long-tailed macaque to zoologists—and the larger, more cold-adapted, Japanese macaque (*M. fuscata*).

Rhesus macaques have become popular for biomedical research because they adapt particularly well to captivity. As a consequence, some 200,000 rhesus macaques *per year* (!) were imported into the United States from India in the late 1950s, leading to such a population decline in India that their exportation was banned in 1978. Since that ban, China has been a source of smaller numbers of rhesus imported for research. The Chinese rhesus line separated from Indian rhesus 160,000 years ago (Hernandez et al., 2007). Although differing in various morphological and behavioral traits, they have roughly similar life histories (Kubisch, Falkenstein, Deroche, & Franke, 2012).

As with most captive primate species including chimpanzees, rhesus macaques in research colonies weigh considerably more than their wild relatives. For instance, rhesus average 50%–75% more in captivity than in the wild: males 7.7 kg in the wild versus 11.0–13.0 kg in captivity; females 5.4 kg in the wild versus 7.0–9.0 kg in captivity (Smith & Jungers, 1997; Mattison et al., 2012). In captivity, both Indian- and Chinese-derived rhesus females have first births at 4–5 years of age, and over the course of their lifetime, produce single young at intervals of just over 1 year (Kubisch et al., 2012). In the healthiest colonies, rhesus life expectancy is about 27 years, with a maximum of about 40 years (see Figure 5.3; Colman & Kemnitz, 1998). However, recently older males (16–23 years) entered into a formal aging study at the U.S. National Institute on Aging (NIA) rhesus colony lived 35 years on average (Mattison et al., 2012), considerably longer than previous reports (see Figure 5.3). Note, because animals were entered into the study later in life, early deaths were censored, which increased calculated life expectancy.

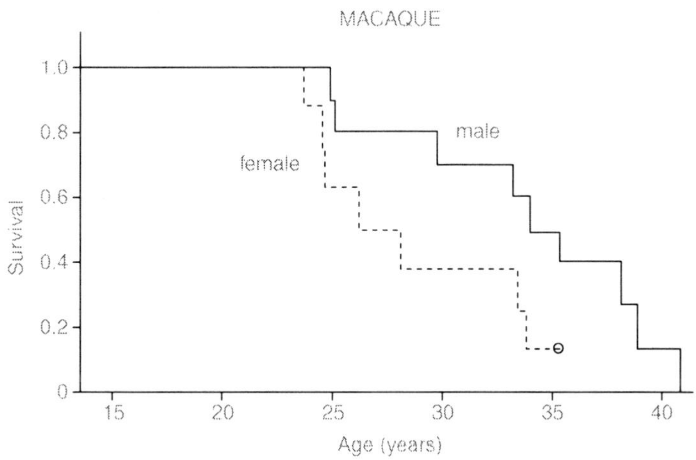

FIGURE 5.3 Survival of rhesus macaques in an extremely healthy colony. Mean longevity females: 27.8 years; males: 35.4 years. Note that animals were not entered into the study until age 16–23 years: thus deaths before these ages are censored, which increases mean longevity but not the pattern of deaths among older individuals. Redrawn from Mattison et al., 2012.

Captive rhesus macaques are prone to some of the human diseases of aging. For instance, on some diets, the prevalence of type II diabetes nears 40% of older individuals (Bodkin, Alexander, Ortmeyer, Johnson, & Hansen, 2003; Colman et al., 2009). As with most mammals, sarcopenia is a common feature of aging (Colman, Beasley, Allison, & Weindruch, 2008). The most common cause of death appears to be neoplasia, particularly in the gastrointestinal tract. Among these, the most prevalent in several North American colonies was adenocarcinoma of the large intestine (Simmons & Mattison 2011). Rhesus also develop spontaneous cardiovascular disease, although it is very mild compared to humans in economically developed countries. However, macaques fed high-fat diets have dramatically increased prevalence of cardiovascular disease (Cefalu & Wagner, 1997).

As noted earlier, other species of macaques—in particular, cynomolgus macaques which are frequently used in studies of cardiovascular disease—have had a smattering of use in aging research, as have other Old World monkeys.

Baboons

Excellent demography and emerging genetics of several diseases and conditions such as obesity, for instance, are available for the baboon. In the largest captive baboon colony, mean longevity of adults (those reaching at least 5 years of age) is 21 years with the oldest individual surviving to 33 years. By comparison, mean adult longevity in two long-term field studies is 12.1 years in a completely natural population (Amboseli, Kenya) and 19.7 years in a population that is food-provisioned (Gombe, Tanzania). In both field populations, the oldest individual was 27 years old (Bronikowski et al., 2002). Interestingly, the slope of the age-specific increase in mortality, as modeled by a Gompertz function, was roughly similar among captive and wild populations. In terms of aging pathologies, analysis of 23 years of mortality records from the largest captive baboon colony ($N > 4{,}000$) found the leading causes of death among those aged >15 years to be euthanasia because of spondylosis and arthritis, followed somewhat distantly by amyloidosis, endometriosis, and several types of cancer (Dick et al., in press). The survival curves of females show strong associations with social class (Silk et al., 2010) as in humans (Crimmins, Kim, & Seeman, 2009). Alpha males also have enhanced wound healing (Archie, Altmann, & Alberts 2012).

Despite the fact that chimpanzees and Old World monkeys are our most closely primate relatives (see Figure 5.1), there are many merits of the smaller, more rapidly aging, shorter lived primate species for aging research, the common marmoset and the grey mouse lemur, described below (Fischer & Austad, 2011). First, their shorter life makes experimental evaluation of potential aging interventions more feasible. Second, the smaller species are less expensive to feed and house. Third, smaller animals often reproduce more rapidly, allowing for the relatively fast build-up of numbers in research colonies. Fourth, smaller animals are more plausibly housed in groups that reflect the social environment of natural populations. In nature, chimpanzees and macaques live in large, complex social groups of up to 100 individuals with varying degrees of kinship among varying subgroups. For these species, it is impossible to mimic under captive conditions the type or complexity of natural social groups experienced in the wild. The social environment is highly likely to affect overall cognitive properties as well as brain aging. From this perspective, these two additional primate species deserve special consideration.

Common Marmoset

Marmosets are members of the New World monkey family Callitrichidae, which comprises about 35 species of small, tropical rainforest living species in Central and South America (Nowak, 1999). Like chimpanzees and macaques, callitrichid monkeys are diurnally active. Unlike chimpanzees and macaques, however, callitrichids live in small family groups and subsist on insects, soft fruit, nectar, and plant exudates. Callitrichids diverged from the human lineage roughly 35 million years ago (Glazko & Nei, 2003). Recently, the common marmoset (*Callithrix jacchus*), here called simply the marmoset, has gained attention as a particularly useful primate model for aging research (Tardif, Mansfield, Ratnam, Ross, & Ziegler, 2011). Because of its healthy conservation status (International Union for Conservation of Nature [IUCN], "Least Concern") compared with other callitrichids, it is subject to minimal conservation-based regulations and consequently is the only callitrichid frequently used in biomedical research. Stereotaxic brain atlases are available.

In a captive setting, marmoset reproduction begins by the age of 1 year. However, because early reproduction compromises survival (see Figure 5.4A), it is recommended not to breed females until at least 1.5 years of age (Tardif et al., 2003). Marmosets typically give birth to nonidentical twins or triplets after a gestation of about 4–5 months. Callitrichids are the only primate group to lack postpartum anovulation, thus marmosets can produce four to six offspring per female per year under optimal conditions. Because they share an in utero blood supply, the littermates are hematopoietic chimeras. Conventional wisdom about marmoset aging is that life expectancy of adults is 5–7 years, with males living slightly longer than females. Maximum longevity was reported to be about 16 years and animals 8 years old or older should be considered "aged" (Tardif et al., 2011). Recently, however, considerably greater longevity was reported in a Japanese marmoset colony spread across two facilities (see Figure 5.4B; Nishijima et al., 2012). Specifically, in that colony, the life expectancy for males was 12.4 years, females 9.3 years, and maximum longevity of just younger than 22 years. These were in a semibarrier facility in which offspring did not remain with parents beyond weaning. In fact, an indeterminate fraction of the young were fostered by

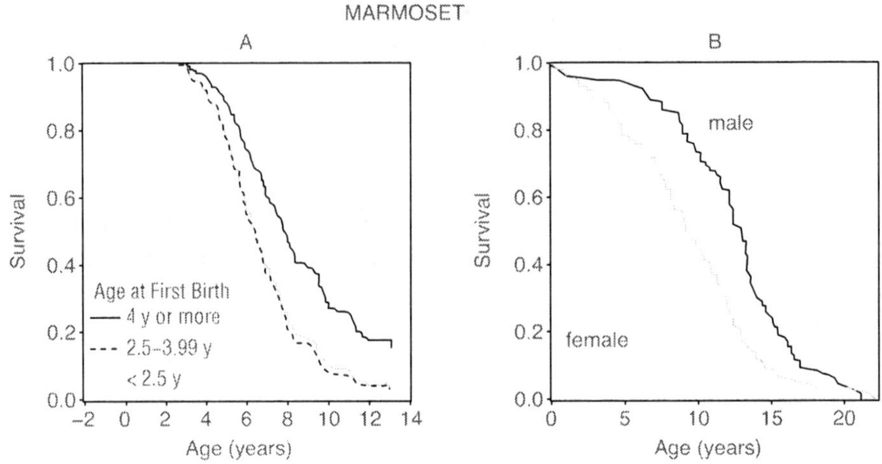

FIGURE 5.4 Survival in two marmoset colonies. A: Female survival in colony of 400. Redrawn from Smucny et al., 2004. Note that those females still reproducing at older ages are longer lived. B: An exceptionally long-lived colony (redrawn from Nishijima et al., 2012). Note that males are longer lived than females.

another female or hand reared. Whether these practices, or some other aspect of the husbandry, were responsible for the longer life is unknown and bears further investigation. In any case, what is considered an "aged" animal is somewhat arbitrary and is likely to be contextual and may best be defined by the life expectancy in a particular colony.

The most thorough analysis of causes of mortality in marmosets is from the New England National Primate Research Center (Tardif et al., 2011). In that colony, mortality at >10 years of age was dominated by amyloidosis (29%) and neoplasia (22%). Clinical grade diabetes mellitus was also observed in these elderly animals. Enteric infections were responsible for 7% of deaths. In younger animals, infection played a greater role in mortality, suggesting that improved control of infectious diseases may be critical to further development of this species as an aging model.

Gray Mouse Lemur

The gray mouse lemur (*Microcebus murinus*, family Cheirogaleidae), as all other lemur species, are found only on the island of Madagascar. Lemurs are primates that diverged from future monkeys, apes, and human some 65–75 million years ago (see Figure 5.1; Fabre et al. 2009). Unlike the other species we discuss, *M. murinus* is nocturnally active. This solitary forager subsists on a broad range of dietary items from insects and spiders to small lizards, fruits, flowers, nectar, and tree exudates (Nowak, 1999). Males are solitary throughout life, but female kin typically share a home range and sleep together in groups of two to nine. In the wild, animals are highly seasonal. In the dry season, they often enter daily torpor and breeding is confined to the long day photoperiod of wet season. Consequently, this species cannot breed in the wild until at least 9 months of age.

In the wild, mean survival is less than about 10 months, which means that nearly half of both sexes do not survive to first breeding; no female is known to reach even 4 years, whereas one male survived to 6 years (Lutermann, Schmelting, Radespiel, Ehresmann, & Zimmermann, 2006).

A captive colony in France, founded in the 1950s, has been well-developed in recent years as a new model for aging research. Mouse lemurs are among the smallest (60–120 g), most rapidly developing (puberty at 6–8 months), and shortest lived of primates, with mean longevity around 5–6 year (see Figure 5.5) and a maximum of about 12 years. The current husbandry conditions include semiannual changes in photoperiod to mimic that of their natural habitat (Weigl, 2005). They breed and are most active under long day photoperiod. In other colonies, gray mouse lemurs have survived as long as 18 years (Weigl, 2005). Like marmosets, mouse lemurs are also highly productive for a primate. Litters of one to three are produced after 2 months gestation, with one litter produced per year (Bons, Rieger, Prudhomme, Fisher, & Krause, 2006).

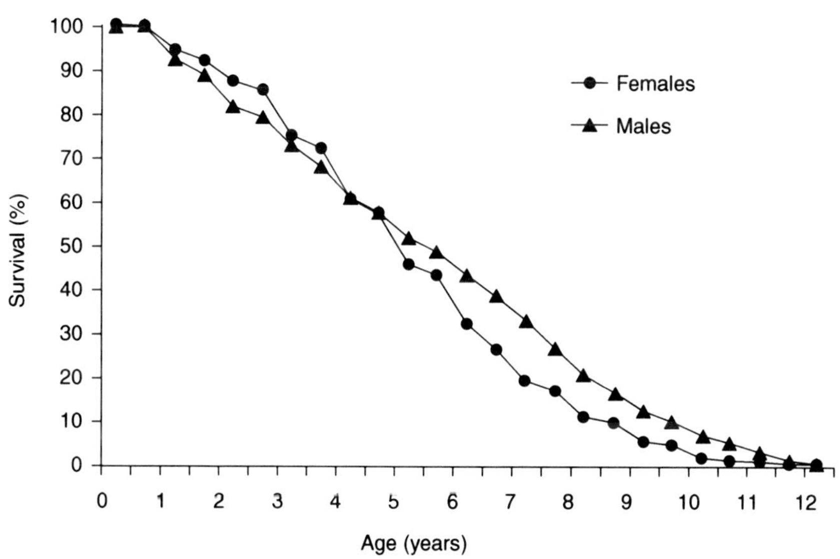

FIGURE 5.5 Survival of gray mouse lemurs in a Brunoy, France colony. N = 361 females, 282 males. Redrawn from Languille et al., 2012.

Older mouse lemurs are prone to many of the maladies of human aging, including cataracts (more than half of animals are affected by ages 7–8 years), loss of olfactory acuity, diminished motor and cognitive abilities, and development of various neurological lesions (discussed below). Frustratingly, we do not have details on the common diseases of aging or causes of death. For further details, see the excellent recent review of Languille and colleagues (2012).

Summary

Our closest relatives among extant primates—the great apes such as the chimpanzees and the Old World monkeys such as the macaques—no doubt have the most to teach us about the evolutionary forces and physiological processes shaping human aging. However, they share several drawbacks as models for brain aging among which are their long lives, their expense, the serious infectious diseases transmissible between them and humans, ethical issues about invasive research, and the impossibility of maintaining them in anything close to natural social groups. By contrast, our more distant primate relatives such as marmosets and mouse lemurs have several advantages to offer, not the least of which is their small size, rapid development, our ability to maintain them in social conditions close to what they experience in the wild, and their comparatively short lives (see Figure 5.6).

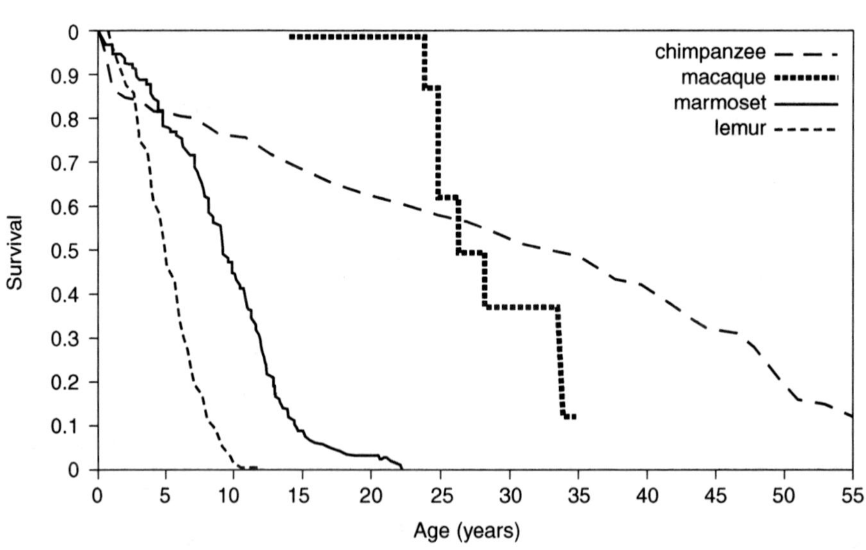

FIGURE 5.6 Comparative survival in captive females of the four species represented in Figures 5.2 to 5.5. Note that deaths in the macaque data were censored prior to age 23 years.

The advantage of their short lives is that it makes interventional aging studies possible within a reasonably short period corresponding to 3- to 5-year grant cycles and student PhD theses. The continuing crisis of federal research funding threatens to greatly restrict use of macaques for long-term studies that cost roughly an order of magnitude more per individual animal that do marmosets. Both marmosets and mouse lemurs transition from healthy young adults to impaired aged individuals within about a 5-year period. Their validity as models in brain aging research is illustrated below.

BRAIN AGING

The following review of aging changes emphasizes findings from laboratory populations of the species described earlier and gives less emphasis to AD-like changes which we have reviewed in greater detail (Finch & Austad, 2012).

Brain Atrophy and Cognitive Functions

Brain atrophy begins soon after maturation in the human and primates, as measured by the magnetic resonance imaging (MRI) for the volume of grey and white matter (see Figure 5.7). The recent definitive study from the Yerkes National Primate Center used T1-weighted and diffusion-weighted MRI (DW-MRI) scans from the Siemens 3T Trio scanner (Chen et al., 2013). Total grey matter volume declined linearly at about 0.5% per year in chimpanzees (14–57 years) and macaques (9–27 years), similar to rates of normal human aging in this and other studies that excluded elderly with indications of AD.

The DW-MRI scans of white matter (myelin) showed increasing disorganization by the MRI parameter of fractional anisotropy (FA). Humans may have a later onset of white matter change. These changes are consistent with histological findings in macaques that showed scattered myelin fraying and patchy erosion in major white matter tracts (Peters, 2002). These findings confirm postmortem brain weight age changes in chimpanzees (Herndon, Tigges, Anderson, Klumpp, & McClure, 1999) and MRI findings on macaques (Andersen, Zhang, Zhang, Gash, & Avison, 1999). However, another recent MRI study did not find grey matter atrophy in a different colony of aging chimpanzees (Sherwood et al., 2011), which may be attributed to lower resolution from a 50% smaller MRI field strength.

Modest cognitive changes were observed in pilot studies of captive bonobos, gorillas, and orangutans (Anderson et al., 2005; Anderson, Stoinski, Bloomsmith, & Maple, 2007). Scattered observations from field studies of chimpanzees suggests that some elderly individuals maintain high-level social and cognitive capacity, despite physical infirmities, as described in Goodall's (1989)

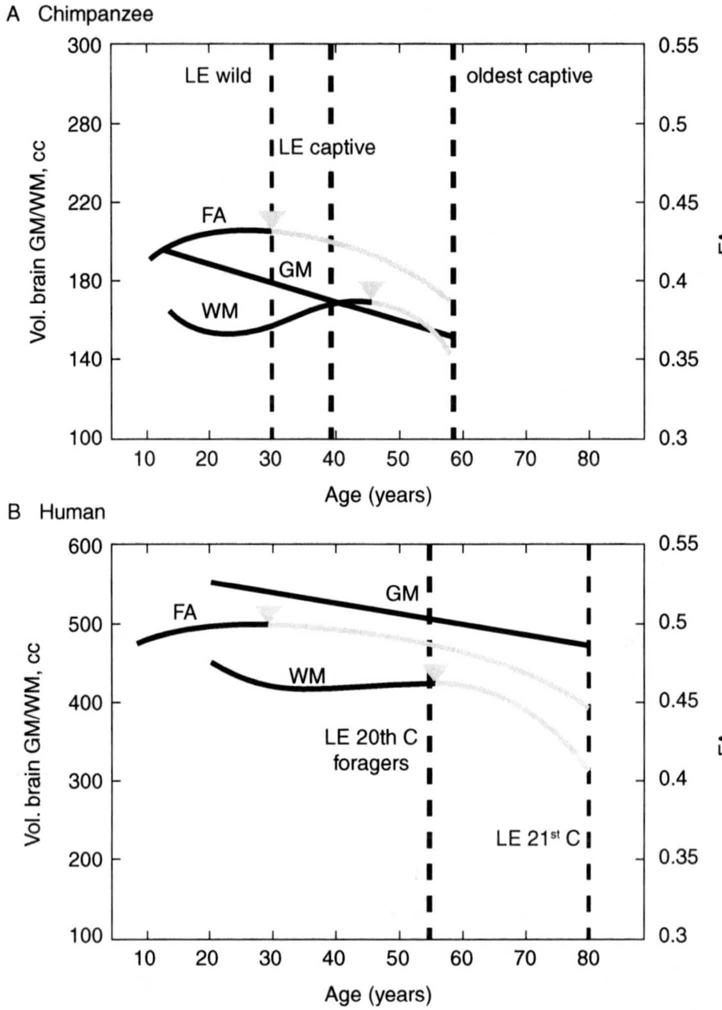

FIGURE 5.7 Comparison of chimpanzees and human for macroscopic parameters of brain aging and in relation to life expectancy (LE). Redrawn from Chen et al. (2013) with additional demographic information. Brain volume measurements from MRI for grey matter (GM; mainly neuron cell bodies and synaptic fields), white matter (WM; myelin pathways providing fast traffic of electrical impulses between brain regions), and fractional anisotropy (FA; a measure of WM organization). The LE at age 15 years for chimpanzees from wild and captive populations is consistently less than for human 20th C foragers with limited access to modern medicine, or preindustrial European populations (not shown; Finch, 2010; Kaplan, Hill, Lancaster, & Hurtado, 2000). Chimpanzees appear to show later onset of myelin decline relative to their lifespan, which implies delayed or slower neurological decline (Chen et al., 2013).

classic studies of the Gombe population in Tanzania. For example, Evered, a toothless male of 40 years, was still one of the best hunters of small monkeys in his community, even though he could not gnaw through the skin of his prey (Finch & Stanford, 2004: Table 5.1 and Appendix Table 1). A review is needed of the scattered reports from field studies on activities of elderly chimps and bonobos. How frustrating that current politics on behalf of laboratory chimps are likely to block further study of cognition and behavior of the elderly individuals in laboratory settings!

White matter FA increases are well-defined in humans (Bartzokis et al., 2012; Wu, Field, Whalen, & Alexander, 2011) and are associated with slower cognitive processing in healthy elderly (Lu et al., 2013). For humans, cognitive processing capacity peaks by age 30 years, with progressive declines across the lifespan, from middle-age into the later years (McArdle, Ferrer-Caja, Hamagami, & Woodcock,,2002). These functional declines proceed at rates of 0.5%–1.0% per year, which approximate the parallel progressive decline in synapse number (Finch, 2009; Masliah, Mallory, Hansen, De Teresa, & Terry, 1993; Morgan, May, & Finch, 1987; Severson, Marcusson, Winblad, & Finch, 1982).

Prefrontal cortex atrophy in macaques was correlated with impaired spatial and recognition memory (Shamy et al., 2011). Macaques and other monkeys show mild age-related impairments of executive functions, visuospatial learning, and slowed motor functions after the age of 15 years (Castner & Goldman-Rakic, 2004; Moore et al., 2006; Nagahara, Bernot, & Tuszynski, 2010; Peters et al., 1996; Zeamer, Decamp, Clark, & Schneider, 2011). Atrophy of the amygdala was also correlated with exploratory activity, a measure of anxiety which varied widely between individuals in middle-aged females ages 18–19 years (Haley et al., 2012). The increase in individual variation in executive function with age (Zeamer et al., 2011) is consistent with the individual variation in white matter degeneration, suggesting sporadic inflammatory causes.

Several studies show altered social interactions. Of particular interest are the studies of macaques on the island of Cayo Santiago, Puerto Rico, which has a large, free-ranging, food-provisioned, population descended from 409 founders imported to the island in 1938. Individuals 20 years of age and older showed gender differences in social network size (males increased with age, female decreased) and social contact time (vice versa; Corr, 2003). In more artificial social conditions at Yerkes National Primate Research Center, the seasonal variation in social interactions (Williams, 1986) render comparison with Cayo Santiago difficult. Both studies, although, reported differences in social interactions between young adults and the middle-aged.

The grey mouse lemur also shows many changes observed in monkeys, including grey matter atrophy (Bons, Mestre, & Petter, 1992, 2006;

Languille et al., 2012). Spatial memory and executive functions become markedly impaired in association with regionally selective atrophy (Picq, Aujard, Volk, & Dhenain, 2012). A subgroup with advanced neuropathology discussed below developed aggressive behaviors requiring social isolation (Bons et al., 2006), for which there was no parallel in the modest shifts of social interactions in older versus middle-aged macaques, noted earlier. No comparable data are available for the aging marmoset.

Synapse and Cell Changes

Aging macaques undergo selective loss of some types of synapses and dendritic spines, reaching nearly 50% in some cerebral cortex regions (Morrison & Baxter, 2012). Importantly, there is no indication that these atrophic changes are linked to neuronal death. Detailed studies have not detected neuron loss in the macaque cerebral cortex and hippocampus up to advanced ages (Tigges et al., 1990; Hof et al., 2000; Duan et al., 2003). For chimpanzees, as well as marmosets and lemurs, the few detailed neuropathological studies did not evaluate synapse or neuron loss. Provisionally, primate brain aging may be considered a mild indolent pathological process that does not model the distinctly more aggressive neurodegeneration of AD.

Amyloid-Beta (Aβ) Deposits in Cerebral Arteries and Brain

The underlying causes of cerebral atrophy and synapse loss during normal aging are poorly understood. At a molecular level, much attention is given to deposits of the 42 amino acid amyloid β-peptide (Aβ42), a neurotoxic peptide that has an identical sequence in primates and humans. Rodent Aβ differs in three amino acids, which reduce its aggregation and neurotoxicity (Boyd-Kimball, Sultana, Mohmmad-Abdul, & Butterfield, 2004; Finch & Austad, 2012). These species' differences enabled the success of AD-transgenic mice, and recently ADtg rats (Cohen et al., 2013), with human Aβ42 in associating neuronal impairments with the Aβ42 load.

Unlike wild-type rodents, which do not accumulate solid deposits of Aβ42 during normal aging, all primates examined accumulate Aβ42 deposits from midlife onwards, as do healthy humans after 30–40 years (Fukumoto et al., 2004). Histologically, the Aβ42 deposits are diffuse and nonfibrillar, differing from the fibrillar thioflavin-positive senile plaques of AD. Diffuse brain Aβ42 deposits increase progressively during aging in the grey mouse lemur and in monkeys of both phyletic branches (see Figure 5.1): the Old World baboon, macaque, and vervet monkey (African green monkey) and the New World common marmoset and squirrel monkey. The great apes, however, accumulate much less Aβ42 in brain parenchyma than monkeys and mouse lemurs (Gearing,

Rebeck, Hyman, Tigges, & Mirra, 1994; Gearing, Tigges, Mori, & Mirra, 1996, 1997). Cerebrovascular Aβ40 may be more regularly accumulated than in brain parenchyma in great apes, but we do not know of quantitative studies.

The marmoset and the grey mouse lemur develop brain Aβ deposits a decade earlier than in macaques. Aβ immunoreactive plaques were detected in several marmoset colonies by 7 years (Geula et al., 2002; Palazzi et al., 2006); the latter reported scattered plaques by age 3 years. These Aβ deposits in brain parenchyma (neuropil) are described as diffuse and nonfibrillar, and are not accompanied by neurofibrillary tangles; most brains also had Aβ40 in cerebral arteries. Marmosets aged 10 years also have plaque-like aggregates of reelin, an extracellular glycoprotein that is associated with ApoE receptor signaling and amyloid precursor protein (APP) processing.

Two marmoset colonies had intriguing differences in age of Aβ onset that imply environmental factors. In contrast to the >90% incidence of brain Aβ deposits in plaques or arteries by age 7 years in Geula et al. (2002), a much lower incidence was found in another colony: Aβ was not detected in those younger than age 10 years, and only reached 17% from 10 to 19 years (Ridley et al., 2006). These two colonies differed in longevity, with the longer lived having less Aβ even at later ages. Other colonies with different LE were shown earlier in Figure 5.4. As emphasized by Ridley et al. (2006), these differences imply the importance of local environment in the progression of brain amyloidosis, possibly involving diet and social interactions. The potential for earlier amyloidosis in the long-lived colony was experimentally shown in vervets injected with human or marmoset brain homogenates that contained Aβ; after 3.5 years or more of "incubation," >90% of injected when young or middle-aged had Aβ deposits (brain plaques and small vessels had stronger immunoreactivity for Aβ42 than Aβ40; conversely for large vessels).

The grey mouse lemur also develops diffuse plaques with Aβ42 (Bons et al., 1992; Bons et al., 2006; Languille et al., 2012). A neuropathological subgroup of about 20% undergo extreme neurodegeneration with major cerebral atrophy, abundant plaques and tauopathy, and loss of cholinergic neurons. Iron deposits also accumulated progressively in the substantia nigra (Dhenain et al., 1998). This neuropathological subgroup also had impaired cognition and altered social interactions noted earlier.

Hyperphosphorylated Tau and Neurofibrillary Degeneration

Neurofibrillary tangles (NFT) with hyperphosphorylated tau, Alzheimer's classic neuropathological marker, vary widely across species. In Braak's classic studies of humans, NFT appeared as scattered tangled neurons before 50 years in random brain autopsies and progressively increased in the brain regions vulnerable to AD neurodegeneration (Braak & Del Tredici, 2012; Braak, Zetterberg, Del Tredici, & Blennow, 2013).

Monkeys and lemurs also develop hyperphosphorylated tau, but not classical neurofibrillary tangles. The baboon progressively accumulates hyperphosphorylated tau after age 10 years, with accelerating incidence after 20 years to involve nearly all 30 years (Schultz, Hubbard, Rüb, Braak, & Braak, 2000). Aged macaques and cynomolgus monkeys also develop hyperphosphorylated tau (Oikawa et al., 2010; Shah et al., 2010). In macaques, the hyperphosphorylated tau in swollen neurites was associated with adjacent Aβ42 compact plaques, but not with diffuse (nonfibrillar) Aβ42 (Shah et al., 2010). The swollen neurites were diverticula (bulges) with abnormal microtubules and degenerating mitochondria that suggest impaired axonal flow (Fiala, Feinberg, Peters, & Barbas, 2007). The aging grey mouse lemur also has tauopathies (Bons et al., 1992; Bons et al., 2006; Languille et al., 2012).

In contrast to these species, great apes typically have negligible tau pathology (Gearing et al., 1997). Although this is remarkable, even more unexpected is one tantalizing exception: an obese hypercholesterolemic 41-year-old chimpanzee that incurred a stroke (R. F. Rosen et al., 2008). Exacting postmortem analysis showed abundant classical NFT in the neocortex on both sides beyond the infarcted zone, but no NFT in the hippocampus, a major site in AD. Although there were moderate Aβ deposits, classical neuritic plaques were fewer than in typical AD. We may conclude that chimpanzees, and possibly other great apes, have the potential for human-like tauopathy with NFTs, depending on individual systemic pathophysiology. Why only humans develop AD-neurodegeneration with plaques, tangles, and neuron loss remains a great mystery.

Motor Functions

No aging primate has shown the full clinical Parkinson's syndrome with all of the clinical traits: bradykinesia, muscular rigidity, postural instability, and tremor. However, various PD phenotypes are recognized in aging macaques, which develop motor dysfunctions and dystrophic neuronal changes in the substantia nigra that may be a model for preclinical-PD. Several studies document decreased spontaneous daytime "home-cage" movements by age 20 years (Ovadia, Zhang, & Gash, 1995; Zhang et al., 2000). Fine motor control worsened progressively, for example, time to reach a food reward that required fine motor control of arm and hand (see Figure 5.8; Zhang et al., 2000). After age 25 years, about 35% showed two or more PD symptoms: bradykinesia and lower limb rigidity were the most common, but one only had tremor (Chu & Kordower, 2007; Hurley, Elsworth, Whittaker, Roth, & Redmond, 2011; Zhang et al., 2000).

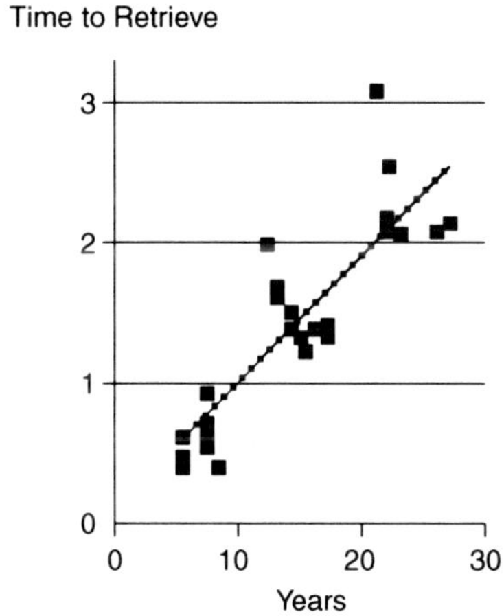

FIGURE 5.8 Fine motor control was assessed as the time (seconds) to retrieve a food reward by movements that required careful coordination of hand, arm, and eye in reaching around through two orthogonal gates (Zhang et al., 2000).

A relationship to underlying changes in dopaminergic functions was shown in a study of cynomolgus monkeys ages 3.5, 10.0, and 15.0 years, which also had progressively slower retrieval of a food award requiring arm extension (Yue et al., 2012). Moreover, declines in food retrieval and total home cage activity were directly correlated with dopamine uptake by single photon emission computed tomography (SPECT) imaging of ^{99m}Tc-TRODAT-1, a measure of striatal dopamine transport functions.

The neurotoxin MPTP which damages dopaminergic neurons of the substantia nigra showed clear age increase in neuronal vulnerability to its effects. In a well-designed experiment of unilateral MPTP that induced hemi-Parkinsonism, lower doses of MPTP induced more PD symptoms in the older group, with high correlation between age and PD rating (Ovadia et al., 1995). At a cellular level, age changes in the loss of dopaminergic neurons in the substantia nigra vary between studies (Collier, Kanaan, & Kordower, 2011; Emborg et al., 1998). Several studies also showed that neurons with low tyrosine or dopamine hydroxylase immunoreactivity also had higher α-synuclein, a marker for PD (Chu & Kordower, 2007; Collier et al., 2011). Together, the motor and neuronal changes suggest that a subset of aging monkeys may be informative as pre-Parkinsonian models.

The grey mouse lemur also had increased α-synuclein aggregates in dopaminergic neurons (Canron, Perret, Vital, Bézard, & Dehay, 2012) and iron deposits as noted earlier (Dhenain et al., 1998). Rotorod performance also declined progressively after 4 years (Némoz-Bertholet & Aujard, 2003);

this age change was sensitive to the photoperiod (Némoz-Bertholet, Menaker, & Aujard, 2004), which should not be surprising for a highly seasonal species exhibiting regular torpor during short day length. Nocturnal primates are typically observed for the usual experimenters' convenience during daytime hours (Finch & Austad, 2012).

Dietary Restriction

Two long-term studies of 30% dietary restriction (DR) in rhesus macaques have been underway for 20 years and older, one at the University of Wisconsin (summarized in Colman et al., 2009), the other at the National Institute on Aging (NIA) colony in Poolesville, Maryland (Mattison et al., 2012). In the Wisconsin colony, control animals were fed a semisynthetic ad lib diet and were obese by the standard of the weights of free-living animals (Austad, 2012). Under the current housing protocols at NIH-supported primate centers, no exertion is required to access food for ad lib feeding. This contrasts with the extensive foraging required in their natural habitat, which is partly restored with greater foraging such as required in the free-living colony at Cayo Santiago. Notably, at the NIA colony, control animals are fed an apportioned amount of a natural ingredient-based diet. Both control and DR animals weighed substantially less in the NIA study.

To no surprise, DR reduced body weight in both studies. However, the studies differ significantly in the impact of DR on survival. Although lifespan was increased in the Wisconsin study, there was no effect in the NIA colony. The colonies also differed in disease patterns, which are likely caused by different dietary strategies and composition (Austad, 2012).

For brain morphology and function, in the NIA study, DR did not alter the age-related decline in striatal volume (Matochik et al., 2004) or hearing sensitivity (Torre et al., 2004). Or did DR consistently alter spontaneous physical activity (Ingram et al. 2001). However, in the Wisconsin study, DR reduced age-associated macaque brain atrophy in key regions subserving motor function and aspects of executive function (Colman et al., 2009) improved fine motor control and decreased iron accumulation in basal ganglia by an equivalent of 10 years of retardation (see Figure 5.9; Kastman et al., 2012). In a separate study of the squirrel monkey (*Saimiri sciureus*, New world), lifelong DR slowed the accumulation of both Aβ40 and Aβ42 peptides in the temporal cortex (Qin et al., 2006). This important finding shows that brain amyloid metabolism is subject to systemic physiological influences, as in lab rodents (Patel et al., 2005).

Short-term DR can also alter brain function. In a 6-month study of induced Parkinsonism, DR improved neurotrophic factors and behavioral deficits (Maswood et al., 2004). Effects of DR on gene expression in brain regions are anticipated because even 2 months of high-fat diet increased mRNA of genes

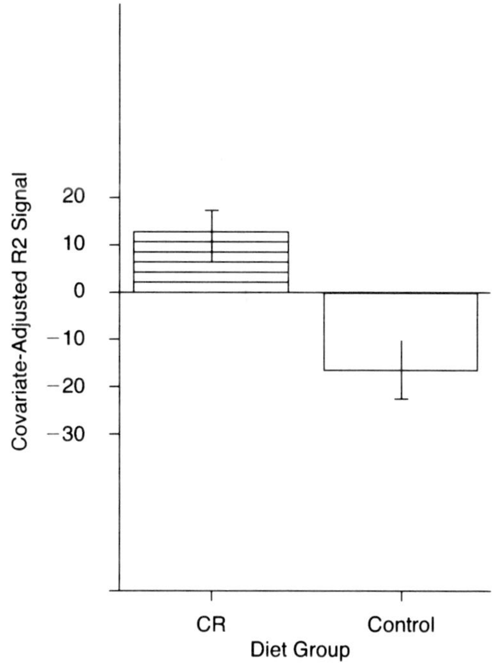

FIGURE 5.9 In the rhesus brain, the age-related increase of iron (MRI R2 signal, a measure of ferritin) was attenuated in the globus pallidus (basal ganglia) by diet restriction (CR). Redrawn from Kastman et al., 2010.

for metabolic signaling and apoptosis with regional differences (Mitchell, Leak, Zigmond, Cameron, & Mirnics, 2012).

OPEN QUESTIONS

Captive Versus Wild

There is little doubt that current primate husbandry is suboptimized for social interactions. To approach the complex issues of social status in outcomes of human brain aging (see "Introduction"), the social context of primate models needs as serious consideration as diet and exercise are now being given. The conventional macaque laboratory housing does not allow natural group associations, which differ by gender and age within each species, as briefly noted earlier. The free-ranging macaques at Cayo Santiago may give opportunity for studying behavioral aging in a more natural social setting, with the caveat that food is still provided.

Because further studies of aging on captive great apes have been sharply curtailed (see below), we suggest collaboration with ongoing field studies of natural chimpanzee populations, which have longitudinal data for some individuals over several or more decades. The benchmark is the Gombe studies in Tanzania begun 50 years ago by Jane Goodall. Her classic monograph (Goodall, 1989) describes other elderly individuals besides Evered noted earlier. However, ongoing studies of chimpanzees could be informative to biomedically oriented researchers. A review is needed of the scattered reports from field studies on activities of elderly chimps and bonobos.

Unknowns in Primate Brain Aging

Despite the rich detail on synapse changes during aging in macaques (see earlier discussion), we know little about neuron cell loss during aging in any primate aging model. This critical gap can be addressed with recent advances in automated stereological cell density methods, for example, serial 2-photon tomography, to comprehensively assess neuron and synapse density by brain systems from olfactory bulb to medulla. Sex differences and social interactions are also undefined for outcomes of primate brain aging. It would not be a surprise if brain amyloid deposits and cognitive changes in lemur and marmoset were sensitive to environmental enrichment and to social interactions as indicated for Alzheimer transgenic mice (Gerenu, Dobarro, Ramirez, & Gil-Bea, 2013; Jankowsky, Xu, Fromholt, Gonzales, & Borchelt, 2003).

Another gap is age effects on neurogenesis, which are known only for the marmoset, in which neuronal stem cell generation declines linearly starting before middle-age (Leuner, Kozorovitskiy, Gross, & Gould, 2007). In adult macaques, neurogenesis is about 90% lower than adult rodents (Kornack & Rakic, 1999), but we do not know the age changes. Wild versus captive conditions may be an influence on primate neurogenesis, as observed in rats (Epp, Barker, & Galea, 2009) and birds (Barnea & Nottebohm, 1994), giving another reason for biomedical researchers to usefully collaborate with field researchers.

Is Chimp Aging a Lost Cause?

Access to aging chimpanzees for noninvasive studies of brain and cognition in current U.S. research facilities is being drastically curtailed (Kaiser, 2013). The process started in 2000 with congressional approval of "The Chimpanzee Health Improvement, Maintenance, and Protection Act" (CHIMP Act). No breeding of chimpanzees has been allowed, although some bonobo breeding continues in municipal zoological facilities. On July 26, 2013, NIH Director Francis Collins announced the NIH policy to retire from research 85% of the remaining 350 chimps in research facilities supported by the NIH. Many of these are older than the age of 25 years, the life expectancy in the wild (see Figure 5.2). It is unclear if their relocation to sanctuaries will eliminate the possibility of behavioral observations.

Alternatively, and perhaps for the better, we suggest collaboration with ongoing field studies of natural chimpanzee populations that have longitudinal data for some individuals over several or more decades. At least 10 other populations of wild chimpanzees and of bonobos have been studied longitudinally and many are ongoing. The accumulated data, largely unpublished, could help assess the extent of cognitive resilience and impairment in older individuals, despite the inevitably accumulating physical injuries during their long lives. Future studies could incorporate an even more targeted approach to investigating how aging affects behavior in the wild. Whether or not noninvasive observations are allowed in the sanctuaries for retired chimpanzees, field studies of wild populations offer rich opportunities to study behavior in a Darwinian context.

ACKNOWLEDGMENTS

CEF is supported by NIA P01 AG026572-06 (RD Brinton, Dir.); Project 2 (CEF). SNA acknowledges support by the Office of the NIH Director grant R24 OD010933 and the National Institute on Aging Nathan Shock Center Comparative Aging Core (P30 AG13319).

REFERENCES

Adler, C. H., Shill, H. A., & Beach, T. G. (2011). Essential tremor and Parkinson's disease: Lack of a link. *Movement Disorders*, *26*, 372–377.

Andersen, A. H., Zhang, Z., Zhang, M., Gash, D. M., & Avison, M. J. (1999). Age-associated changes in rhesus CNS composition identified by MRI. *Brain Research*, *829*, 90–98.

Anderson, U. S., Stoinski, T. S., Bloomsmith, M. A., Marr, M. J., Smith, A. D., & Maple, T. L. (2005). Relative numerousness judgment and summation in young and old Western lowland gorillas. *Journal of Comparative Psychology*, *119*, 285–295.

Anderson, U. S., Stoinski, T. S., Bloomsmith, M. A., & Maple, T. L. (2007). Relative numerousness judgment and summation in young, middle-aged, and older adult orangutans (Pongo pygmaeus abelii and Pongo pygmaeus pygmaeus). *Journal of Comparative Psychology*, *121*, 1–11.

Archie, E. A., Altmann, J., & Alberts, S. C. (2012). Social status predicts wound healing in wild baboons. *Proceedings of the National Academy of Sciences USA*, *109*, 9017–9022.

Austad, S. N. (2012). Ageing: Mixed results for dieting monkeys. *Nature*, *489*, 210–211.

Barnea, A., & Nottebohm, F. (1994). Seasonal recruitment of hippocampal neurons in adult free-ranging black-capped chickadees. *Proceedings of the National Academy of Sciences*, *91*, 11217–11221.

Bartzokis, G., Lu, P. H., Heydari, P., Couvrette, A., Lee, G. J., Kalashyan, G., . . . Altshuler, L. L. (2012). Multimodal magnetic resonance imaging assessment of white matter aging trajectories over the lifespan of healthy individuals. *Biological Psychiatry*, *72*, 1026–1034.

Bodkin, N. L., Alexander, T. M., Ortmeyer, H. K., Johnson, E., & Hansen, B. C. (2003). Mortality and morbidity in laboratory-maintained Rhesus monkeys and effects of long-term dietary restriction. *Journals of Gerontology Series A: Biological Sciences and Medical Sciences*, *58*, 212–219.

Bons, N., Mestre, N., & Petter, A. (1992). Senile plaques and neurofibrillary changes in the brain of an aged lemurian primate, Microcebus murinus. *Neurobiology of Aging*, *13*, 99–105.

Bons, N., Rieger, F., Prudhomme, D., Fisher, A., & Krause, K. H. (2006). Microcebus murinus: A useful primate model for human cerebral aging and Alzheimer's disease? *Genes, Brain and Behavior*, *5*, 120–130.

Boyd-Kimball, D., Sultana, R., Mohmmad-Abdul, H., & Butterfield, D. A. (2004). Rodent Abeta (1-42) exhibits oxidative stress properties similar to those of human Abeta (1-42): Implications for proposed mechanisms of toxicity. *Journal of Alzheimer's Disease*, *6*, 515–525.

Braak, H., & Del Tredici, K. (2012). Where, when, and in what form does sporadic Alzheimer's disease begin? *Current Opinion in Neurology*, *25*, 708–714.

Braak, H., Zetterberg, H., Del Tredici, K., & Blennow, K. (2013). Intraneuronal tau aggregation precedes diffuse plaque deposition, but amyloid-β changes occur before increases of tau in cerebrospinal fluid. *Acta Neuropathologica*, *126*(5), 631–641.

Bronikowski, A. M., Alberts, S. C., Altmann, J., Packer, C., Carey, K. D., & Tatar, M. (2002). The aging baboon: Comparative demography in a non-human primate. *Proceedings of the National Academy of Sciences USA*, *99*, 9591–9595.

Brown, S. L., Anderson, D. C., Dick, E. J., Jr., Guardado-Mendoza, R., Garcia, A. P., & Hubbard, G. B. (2009). Neoplasia in the chimpanzee (Pan spp.). *Journal of Medical Primatology*, *38*, 137–144.

Canron, M. H., Perret, M., Vital, A., Bézard, E., & Dehay, B. (2012). Age-dependent α-synuclein aggregation in the Microcebus murinus lemur primate. *Scientific Reports*, 2, 910. http://dx.doi.org/10.1038/srep00910

Castner, S. A., & Goldman-Rakic, P. S. (2004). Enhancement of working memory in aged monkeys by a sensitizing regimen of dopamine D1 receptor stimulation. *The Journal of Neuroscience*, *24*, 1446–1450.

Cefalu,W. T., & Wagner, J. D. (1997). Aging and atherosclerosis in human and nonhuman primates. *Age* (Omaha.), *20*, 15–28.

Chatterjee, H. J., Ho, S. Y., Barnes, I., & Groves, I. (2009). Estimating the phylogeny and divergence times of primates using a supermatrix approach. *BMC Evolutionary Biology*, *9*, 259.

Chen, X., Errangi, B., Li, L., Glasser, M. F., Westlye, L. T., Fjell, A. M., . . . Rilling, J. K. (2013). Brain aging in humans, chimpanzees (Pan troglodytes), and rhesus macaques (Macaca mulatta): Magnetic resonance imaging studies of macro- and microstructural changes. *Neurobiology of Aging, 34,* 2248–2260.

Chimpanzee Sequencing & Analysis Consortium. (2005). Initial sequence of the chimpanzee genome and comparison with the human genome. *Nature, 437,* 69–87.

Christensen, K., Thinggaard, M., Oksuzyan, A., Steenstrup, T., Andersen-Ranberg, K., Jeune, B., McGue, M., & Vaupel, J. W. (2013). Physical and cognitive functioning of people older than 90 years: A comparison of two Danish cohorts born 10 years apart. *Lancet, 382,* 1507–1513.

Chu, Y., & Kordower, J. H. (2007). Age-associated increases of alpha-synuclein in monkeys and humans are associated with nigrostriatal dopamine depletion: Is this the target for Parkinson's disease? *Neurobiology of Disease, 25*(1), 134–149.

Cohen, R. M., Rezai-Zadeh, K., Weitz, T. M., Rentsendorj, A., Gate, D., Spivak, I., . . . Town, T. (2013). A transgenic Alzheimer rat with plaques, tau pathology, behavioral impairment, oligomeric aβ, and frank neuronal loss. *The Journal of Neuroscience, 33,* 6245–6256.

Colman, R. J., & Kemnitz, J. W. (1998). Aging experiments using nonhuman primates. In *Methods in aging research* (Ed., B. P. Yu, pp. 249–267). Boca Raton, FL: CRC Press.

Colman, R. J., Anderson, R. M., Johnson, S. C., Kastman, E. K., Kosmatka, K. J., Beasley, T. M., . . . Weindruch, R. (2009). Caloric restriction delays disease onset and mortality in rhesus monkeys. *Science, 325,* 201–204.

Colman, R. J., Beasley, T. M., Allison, D. B., & Weindruch, R. (2008). Attenuation of sarcopenia by dietary restriction in rhesus monkeys. *Journals of Gerontology Series A: Biological Sciences and Medical Sciences, 63*(6), 556–559.

Collier, T. J., Kanaan, N. M., & Kordower, J. H. (2011). Ageing as a primary risk factor for Parkinson's disease: Evidence from studies of non-human primates. *Nature Reviews Neuroscience, 12,* 359–366.

Corr, J. (2003). Social behavior in aged rhesus macaques. *Collegium Antropologicum, 27*(1), 87–94.

Crimmins, E. M., Kim, J. K., & Seeman, T. E. (2009). Poverty and biological risk: The earlier "aging" of the poor. *Journals of Gerontology Series A: Biological Sciences and Medical Sciences, 64,* 286–292.

De Lathouwers, M., &Van Elsacker, L. (2005). Reproductive parameters of female Pan paniscus and P. troglodytes: Quality versus quantity. *International Journal of Primatology, 26,* 55–71.

Dhenain, M., Duyckaerts, C., Michot, J. L., Volk, A., Picq, J. L., & Boller, F. (1998). Cerebral T2-weighted signal decrease during aging in the mouse lemur primate reflects iron accumulation. *Neurobiology of Aging, 19,* 65–69.

Dick, E. J., Jr., Owston, M. A., David, J. M., Sharp, R. M., Rouse, S., & Hubbard, G. B. (in press). Mortality in captive baboons (Papio spp.): A 23 year study. *Veterinary Pathology.*

Duan, H., Wearne, S. L., Rocher, A. B., Macedo, A., Morrison, J. H., & Hof, P. R. (2003). Age-related dendritic and spine changes in corticocortically projecting neurons in macaque monkeys. *Cerebral Cortex, 13,* 950–961.

Emborg, M. E., Ma, S. Y., Mufson, E. J., Levey, A. I., Taylor, M. D., Brown, W. D., . . . Kordower, J. H. (1998). Age-related declines in nigral neuronal function correlate with motor impairments in rhesus monkeys. *Journal of Comparative Neurology*, *401*, 253–265.

Epp, J. R., Barker, J. M., & Galea, L. A. (2009). Running wild: Neurogenesis in the hippocampus across the lifespan in wild and laboratory-bred Norway rats. *Hippocampus*, *19*, 1040–1049.

Evans, D. A., Hebert, L. E., Beckett, L. A., Scherr, P. A., Albert, M. S., Chown, M. J., . . . Taylor, J. O. (1997). Education and other measures of socioeconomic status and risk of incident Alzheimer disease in a defined population of older persons. *Archives of Neurology*, *54*, 1399–1405.

Fabre, P. H., Rodrigues, A., & Douzery, E. J. (2009). Patterns of macroevolution among Primates inferred from a supermatrix of mitochondrial and nuclear DNA. *Molecular Phylogenetics and Evolution*, *53*, 808–825.

Fiala, J. C., Feinberg, M., Peters, A., & Barbas, H. (2007). Mitochondrial degeneration in dystrophic neurites of senile plaques may lead to extracellular deposition of fine filaments. *Brain Structure and Function*, *212*, 195–207.

Finch, C. E. (2009). The neurobiology of middle-age has arrived. *Neurobiology of Aging*, *30*, 515–520.

Finch, C. E. (2010). Evolution of the human lifespan and diseases of aging: Roles of infection, nutrition, and nutrition. *Proceedings of the National Academy of Sciences*, *107*(suppl. 1), 1718–1724.

Finch, C. E., & Austad, S. A. (2012). Primate aging in the mammalian scheme: The puzzle of extreme variation in brain aging. *AGE* (Special Issue) Nonhuman Primate Models of Aging. *Journal of the American Aging Association*, *34*(5), 1075–1091. http://dx.doi.org/10.1007/s11357-011-9355-9

Finch, C. E., & Loehlin, J. (1998). Environmental influences that may precede fertilization: A first examination of the prezygotic hypothesis from maternal age influences on twins. *Behavior Genetics*, *28*, 101–106.

Finch, C. E., & Stanford, C. B. (2004). Meat adaptive genes and the evolution of slower aging in humans. *The Quarterly Review of Biology*, *79*(1), 3–50.

Fischer, K. E., & Austad, S. N. (2011). The development of small primate models for aging research. *Institute of Laboratory Animal Resources Journal*, *52*, 78–88.

Freire, C., & Koifman, S. (2012). Pesticide exposure and Parkinson's disease: Epidemiological evidence of association. *Neurotoxicology*, *33*, 947–971.

Fukumoto, H., Rosene, D. L., Moss, M. B., Raju, S., Hyman, B. T., & Irizarry, M. C. (2004). Beta-secretase activity increases with aging in human, monkey, and mouse brain. *American Journal of Pathology*, *164*, 719–725.

Gage, T. B. (1998). The comparative demography of primates: With some comments on the evolution of life histories. *Annual Review of Anthropology*, *27*, 197–221.

Gearing, M., Rebeck, G. W., Hyman, B. T., Tigges, J., & Mirra, S. S. (1994). Neuropathology and apolipoprotein E profile of aged chimpanzees: Implications for Alzheimer disease. *Proceedings of the National Academy of Sciences*, *91*, 9382–9386.

Gearing, M., Tigges, J., Mori, H., & Mirra, S. S. (1996). A beta40 is a major form of beta-amyloid in nonhuman primates. *Neurobiology of Aging, 17*, 903–908.

Gearing, M., Tigges, J., Mori, H., & Mirra, S. S. (1997). A beta-amyloid (A beta) deposition in the brains of aged orangutans. *Neurobiology of Aging, 18*, 139–146.

Gerenu, G., Dobarro, M., Ramirez, M. J., & Gil-Bea, F. J. (2013). Early cognitive stimulation compensates for memory and pathological changes in Tg2576 mice. *Biochimica et Biophysica Acta, 1832*, 837–847.

Geula, C., Nagykery, N., & Wu, C. K. (2002). Amyloid-beta deposits in the cerebral cortex of the aged common marmoset (Callithrix jacchus): Incidence and chemical composition. *Acta Neuropathologica, 103*, 48–58.

Glazko, G. V., & Nei, M. (2003). Estimation of divergence times for major lineages of primate species. *Molecular Biology and Evolution, 20*, 424–434.

Goldstein, L. B., Bushnell, C. D., Adams, R. J., Appel, L. J., Braun, L. T., Chaturvedi, S., . . . Council on Peripheral Vascular Disease, and Interdisciplinary Council on Quality of Care and Outcomes Research. (2011). Guidelines for the primary prevention of stroke: A guideline for healthcare professionals from the American Heart Association/American Stroke Association. *Stroke, 42*, 517–584.

Goodall, J. (1989). *The chimpanzees of Gombe. Patterns of behavior*. Cambridge, MA: Harvard University Press.

Haber, C. (2004). Life extension and history: The continual search for the fountain of youth. *Journals of Gerontology, Series A Biological Sciences Medical Sciences, 59*, B515–B522.

Haley, G. E., McGuire, A., Berteau-Pavy, D., Weiss, A., Patel, R., Messaoudi, I., . . . Raber, J. (2012). Measures of anxiety, amygdala volumes, and hippocampal scopolamine phMRI response in elderly female rhesus macaques. *Neuropharmacology, 62*, 385–390.

Hernandez, R. D., Hubisz, M. J., Wheeler, D. A., Smith, D. G., Ferguson, B., Rogers, J., . . . Bustamante, C. D. (2007). Demographic histories and patterns of linkage disequilibrium in Chinese and Indian rhesus macaques. *Science, 316*, 240–243.

Herndon, J. G., Tigges, J., Anderson, D. C., Klumpp, S. A., & McClure, H. M. (1999). Brain weight throughout the life span of the chimpanzee. *Journal of Comparative Neurology, 409*, 567–572.

Hill, K., Boesch, C., Goodall, J., Pusey, A., Williams, J., & Wrangham, R. (2001). Mortality rates among wild chimpanzees. *Journal of Human Evolution, 40*, 437–450.

Hill, K. H., & Hurtado, A. M. (1996). *Ache life history: The ecology and demography of a foraging people*. New York, NY: Aldine de Gruyter.

Hof, P. R., Nimchinsky, E. A., Young, W. G., & Morrison, J. H. (2000). Numbers of meynert and layer IVB cells in area V1: A stereologic analysis in young and aged macaque monkeys. *Journal of Comparative Neurology, 420*, 113–126.

Hurley, P. J., Elsworth, J. D., Whittaker, M. C., Roth, R. H., & Redmond D. E., Jr. (2011). Aged monkeys as a partial model for Parkinson's disease. *Pharmacology Biochemistry and Behavior, 99*, 324–332.

Ingram, D. K., Chefer, S., Matochik, J., Moscrip, T. D., Weed, J., Roth, G. S., & Lane, M. A. (2001). Aging and caloric restriction in nonhuman primates: Behavioral and in vivo brain imaging studies. *Annals of the New York Academy of Sciences*, *928*, 316–326.

Jankowsky, J. L., Xu, G., Fromholt, D., Gonzales, V., & Borchelt, D. R. (2003). Environmental enrichment exacerbates amyloid plaque formation in a transgenic mouse model of Alzheimer disease. *Journal of Neuropathology & Experimental Neurology*, *62*, 1220–1227.

Kaiser, J. (2013). Biomedical research. NIH to phase out most chimp research. *Science*, *341*, 17–18.

Kaplan, H., Hill, K., Lancaster, J., & Hurtado, A. M. (2000). A theory of life history evolution: Diet, intelligence, and longevity. *Evolutionary Anthropology*, *9*, 156–185.

Kastman, E. K., Willette, A. A., Coe, C. L., Bendlin, B. B., Kosmatka, K. J., McLaren, D. G., . . . Johnson, S. C. (2010). A calorie-restricted diet decreases brain iron accumulation and preserves motor performance in old rhesus monkeys. *The Journal of Neuroscience*, *32*, 11897–11904.

Kokubo, Y. (2012). Traditional risk factor management for stroke: A never-ending challenge for health behaviors of diet and physical activity. *Current Opinion in Neurology*, *25*, 11–17.

Kornack, D. R., & Rakic, P. (1999). Continuation of neurogenesis in the hippocampus of the adult macaque monkey. *Proceedings of the National Academy of Sciences*, *96*, 5768–5773.

Kubisch, H. M., Falkenstein, K. P., Deroche, C. B., & Franke, D. E. (2012). Reproductive efficiency of captive Chinese- and Indian-origin rhesus macaque (Macaca mulatta) females. *American Journal of Primatology*, *74*, 174–184.

Languille, S., Blanc, S., Blin, O., Canale, C. I., Dal-Pan, A., Devau, G., . . . Aujard, F. (2012). The grey mouse lemur: A non-human primate model for ageing studies. *Ageing Research Reviews*, *11*, 150–162.

Leuner, B., Kozorovitskiy, Y., Gross, C. G., & Gould, E. (2007). Diminished adult neurogenesis in the marmoset brain precedes old age. *Proceedings of the National Academy of Sciences of the United States of America*, *104*, 17169–17173.

Louis, E. D. (2011). Essential tremor. *Handbook of Clinical Neurology*, *100*, 433–448.

Lu, P. H., Lee, G. J., Tishler, T. A., Meghpara, M., Thompson, P. M., & Bartzokis, G. (2013). Myelin breakdown mediates age-related slowing in cognitive processing speed in healthy elderly men. *Brain and Cognition*, *81*, 131–138.

Lutermann, H., Schmelting, B., Radespiel, U., Ehresmann, P., & Zimmermann, E. (2006). The role of survival for the evolution of female philopatry in a solitary forager, the grey mouse lemur (Microcebus murinus). *Proceedings of the Royal Society B: Biological Sciences*, *273*, 2527–2533.

Manning, G. W. (1943). Coronary disease in the ape. *American Heart Journal*, *23*, 719–724.

Masliah, E., Mallory, M., Hansen, L., De Teresa, R., & Terry, R. D. (1993). Quantitative synaptic alterations in the human neocortex during normal aging. *Neurology*, *43*, 192–197.

Maswood, N., Young, J., Tilmont, E., Zhang, Z., Gash, D. M., Gerhardt, G. A., . . . Ingram, D. K. (2004). Caloric restriction increases neurotrophic factor levels and attenuates neurochemical and behavioral deficits in a primate model of Parkinson's disease. *Proceedings of the National Academy of Sciences of the United States of America, 101*, 18171–18176.

Matochik, J. A., Chefer, S. I., Lane, M. A., Roth, G. S., Mattison, J. A., & Ingram, D. K. (2004). Age-related decline in striatal volume in rhesus monkeys: Assessment of long-term calorie restriction. *Neurobiology of Aging, 25*, 193–200.

Mattison, J. A., Roth, G. S., Beasley, T. M., Tilmont, E. M., Handy, A. M., Herbert, R. L., . . . de Cabo, R. (2012). Impact of caloric restriction on health and survival in rhesus monkeys from the NIA study. *Nature, 489*, 318–321.

McArdle, J. J., Ferrer-Caja, E., Hamagami, F., & Woodcock, R. W. (2002). Comparative longitudinal structural analyses of the growth and decline of multiple intellectual abilities over the life span. *Developmental Psychology, 38*, 115–142.

Mitchell, A. C., Leak, R. K., Zigmond, M. J., Cameron, J. L., & Mirnics, K. (2012). Gene transcripts associated with BMI in the motor cortex and caudate nucleus of calorie restricted rhesus monkeys. *Genomics, 99*, 144–151.

Moore, T. L., Killiany, R. J., Herndon, J. G., Rosene, D. L., & Moss, M. B. (2006). Executive system dysfunction occurs as early as middle-age in the rhesus monkey. *Neurobiology of Aging, 27*, 1484–1493.

Morgan, D. G., May, P. C., & Finch, C. E. (1987). Dopamine and serotonin systems in human and rodent brain: Effects of age and degenerative disease. *Journal of the American Geriatrics Society, 35*, 334–345.

Morrison, J. H., & Baxter, M. G. (2012). The ageing cortical synapse: Hallmarks and implications for cognitive decline. *Nature Reviews Neuroscience, 13*, 240–250.

Nagahara, A. H., Bernot, T., & Tuszynski, M. H. (2010). Age-related cognitive deficits in rhesus monkeys mirror human deficits on an automated test battery. *Neurobiology of Aging, 31*, 1020–1031.

Némoz-Bertholet, F., & Aujard, F. (2003). Physical activity and balance performance as a function of age in a prosimian primate (Microcebus murinus). *Experimental Gerontology, 38*, 407–414.

Némoz-Bertholet, F., Menaker, M., & Aujard, F. (2004). Are age-related deficits in balance performance mediated by time of day in a prosimian primate (Microcebus murinus)? *Experimental Gerontology, 39*, 841–848.

Nishijima, K., Saitoh, R., Tanaka, S., Ohsato-Suzuki, M., Ohno, T., & Kitajima, S. (2012). Life span of common marmoset (Callithrix jacchus) at CLEA Japan breeding colony. *Biogerontology, 13*, 439–443.

Nowak, R. M. (1999). *Walker's mammals of the world*. Baltimore, MD: Johns Hopkins University Press.

Oikawa, N., Kimura, N., & Yanagisawa, K. (2010). Alzheimer-type tau pathology in advanced aged nonhuman primate brains harboring substantial amyloid deposition. *Brain Research, 1315*, 137–149.

Ovadia, A., Zhang, Z., & Gash, D. M. (1995). Increased susceptibility to MPTP toxicity in middle-aged rhesus monkeys. *Neurobiology of Aging, 16*, 931–937.

Palazzi, X., Switzer, R., & George, C. (2006). Natural occurrence of amyloid-Abeta deposits in the brain of young common marmosets (Callithrix jacchus): A morphological and immunohistochemical evaluation. *Veterinary Pathology, 43,* 777–779.

Patel, N. V., Gordon, M. N., Connor, K. E., Good, R. A., Engelman, R. W., Mason, J., . . . Finch, C. E. (2005). Caloric restriction attenuates Aβ-deposition in Alzheimer transgenic models. *Neurobiology of Aging, 26,* 995–1000.

Peters, A. (2002). Structural changes in the normally aging cerebral cortex of primates. *Progress in Brain Research, 136,* 455–465.

Peters, A., Rosene, D. L., Moss, M. B., Kemper, T. L., Abraham, C. R., Tigges, J., & Albert, M. S. (1996). Neurobiological bases of age-related cognitive decline in the rhesus monkey. *Journal of Neuropathology and Experimental Neurology, 55,* 861–874.

Picq, J. L., Aujard, F., Volk, A., & Dhenain, M. (2012). Age-related cerebral atrophy in nonhuman primates predicts cognitive impairments. *Neurobiology of Aging, 33,* 1096–1109.

Prüfer, K., Munch, K., Hellmann, I., Akagi, K., Miller, J. R., Walenz, B., . . . Paabo, S. (2012). The bonobo genome compared with the chimpanzee and human genomes. *Nature, 486,* 527–531.

Pusey, A., Williams, J., & Goodall, J. (1997). The influence of dominance rank on the reproductive success of female chimpanzees. *Science, 277,* 828–831.

Qin, W., Chachich, M., Lane, M., Roth, G., Bryant, M., de Cabo, R., . . . Pasinetti, G. M. (2006). Calorie restriction attenuates Alzheimer's disease type brain amyloidosis in Squirrel monkeys (Saimiri sciureus). *Journal of Alzheimer's Disease, 10,* 417–422.

Quik, M., Perez, X. A., & Bordia, T. (2012). Nicotine as a potential neuroprotective agent for Parkinson's disease. *Movement Disorders, 27,* 947–957.

Ridley, R. M., Baker, H. F., Windle, C. P., & Cummings, R. M. (2006). Very long term studies of the seeding of beta-amyloidosis in primates. *Journal of Neural Transmission, 113,* 1243–1251.

Rosen, R. D. (2008, December 7). The lie of the jungle. *The Washington Post,* p. W14.

Rosen, R. F., Farberg, A. S., Gearing, M., Dooyema, J., Long, P. M., Anderson, D. C., . . . Walker, L. C. (2008). Tauopathy with paired helical filaments in an aged chimpanzee. *Journal of Comparative Neurology, 509,* 259–270.

Schultz, C., Hubbard, G. B., Rüb, U., Braak, E., & Braak, H. (2000). Age related progression of tau pathology in brains of baboons. *Neurobiology of Aging, 21,* 905–912.

Severson, J. A., Marcusson, J., Winblad, B., & Finch, C. E. (1982). Age correlated loss of dopaminergic binding sites in human basal ganglia. *Journal of Neurochemistry, 39,* 1623–1631.

Shah, P., Lal, N., Leung, E., Traul, D. E., Gonzalo-Ruiz, A., & Geula, C. (2010). Neuronal and axonal loss are selectively linked to fibrillar amyloid-β within plaques of the aged primate cerebral cortex. *American Journal of Pathology, 177,* 325–333.

Shamy, J. L., Habeck, C., Hof, P. R., Amaral, D. G., Fong, S. G., Buonocore, M. H., . . . Rapp, P. R. (2011). Volumetric correlates of spatiotemporal working and recognition memory impairment in aged rhesus monkeys. *Cerebral Cortex, 21,* 1559–1573.

Sharp, E. S., & Gatz, M. (2011). Relationship between education and dementia: An updated systematic review. *Alzheimer Disease and Associated Disorders, 25*, 289–304.

Sherwood, C. C., Gordon, A. D., Allen, J. S., Phillips, K. A., Erwin, J. M., Hof, P. R., & Hopkins, W. D., (2011). Aging of the cerebral cortex differs between humans and chimpanzees. *Proceedings of the National Academy of Sciences of the United States of America, 108*, 13029–13034.

Silk, J. B., Beehner, J. C., Bergman, T. J., Crockford, C., Engh, A. L., Moscovice, L. R., . . . Cheney, D. L. (2010). Strong and consistent social bonds enhance the longevity of female baboons. *Current Biology, 20*, 1359–1361.

Simmons, H. A., & Mattison, J. A. (2011). The incidence of spontaneous neoplasia in two populations of captive rhesus macaques (Macaca mulatta). *Antioxidants & Redox Signaling, 14* 221–227.

Smith, R. J., & Jungers, W. L. (1997). Body mass in comparative primatology. *Journal of Human Evolution, 32*, 523–559.

Smucny, D. A., Abbott, D. H., Mansfield, K. G., Schultz-Darken, N. J., Yamamoto, M. E., Alencar, A. I., & Tardif, S. D. (2004). Reproductive output, maternal age, and survivorship in captive common marmoset females (Callithrix jacchus). *American Journal of Primatology, 64*, 107–121.

Tardif, S. D., Mansfield, K. G., Ratnam, R., Ross, C. N., & Ziegler, T. E. (2011). The marmoset as a model of aging and age-related diseases. *Institute of Laboratory Animal Resources Journal, 52*, 54–65.

Tardif, S. D., Smucny, D. A., Abbott, D. H., Mansfield, K., Schultz-Darken, N., & Yamamoto, M. E. (2003). Reproduction in captive common marmosets (Callithrix jacchus). *Comparative Medicine, 53*, 364–368.

Thomas, M. (2006). Yerkes, Hamilton and the experimental study of the ape mind: from evolutionary psychiatry to eugenic politics. *Studies in History and Philosophy of Biological and Biomedical Sciences, 37*, 273–294.

Tigges, J., Herndon, J. G., & Peters, A. (1990). Neuronal population of area 4 during the life span of the rhesus monkey. *Neurobiology of Aging, 11*, 201–208.

Torre, P., III, Mattison, J. A., Fowler, C. G., Lane, M. A., Roth, G. S., & Ingram, D. K. (2004). Assessment of auditory function in rhesus monkeys (Macaca mulatta): Effects of age and calorie restriction. *Neurobiology of Aging, 25*, 945–954.

Van Maele-Fabry, G., Hoet, P., Vilain, F., & Laison, D. (2012). Occupational exposure to pesticides and Parkinson's disease: A systematic review and meta-analysis of cohort studies. *Environment International, 46*, 30–43.

Varki, N., Anderson, D., Herndon, J. G., Pham, T., Gregg, C. J., Cheriyan, M., . . . Varki, A. (2009). Heart disease is common in humans and chimpanzees, but is caused by different pathological processes. *Evolutionary Applications*, 2(1), 101–112.

Weigl, R. (2005). *Longevity of mammals in captivity; from the living collections of the world.* Stuttgart, Germany: Schweizerbart.

Wich, S. A., Shumaker, R. W., Perkins, L., & de Vries, H. (2009). Captive and wild orangutan (Pongo sp.) survivorship: A comparison and the influence of management. *American Journal of Primatology, 71*, 680–686.

Wich, S. A., Utami-Atmoko, S. S., Mitra Setia, T., Rijksen, H. D., Schurmann, C., van Hooff, J. A., & van Schaik, C. P. (2004). Life history of wild Sumatran orangutans (Pongo abelii). *Journal of Human Evolution, 47*, 385–398.

Williams, L. (1986). Partner preferences in different aged female rhesus macaques (Macaca mullata). *The Journals of Gerontology, 41*, 623–628.

Wu, Y. C., Field, A. S., Whalen, P. J., & Alexander, A. L. (2011). Age- and gender-related changes in the normal human brain using hybrid diffusion imaging. *Neuroimage, 54*, 1840–1853.

Yue, F., Zeng, S., Wu, D., Yi, D., Alex Zhang, Y., & Chan, P. (2012). Age-related decline in motor behavior and striatal dopamine transporter in Cynomolgus monkeys. *Journal of Neural Transmission, 119*, 943–952.

Zeamer, A., Decamp, E., Clark, K., & Schneider, J. S. (2011). Attention, executive functioning and memory in normal aged rhesus monkeys. *Behavioural Brain Research, 219*, 23–30.

Zhang, Z., Andersen, A., Smith, C., Grondin, R., Gerhardt, G., & Gash, D. (2000). Motor slowing and parkinsonian signs in aging rhesus monkeys mirror human aging. *Journals of Gerontology Series A: Biological Sciences and Medical Sciences, 55*, B473–B480.

CHAPTER 6

Genes for Exceptional Longevity

Nir Barzilai and Gil Atzmon

ABSTRACT

Families with exceptional longevity may inherit biological factors that favorably modulate aging processes and disease susceptibility. This inheritance has been demonstrated across generations in families with exceptional long-lived individuals. However, the genetic/biological pathways responsible for such phenotypes are still under active investigation.

When studying genes that may be associated with human longevity, one must consider several approaches:

1. Infer that genes that modulate lifespan in lower species are conserved and have similar role in human aging. Such aging associated systems might have originated from a very early common ancestor. An example of such a lineage associated with aging is the insulin/insulin-like growth factor (IGF1) signaling pathway, which involves in many functions that are necessary for metabolism, growth, and fertility in animal models including flies, nematodes, and mammals. Mutations in genes that are part of this pathway in lower species led to significant increases in lifespan. This observation, coupled with the homology to the human pathway, raised special interest in studying genetic alterations in the insulin/IGF1 signaling that may contribute to human's longevity.
2. Study genetic factors associated or causative to age-related diseases, namely cardiovascular disease, diabetes mellitus, cancer, and Alzheimer's disease. Because those diseases account for most age-dependent mortality, it was proposed that the more "perfect" (the one depleted from genotypes associated with age-related disease), the longer and healthier one would live.

http://dx.doi.org/10.1891/0198-8794.34.171

However, extremely old individuals that have genetic factors for these diseases seem to be protected from such diseases. Discovering such genomic mechanisms may provide another avenue to discover genetic protective mechanisms against known disease genotypes.

3. Discover protective genes in centenarians and their families. Centenarians and their family members seem to share certain biological protective factors that could be more easily discerned when looking beyond the centenarian index case. The survival advantage of these families is highly heritable, with siblings and offspring of centenarians also living long lives. Identifying which genes confer this unique advantage is also critical in understanding what controls human lifespan.

INTRODUCTION

From evolutionary perspective, aging as a trait has been exposed to natural selection simply because in most species, including humans, very few lived beyond reproductive maturity, with no fitness advantages. However, evidence for aging mechanisms that were genetically predisposed have been heavily cited during the last decades. Examples are protective, adaptive, and stress responses against aging breakdown and insults that can play a major role in influencing the rate of aging, all of which are regulated by genetic networks (Barzilai et al., 2012). In addition, each individual cell's DNA is being exposed to somatic mutations and epigenetic modulations, which may contribute to decline in organ size, function, and health, and which will promote body aging. We chose to discuss subjects with exceptional longevity in this chapter for several reasons. First, there is overwhelming evidence for genetic predisposition associated with increased lifespan and health span in many species, supporting these links. Second and relevant to humans, people age at different rates, and biological and chronological ages do not seem to be the same. Choosing exceptionally long-lived subjects may increase the chances to discover the genetic makeup for delayed aging. Third, there are increasing amounts of data demonstrating the existence of longevity genotypes. Finally, we chose to discuss genetic factors that are associated with increased rather than limited lifespan because this approach deals with the whole process of aging as opposed to focus on a specific disease relevant to one or few organs.

This chapter will review several genetic pathways that appear to be modulating aging from lower species to humans, discuss genes involved in age-related diseases and their possible relation to longevity regulation, and longevity genes that have already been discovered in human studies. Throughout the chapter, there is a thorough description of the metabolic phenotype of centenarians because it pertains to the genes and pathways being discussed.

Exceptional Longevity Heritability

The contribution of gene(s) to survival to extreme old age compared with environmental influences is not clear (Cournil & Kirkwood, 2001). Although there is a definite contribution of genes to determining lifespan across different species, genes seem to explain only about 25% of human longevity variation (Herskind et al., 1996; McGue, Vaupel, Holm, & Harvald, 1993). However, strong emerging evidence provides the link between parent/parents longevity and the delay in the occurrence of age-related diseases in their offspring. Having either father or mother living pass the age of 80 years delayed diabetes by ~30% in their offspring (Florez et al., 2011). Similarly, having one parent living pass the age of 85 years delayed cognitive decline or Alzheimer's disease (AD) by ~30% in their offspring (Lipton et al., 2010). Strong heritable effects of longevity and the delayed onset of major age-associated diseases is shown in the offspring of two centenarian parents who have been generally spared from the major age-related diseases (e.g., cardiovascular disease [CVD], diabetes mellitus [DM], AD, and cancer) that are responsible for most deaths among the elderly persons. As a group, centenarians are relatively rare, accounting for only 1 in 5,000 individuals in the general population (Barzilai et al., 2003). This phenomenon is more likely to be manifested among their close relatives than in unrelated individuals. In the Framingham centenarian study, siblings of centenarians showed a lifelong reduction in risk for death of approximately one-half (Perls et al., 2002). This relative risk for death remains stable as they became older, suggesting that the siblings' survival advantage is caused by genetic factors because the environment is likely to differ during adulthood (Perls et al., 2002).

Families of Centenarians as a Study Group

Family members of centenarians may share certain biological protective factors that can be modulated by genetic elements and could be more easily discerned when using such a structure. Offspring of long-lived parents have an approximately 50% lower prevalence of hypertension, DM, myocardial infarction, and stroke/transient ischemic attacks compared with age-matched control groups (Atzmon et al., 2004). This group of subjects from families with exceptional longevity may contribute to our understanding of aging in several ways. First, by serving as a group for the search for inherited biological factors (with genetic predisposition) that modulates lifespan. Because centenarians are at the end of their lives, biological factors that could have sustained their health until this moment may be on the decline and may limit the discovery of biological markers. However, their DNA is a precious resource that can be used for discovery of the genetic component of the biological factors simply by applying case-control analysis. If significant longevity factors are inherited, it might be more apparent in the offspring or relatives of centenarians. This unique group of exceptionally long-lived families appear to be unusually healthy and have proved to be worthwhile to study for both phenotypic and genetic determinants of exceptionally long life (Atzmon, Rincon, Rabizadeh, & Barzilai, 2005; Atzmon et al., 2004; Barzilai et al., 2003).

Second, studies mainly focus on a disease of interest, thus selection is being targeted to either subjects with or without the disease. In such cases, groups selected for good health are left aside. The offspring of centenarians may be an ideal group in which to characterize a disease-free aging phenotype because their aging process is half as likely to be delayed or modulated by disease. Choosing a potential healthy group (such as offspring of centenarians) is an advantage in aging research, in particular when comparing their clinical phenotype and biological/genetic characteristics to those of groups with a high risk for a certain disease and usual survival.

Third, epidemiological studies may consider acquiring data regarding family history of longevity and adjusting for this variable. Indeed, recent evidence suggests that a subtle "dose-response" effect of age of parents versus the risk for better health in their offspring exists (Adams, Nolan, Andersen, Perls, & Terry, 2008; Atzmon et al., 2004).

Another compelling reason to study centenarians is that while the genetic component of longevity assessed by twin study and sib pair analysis is relatively small and environment seems to have limited effect (Rajpathak et al., 2011), the interaction between the two would be predicted to have a large impact. As for lifestyle, a study by Rajpathak et al. (2011) reported that almost half of centenarians are overweight or obese, smokers, and practice moderate exercise, which is similar or worse than their birth cohort (National Health and Nutrition Examination Survey 1 [NHANES 1]). Other young unrelated cohort studies report on the high prevalence of smoking, obesity, and low exercise rates. These studies in part led to the hypothesis that individuals who live to extreme old age possess some "protection" either genetic or the interaction between the genetic and the environment that allows them to withstand the deleterious effects of aging process and diseases. To discern the genetic component of extreme longevity, the selection of control groups is also critical. Centenarian's studies today lack an appropriate age-matched control group because DNA of their birth cohort has not been collected. If extreme longevity is genetically predisposed and inherited, then offspring of centenarians can substitute for their parents with the benefit of delaying age-associated processes and disease occurrence as well as the favorable genetic background. Having such a unique group can make the search for longevity genes less conditional with a more appropriate control group (age-matched, sex-matched, socioeconomic-matched, environmentally matched). Studies that used this model of analysis structure, such as the use of spouses of the offspring as controls, were rare but are becoming more and more apparent (Barzilai et al., 2003). This approach allows correction for external factors because the controls share a common environment and household with the offspring. This approach favors the notion that spouses share propensity for similar diseases (Hippisley-Cox, Coupland, Pringle, Crown, & Hammersley, 2002), and a longitudinal study may benefit technically and academically by recruiting couples and following them as they age together (Atzmon et al., 2004).

Centenarians are also a preferable candidate group to study compression-of-morbidity (Mor, 2005). This notion is based on the observation that centenarians have been not only healthier longer but also have less relative and absolute morbidity before dying. Consistent with the compression-of-morbidity hypothesis, several studies report that a significant proportion of centenarians delay or escape age-related diseases. CVD, cancer, and cognitive decline are delayed in proportion to longevity and there is an absolute and relative contraction of morbidity with exceptional longevity (Andersen, Sebastiani, Dworkis, Feldman, & Perls, 2012). Moreover, offspring of centenarians appear to enjoy better physical function and lower rates of frailty than age-matched controls (Adams et al., 2008), suggesting biological benefits that might genetically predispose of longevity traits. Therefore, centenarians may be an ideal population to investigate candidate longevity genes and genes associated with aging mechanisms.

The challenge is to identify and determine these potential genes. One approach is to study genes that have been already associated with lifespan in lower species. Such genes that have human homologs may contribute to phylogenetically conserved pathways (Browner et al., 2004). A second approach is to compare gene frequencies in two different age groups (e.g., centenarians versus younger controls), demonstrating possible candidate survival genes by the observed case-control differences in allele frequencies (Yashin et al., 2000). A third approach is to investigate genes associated with age-related diseases or accelerated aging syndromes (Perls, Kunkel, & Puca, 2002). Regardless of the chosen approach, it is obvious that there are multiple pathways involved in human longevity and that this complexity makes deciphering the involved genes even more difficult.

RELEVANCE OF CONSERVED PATHWAYS OF AGING TO HUMAN LONGEVITY

The evolutionary conservation of the insulin/IGF1 pathway from nematodes and flies to mammals and their relevance to aging strongly suggests that such a pathway could be important for human longevity as well. Studies have shown that growth hormone (GH) secretion and IGF1 levels decrease with age (Elahi, Muller, Tzankoff, Andres, & Tobin, 1982; Rudman et al., 1981). The phenotype of aging includes increased adipose tissue, reduced lean body mass, insulin resistance, and CVD (atherosclerosis, hypertension; Corpas, Harman, & Blackman, 1993). All these features are also present in individuals with GH deficiency (Carter et al., 2002; Goodman-Gruen, Barrett-Connor, & Rosen, 2000; Janssen, Stolk, Pols, Grobbee, & Lamberts, 1998; Khan, Sane, Wannenburg, & Sonntag, 2002). Moreover, GH/IGF1 therapy in the elderly and in GH-deficient patients improves body composition and lipid profile, protein synthesis, and immune functions (Khan et al., 2002; Marcus et al., 1990; Vance & Mauras, 1999). The GH-insensitive or Laron syndrome, in which a mutation of the GH receptor produces accumulation of high levels of GH, with low IGF1, has a phenotype of short stature, obesity, mental retardation, and glucose intolerance. The syndrome is not associated with shorter lifespan but protects from cancer and diabetes (Guevara-Aguirre et al., 2011) as described below. In our longevity study, centenarians probably do not have IGF1 deficiency because their average maximal height is similar to the average maximal height of a control cohort (Suh et al., 2008). Acromegalic patients (overproduction of GH) have an increased mortality risk because of CVD, diabetes, and malignancy (Orme, McNally, Cartwright, & Belchetz, 1998). Similarly, side effects of GH/IGF1 therapy include development of insulin resistance, glucose intolerance, arthralgia, edema, sodium retention, and increased mitogenic activity, probably promoting neoplasia.

The relative GH/IGF1 deficiency during aging does not necessarily mean that old individuals should receive GH replacement to extend their old age because there are high rates of adverse effects with the use of these hormones (Corpas et al., 1993). GH is known to be potentially diabetogenic and IGF1 is considered a risk factor for lung, breast, prostate, and colorectal cancer (Juul, 1999; Khan et al., 2002).

Mutations of the insulin receptor have been described in humans, causing different degrees of insulin resistance and DM (Accili, 1995). It is known that insulin sensitivity declines with age and is associated with increased morbidity and mortality because of atherosclerosis, CVD, obesity, and diabetes (Fontbonne & Eschwege, 1991). It is unclear whether hyperinsulinism alone or abnormalities in glucose and nutrient metabolism are responsible for disease. Studies in healthy centenarians show enhanced insulin sensitivity, demonstrating an important role of a healthy insulin pathway for extreme long life (Bonafe et al., 2003). It is worth mentioning that the longevity genes known to date are, in general, associated with favorable insulin action (Barzilai et al., 2003; Bluher, Kahn, & Kahn, 2003).

AGE-RELATED DISEASES AND LONGEVITY GENES

The precise interaction of all possible determinants of human aging is unknown, but ultimately they would regulate the time of onset of various age-related diseases that are important limiting factors for human life expectancy. CVD, DM, metabolic syndrome, AD, and cancer are the common killers of aging humans. Thus, genes associated with these diseases are good targets for investigation. Despite the exponential increase of mortality with increasing age, extremely old individuals seem to be protected from such diseases and "early death" (Evert, Lawler, Bogan, & Perls, 2003). Other diseases characterized by premature aging, such as the progeroid syndromes, are another possible source of genes for study (Perls & Puca, 2002). All these disorders may be caused by polymorphisms, epigenetic changes (e.g., changes in methylation, decreased telomere length), metabolic dysfunction (e.g., mitochondria genome disturbances), physical deconditioning, or loss of immunological responsiveness (Volkova, Garg, Dick, & Boheler, 2005). Targeting the various genes and pathways that are associated with these diseases has been helpful in the search for determinants of human longevity.

APPROACH AND CHALLENGES FOR GENETIC DISCOVERIES FOR EXCEPTIONAL LONGEVITY

The Conceptual Framework for Discovery of Longevity Genotypes

The conceptual framework for discovery of longevity-associated genotypes is similar to that employed for genetic discovery of other diseases and conditions, and is depicted in Figure 6.1. Subjects are nonagenarians, centenarians or elderly but healthy subjects. Because this trait is uncommon (centenarians are 1/5,000–10,000), and heritability is low, the chances of success in "gene hunt" decrease as the phenotype becomes more rare, thus large sized population sources are needed. Most of the success in the field until now has been derived by using our preexisting knowledge and interrogating genes and networks that are suspected to play role in aging based on studies in animal/organism models, or from a biological phenotype that has been established in the lab. Although this approach provides a better chance to detect longevity-associated genotypes, it is limited in its capacity because it tests few genes at a time. High-throughput genotyping for genome wide association studies (GWAS) is popular because it provides both an unbiased approach for analysis and genome wide screening at once for the entire set of genes. However, there are some biases when searching for longevity genes because most commercial platforms use single nucleotide polymorphisms (SNPs) with minor allele frequency of 5%–49% in the overall population, whereas exceptional longevity is very rare and thus longevity allele prevalence would be estimated

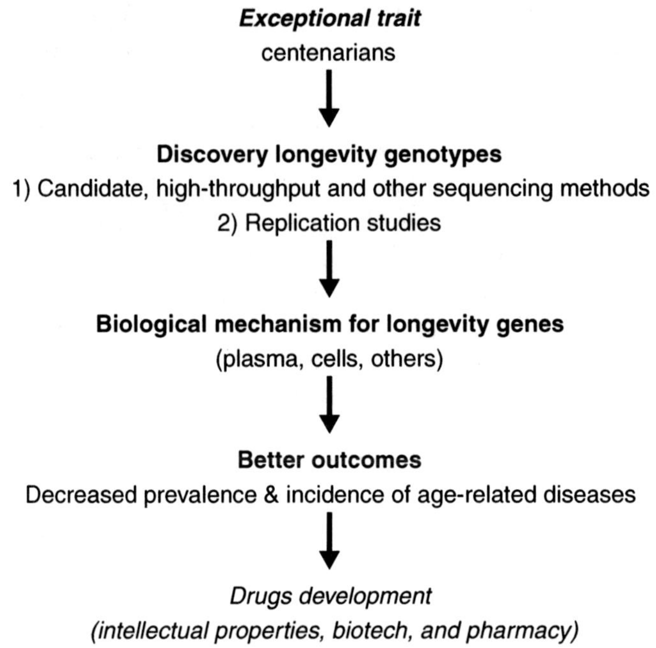

FIGURE 6.1 Conceptual framework for genetic studies on exceptional longevity.

to be far less than common. Exome or whole genome sequencing is available and will become increasingly useful as the technology becomes cheaper and analysis value and cost decreases. Another problem of high-throughput genotyping is that the high statistical demand because of multiple testing (in order of $p<10–8$ for SNP) results in loss of true positive results. The problem that plagues classical genetics today is the need for replications. The analysis in GWAS includes that of one SNP at a time, although we are built from numerous SNPs that are interactive. This is a problem, in particular when you move from one population to another. As general example, common SNPs in the White population may not exist in an Oriental population, yet for a certain conditions either another SNP in the same gene or SNPs in the pathway may result in the same phenotype. Thus, not replicating SNPs in all population does not make any previous discovery necessarily wrong. The way to get simple genotype confirmation is to associate genotype with intermediate phenotype (such as levels in plasma) or functional studies. At the end, these genotypes need to be correlated with health outcomes and for decline in age-related diseases. Discoveries of this sort should lead to drug development that can modulate the action of genes implicated in longevity. Interestingly, as seen below, there are examples for all these.

Innovative Approaches to Determine Longevity Genes

The age axis in Figure 6.2 can be populated in each age group with hundreds of subjects. It is important to note that although we can have hundreds of centenarians, they represent unusual selection because half of the people in the United States die on average at the age of ~80 years. Considering this selection, we can consider methods to identify relevant genes involved in aging/longevity based on the following considerations as exemplified in Figure 6.2 (Barzilai et al., 2012; Bergman, Atzmon, Ye, MacCarthy, & Barzilai, 2007). The relative prevalence of favorable "longevity" genotypes in the population increases as the population ages because mortality will catch up with individuals lacking the favorable genotype, causing the proportion of those endowed with the favorable genotypes to increase (Florez et al. 2011). The relative prevalence of deleterious genotypes in genes associated with age-related diseases decreases as the population ages because mortality reduces the proportion of individuals carrying the deleterious genotype. Those genes can cause organ-system specific diseases and are referred to here as "killing-genes" (Bergman, Atzmon, Ye, MacCarthy, & Barzilai, 2007; Lipton et al., 2010). The relative frequencies of the deleterious genotypes in some killing-genes decrease only within younger age individuals but return to near-initial frequency among the extremely old individuals. At first glance, it appears as if a killing gene becomes a longevity gene after the age of 80 years, a biologically unlikely explanation. In fact, our data supports the notion that this U shape demonstrates how rare and highly selected subjects with genes for exceptional longevity can harbor and be protected from the effects of deleterious killing genes. We will refer to this U shape to gene frequencies of some genes

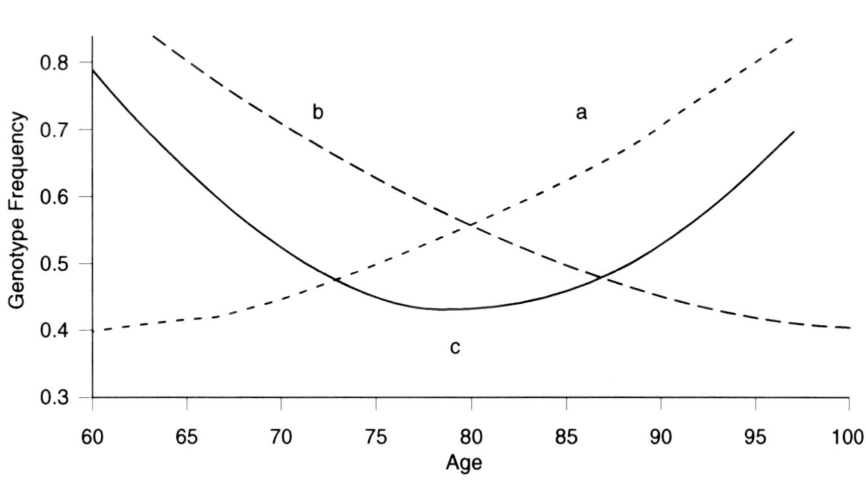

FIGURE 6.2 Possibilities for change in the frequency of a functional genotype with age.

as the effect of "buffered-aging genes." For instance, our studies show that rises in the deleterious lipoprotein [Lp(a)] and microsomal triglyceride transfer protein (MTP) genotype were seen in centenarians with protective cholesteryl ester transfer protein (CETP) genotype, which likely buffered the effect of the Lp(a) and MTP genotypes (Bergman et al., 2007; Huffman et al., 2012). If the whole aging axis is not adequately populated, and if the study population does not have a representation of people younger than 70 years and is lacking the group between 80 and 90 years, an SNP that is U shaped will show up as "longevity gene." For example, the MTP gene was previously thought to be associated with human longevity. However, its increase with exceptional longevity is consistent with a "buffered" aging genotype because it is forming a U-shape pattern (Huffman et al., 2012). Furthermore, the MTP CC genotype was buffered by three validated longevity genotypes. A method to perform whole genome gene to gene int*eraction on the X axis has been suggested (Bergman et al., 2007).

LONGEVITY GENES IN CENTENARIANS

Candidate Gene Approach

Searches for candidate genes based on single gene manipulations in *C. elegans*, Drosophila, and mice, which demonstrated how genes could extend lifespan in a stable environment, were the first and best attempts so far to validate such effects in humans. Several studies in humans have implicated either conserved or new genetically mediated pathways in human longevity.

The GH/insulin IGF1 pathways in human longevity have been investigated most frequently. The most validated (by at least eight groups studying exceptional longevity) is a genotype for the conserved DAF16/FOXO transcription factors (human ortholog FOXO3a), first established in centenarians from Okinawa. Although FOXO3a is the most validated genotype for exceptional longevity, it lags behind in other major requirements. The SNPs have not been functional (intronic, none coding) and although the whole gene was sequenced by several groups, no functional mutations were reported in important areas (or the SNP itself). Assays tests on cells of the individuals have not been associated with functional changes so far. Finally, intermediate phenotype/phenotypes associated with the genotype have not been found for outcomes of diseases (or longevity) associated with the phenotype.

Other significant SNPs in the insulin/IGF1 signaling pathway have been validated for exceptional longevity, but again, no phenotype is apparent, so it is not what types of effects exist in this pathway. This is important because decline in insulin signaling in humans is a hallmark for the metabolic syndrome of aging, which seems to be required for longevity. This paradox needs to be resolved.

A single outstanding example of correlation with function was obtained by target sequencing of the IGF1 and IGF1 receptor (IGF1R) genes of female centenarians. Overrepresentation of heterozygous mutations in the IGF1R gene among centenarians relative to controls is associated with high serum IGF1 levels and reduced activity of the IGF1R as measured in transformed lymphocytes (see below). The functionality of those genotype was later confirmed when examined in cells that did not belong to the carriers (Tazearslan, Huang, Barzilai, & Suh, 2011).

A second example for GH/IGF1 signaling derives from the rare genetic form of Laron dwarfism (GH receptor deficiency). A group with this genotype was studied in Ecuador and seems to have negligible prevalence of type 2 DM (T2DM) and cancer (Guevara-Aguirre et al., 2011). Although they did not live long, clearly they have been protected from major age-related diseases. Other genes that have been implicated in human aging (not necessarily longevity), usually without phenotypic correlates, are updated on http://genomics.senescence.info/genes/.

Genotype-Phenotype-Outcome Correlates for Candidate Genes

One of the early studies in nonagenarians (Leiden) and near-centenarians demonstrated that improved lipid profile, primarily high HDL levels, are common with exceptional longevity. A common homozygosity in the favorable genotypes associated with this lipid for the following were also associated with exceptional longevity: cholesteryl ester transfer protein gene codon 405 (CETP VV; Barzilai et al., 2003), apolipoprotein C-3 gene codon A (−641) C variant (APOC3 CC; Atzmon et al. 2006), a deletion at +2019 in the adiponectin (ADIPOQ; Atzmon et al. 2008) gene. We measured the gene products of the genes noted earlier and showed reduced plasma CETP and APOC3 levels, and increased plasma ADIPOQ levels, according to the relevant homozygosity (Atzmon et al., 2008; Atzmon et al., 2006; Barzilai et al., 2003). Those 3 genotypes increase monotonically with age as indicted in Figure 6.2. Furthermore, we linked the favorable CETP, APOC3, and ADIPOQ genotype with an intermediate favorable lipid phenotype (Barzilai et al., 2003). A most novel and striking example is that of the favorable CETP genotype and cognitive decline (Barzilai, Atzmon, Derby, Bauman, & Lipton, 2006; Sanders et al., 2010). In the case of APOC3, application of Kaplan-Meier survival analysis showed that carriers of the CC variant had a survival advantage (hazard ratio [HR] = 1.81, p = .0001), and the carriers lived 4 years longer (Atzmon et al., 2006). Subjects with high ADIPOQ had a fourfold reduced prevalence of multiple sclerosis (MS; Atzmon et al., 2008) and ADIPOQ genotype and levels are associated with less frailty and cognitive decline in centenarians.

These data were all established by using the homogenous population of Ashkenazi Jews. One advantage of homogenous populations is that genetic analysis is done in family-like population structure, which increases the chance to detect the link between genotype and phenotype. But once the link is established, the search for replication should be based not strictly on the genetic variant but rather on the whole gene. For example, CETP VV homozygosity was validated in one prior study (Lucchi et al., 2005) but not in another (Cellini et al., 2005). Japanese centenarians also have lower CETP levels and increased lipoprotein particle sizes compared to younger Japanese (Arai & Hirose, 2004), but Japanese have different polymorphisms and a tendency to lower incidence of CVD (Curb et al., 2004). The APOC3 genotype was increased by twofold to threefold in Polish centenarians (M. Puzianowska, personal communication, 2008). Another APOC3 genotype with low APOC3 levels is protective against CVD and is associated with longevity in its carriers in the Amish population (Pollin et al., 2008).

Other Genotypes

A thyroid-stimulating hormone (TSH)-receptor mutation is associated with clinically detectable alterations in thyroid hormone metabolism, specifically high TSH and low T3 levels (Atzmon, Barzilai, Hollowell, Surks, & Gabriely, 2009). The TSH-receptor genotype was recently validated by the New England Centenarian Study group. The Leiden study (Rozing et al., 2010) and others (Corsonello et al., 2010) have already published on the heritability of a sub-hypothyroid phenotype of longevity. Because of the intense interest in telomeres and aging, telomere length or mass (Atzmon et al., 2010) assessment showed that centenarians have longer telomeres, that this length is inherited in their offspring, and that this is associated with decreased incidence of MS, T2DM, and cognitive decline and has a genetic "fingerprint" in the telomerase genes in centenarians.

Unbiased Approach to the Genetics Human Longevity

Several GWAS studies (Beekman et al., 2010) have shown that long-lived individuals, surprisingly, harbor the same number or frequencies of genotypes associated with aging diseases as do non-long-lived individuals (Rajpathak et al., 2011). As indicted before, there may be several reasons for these facts including that the tools are not set for discovery on new or uncommon SNPs and the small number of studied subjects. Because the candidate gene approach has resulted in significant genotypes (not presented in the genotyping platform), but is still limited and GWAS is not fruitful as indicated earlier, exome and whole genome sequencing should provide the next DNA pool for variants screening. This approach was successfully tested in centenarians through whole gene sequencing of ~1,000 genes selected for potential impact on longevity (Han et al., 2013).

In this study, 51 novel nonsynonymous SNPs were validated, supporting the potential of next-generation sequencing for discovery of rare but functional genetic variants, which may lead to exceptional longevity in humans.

Epigenetic Mechanisms for Longevity

MicroRNAs (miRNAs) are small, noncoding RNAs that regulate gene expression and play a critical role in development, homeostasis, and disease. From technological point of view, massively parallel sequencing technology is available and used extensively in discovery cohorts and tissues. There are initial studies on B-cells and plasma of centenarian that have both demonstrated that although many miRNA expressions decrease with aging, there are several miRNAs whose expression is higher than in younger controls (Gombar et al., 2012; Serna et al., 2012), suggesting the potential for "longevity miRNAs."

Methylation

Methylation patterns change with aging. In animal models, more hypomethylation then hypermethylation occurs but the change is bidirectional. Initial studies in humans suggest the opposite. The challenge is that in each cell, methylation may or may not occur, prompt us to develop technics that are quantitative. They are tissue-specific, thus no tissue can determine overall methylation pattern but certainly correlated. Lastly, there is a challenge to associate many methylation loci on many genes with gene expression and physiological outcomes.

CONCLUSIONS

The challenges we face in aging as much as in age-related diseases is to translate the concepts learned in animal models to humans. Although genetic manipulations in lower species have been shown to extend lifespan, some pathways may not be relevant to humans because humans may have other mechanisms for longevity that are not relevant in animal models. Because exceptional longevity is heritable, we focused on the proof of concept that centenarian genomic studies have contributed to the field. The challenges include the fact that not enough studies are funded across the world to collect these precious subjects; and for rare phenotypes, a creative genetic approach is needed and the entire genomic data will be needed to discover all components that can lead to delayed aging in humans. Finally, inhibitors for CETP and APOC3 are in Phase 3 studies in major pharmaceutical trials based in large part on data derived from centenarians or from aging studies. This demonstrates that the search is important and is likely to be fruitful in translating knowledge to drug development that will delay aging or its diseases.

ACKNOWLEDGMENTS

Dr. Barzilai's research in animal models is supported by grants from the National Institute of Health (RO1-AG18381, and P01-AG021654), The Nathan Shock Center of Excellence for the Biology of Aging (P30AG038072), and the Glenn Center for the Biology of Human Aging (Paul Glenn Foundation Grant; NB). The longevity study was supported by grants from the Paul Beeson Physician Faculty Scholar in Aging Award, the Ellison Medical Foundation Senior Scholar Award, and RO1 (AG-18728), and the Diabetes Research and Training Center (DK 20541) at the Albert Einstein College of Medicine. Dr. Atzmon is supported by grants from the National Institute of Health (RO1-AG042188).

REFERENCES

Accili, D. (1995). Molecular defects of the insulin receptor gene. *Diabetes/Metabolism Research and Reviews*, *11*, 47–62.

Adams, E. R., Nolan, V. G., Andersen, S. L., Perls, T. T., & Terry, D. F. (2008). Centenarian offspring: Start healthier and stay healthier. *Journal of the American Geriatrics Society*, *56*, 2089–2092. http://dx.doi.org/10.1111/j.1532-5415.2008.01949.x

Andersen, S. L., Sebastiani, P., Dworkis, D. A., Feldman, L., & Perls, T. T. (2012). Health span approximates life span among many supercentenarians: Compression of morbidity at the approximate limit of life span. *The Journals of Gerontology Series A: Biological Sciences and Medical Sciences*, *67*, 395–405. http://dx.doi.org/10.1093/gerona/glr223

Arai, Y., & Hirose, N. (2004). Aging and HDL metabolism in elderly people more than 100 years old. *Journal of Atherosclerosis and Thrombosis*, *11*, 246–252.

Atzmon, G., Barzilai, N., Hollowell, J. G., Surks, M. I., & Gabriely, I. (2009). Extreme longevity is associated with increased serum thyrotropin. *The Journal of Clinical Endocrinology & Metabolism*, *94*, 1251–1254.

Atzmon, G., Cho, M., Cawthon, R. M., Budagov, T., Katz, M., Yang, X., . . . Suh, Y. (2010). Evolution in health and medicine Sackler colloquium: Genetic variation in human telomerase is associated with telomere length in Ashkenazi centenarians. *Proceedings of the National Academy of Sciences of the United States of America*, *107*(Suppl. 1), 1710–1717.

Atzmon, G., Pollin, T. I., Crandall, J., Tanner, K., Schechter, C. B., Scherer, P. E., . . . Barzilai, N. (2008). Adiponectin levels and genotype: A potential regulator of life span in humans. *The Journals of Gerontology Series A: Biological Sciences and Medical Sciences*, *63*, 447–453.

Atzmon, G., Rincon, M., Rabizadeh, P., & Barzilai, N. (2005). Biological evidence for inheritance of exceptional longevity. *Mechanisms of Ageing and Development*, *126*, 341–345.

Atzmon, G., Rincon, M., Schechter, C. B., Shuldiner, A. R., Lipton, R. B., Bergman, A., & Barzilai, N. (2006). Lipoprotein genotype and conserved pathway for exceptional longevity in humans. *PLoS Biology*, *4*, e113.

Atzmon, G., Schechter, C., Greiner, W., Davidson, D., Rennert, G., & Barzilai, N. (2004). Clinical phenotype of families with longevity. *Journal of the American Geriatrics Society*, *52*, 274–277.

Barzilai, N., Atzmon, G., Derby, C. A., Bauman, J. M., & Lipton, R. B. (2006). A genotype of exceptional longevity is associated with preservation of cognitive function. *Neurology*, *67*, 2170–2175.

Barzilai, N., Atzmon, G., Schechter, C., Schaefer, E. J., Cupples, A. L., Lipton, R., . . . Shuldiner, A. R. (2003). Unique lipoprotein phenotype and genotype associated with exceptional longevity. *JAMA: The Journal of the American Medical Association*, *290*, 2030–2040. http://dx.doi.org/10.1001/jama.290.15.2030

Barzilai, N., Guarente, L., Kirkwood, T. B., Partridge, L., Rando, T. A., & Slagboom, P. E. (2012). The place of genetics in ageing research. *Nature Reviews Genetics*, *13*, 589–594. http://dx.doi.org/10.1038/nrg3290

Beekman, M., Nederstigt, C., Suchiman, H. E., Kremer, D., van der Breggen, R., Lakenberg, N., . . . Slagboom, P. E. (2010). Genome-wide association study (GWAS)-identified disease risk alleles do not compromise human longevity. *Proceedings of the National Academy of Sciences of the United States of America*, *107*, 18046–18049. http://dx.doi.org/10.1073/pnas.1003540107

Bergman, A., Atzmon, G., Ye, K., MacCarthy, T., & Barzilai, N. (2007). Buffering mechanisms in aging: A systems approach toward uncovering the genetic component of aging. *PLOS Computational Biology*, *3*, e170. http://dx.doi.org/10.1371/journal.pcbi.0030170

Bluher, M., Kahn, B. B., & Kahn, C. R. (2003). Extended longevity in mice lacking the insulin receptor in adipose tissue. *Science*, *299*, 572–574. http://dx.doi.org/10.1126/science.1078223

Bonafe, M., Barbieri, M., Marchegiani, F., Olivieri, F., Ragno, E., Giampieri, C., . . . Paolisso, G. (2003). Polymorphic variants of insulin-like growth factor I (IGF-I) receptor and phosphoinositide 3-kinase genes affect IGF-I plasma levels and human longevity: Cues for an evolutionarily conserved mechanism of life span control. *The Journal of Clinical Endocrinology & Metabolism*, *88*, 3299–3304.

Browner, W. S., Kahn, A. J., Ziv, E., Reiner, A. P., Oshima, J., Cawthon, R. M., . . . Cummings, S. R. (2004). The genetics of human longevity. *Am J Med*, *117*, 851–860. http://dx.doi.org/10.1016/j.amjmed.2004.06.033

Carter, C. S., Ramsey, M. M., Ingram, R. L., Cashion, A. B., Cefalu, W. T., Wang, Z. Q., & Sonntag, W. E. (2002). Models of growth hormone and IGF-1 deficiency: Applications to studies of aging processes and life-span determination. *The Journals of Gerontology Series A: Biological Sciences and Medical Sciences*, *57*, B177–B188.

Cellini, E., Nacmias, B., Olivieri, F., Ortenzi, L., Tedde, A., Bagnoli, S., . . . Sorbi, S. (2005). Cholesteryl ester transfer protein (CETP) I405V polymorphism and longevity in Italian centenarians. *Mechanisms of Ageing and Development*, *126*, 826–828.

Corpas, E., Harman, S. M., & Blackman, M. R. (1993). Human growth hormone and human aging. *Endocrine Reviews*, *14*, 20–39.

Corsonello, A., Montesanto, A., Berardelli, M., De Rango, F., Dato, S., Mari, V., . . . Passarino, G. (2010). A cross-section analysis of FT3 age-related changes in a group of old and oldest-old subjects, including centenarians' relatives, shows that a down-regulated thyroid function has a familial component and is related to longevity. *Age Ageing*, *39*, 723–727.

Cournil, A., & Kirkwood, T. B. (2001). If you would live long, choose your parents well. *Trends in Genetics*, *17*, 233–235.

Curb, J. D., Abbott, R. D., Rodriguez, B. L., Masaki, K., Chen, R., Sharp, D. S.,& Tall, A. R. (2004). A prospective study of HDL-C and cholesteryl ester transfer protein gene mutations and the risk of coronary heart disease in the elderly. *The Journal of Lipid Research*, *45*, 948–953.

Elahi, D., Muller, D. C., Tzankoff, S. P., Andres, R., & Tobin, J. D. (1982). Effect of age and obesity on fasting levels of glucose, insulin, glucagon, and growth hormone in man. *The Journals of Gerontology*, *37*, 385–391.

Evert, J., Lawler, E., Bogan, H., & Perls, T. (2003). Morbidity profiles of centenarians: Survivors, delayers, and escapers. *The Journals of Gerontology Series A: Biological Sciences and Medical Sciences*, *58*, 232–237.

Florez, H., Ma, Y., Crandall, J. P., Perreault, L., Marcovina, S. M., Bray, G. A., . . . Knowler, W. C. (2011). Parental longevity and diabetes risk in the Diabetes Prevention Program. *The Journals of Gerontology Series A: Biological Sciences and Medical Sciences*, *66*, 1211–1217. http://dx.doi.org/10.1093/gerona/glr114

Fontbonne, A. M., & Eschwege, E. M. (1991). Insulin and cardiovascular disease. Paris Prospective Study. *Diabetes Care*, *14*, 461–469.

Gombar, S., Jung, H. J., Dong, F., Calder, B., Atzmon, G., Barzilai, N., . . . Suh, Y. (2012). Comprehensive microRNA profiling in B-cells of human centenarians by massively parallel sequencing. *BMC Genomics*, *13*, 353. http://dx.doi.org/10.1186/1471-2164-13-353

Goodman-Gruen, D., Barrett-Connor, E., & Rosen, C. (2000). IGF-I and ischemic heart disease in older people. *Journal of the American Geriatrics Society*, *48*, 860–861.

Guevara-Aguirre, J., Balasubramanian, P., Guevara-Aguirre, M., Wei, M., Madia, F., Cheng, C. W., . . . Longo, V. D. (2011). Growth hormone receptor deficiency is associated with a major reduction in pro-aging signaling, cancer, and diabetes in humans. *Science Translational Medicine*, 3, 70ra13. http://dx.doi.org/10.1126/scitranslmed.3001845

Han, J., Ryu, S., Moskowitz, D. M., Rothenberg, D., Leahy, D. J., Atzmon, G., . . . Suh, Y. (2013). Discovery of novel non-synonymous SNP variants in 988 candidate genes from 6 centenarians by target capture and next-generation sequencing. *Mechanisms of Ageing and Development*. Advance online publication. http://dx.doi.org/10.1016/j.mad.2013.01.005

Herskind, A. M., McGue, M., Holm, N. V., Sorensen, T. I., Harvald, B., & Vaupel, J. W. (1996). The heritability of human longevity: A population-based study of 2872 Danish twin pairs born 1870–1900. *Human Genetics*, *97*, 319–323.

Hippisley-Cox, J., Coupland, C., Pringle, M., Crown, N., & Hammersley, V. (2002). Married couples' risk of same disease: Cross sectional study. *British Medical Journal*, *325*, 636.

Huffman, D. M., Deelen, J., Ye, K., Bergman, A., Slagboom, E. P., Barzilai, N., & Atzmon, G. (2012). Distinguishing between longevity and buffered-deleterious genotypes for exceptional human longevity: The case of the MTP gene. *The Journals of Gerontology Series A: Biological Sciences and Medical Sciences*, *67*, 1153–1160. http://dx.doi.org/10.1093/gerona/gls103

Janssen, J. A., Stolk, R. P., Pols, H. A., Grobbee, D. E., & Lamberts, S. W. (1998). Serum total IGF-I, free IGF-I, and IGFB-1 levels in an elderly population: Relation to cardiovascular risk factors and disease. *Arteriosclerosis, Thrombosis, and Vascular Biology*, *18*, 277–282.

Juul, A. (1999). Determination of insulin-like growth factor-I in the monitoring of growth hormone treatment with respect to efficacy of treatment and side effects: Should potential risks of cardiovascular disease and cancer be considered? *Hormone Research*, *51*(Suppl. 3), 141–148. http://dx.doi.org/53177

Khan, A. S., Sane, D. C., Wannenburg, T., & Sonntag, W. E. (2002). Growth hormone, insulin-like growth factor-1 and the aging cardiovascular system. *Cardiovascular Research*, *54*, 25–35.

Laron, Z. (1999). The essential role of IGF-I: Lessons from the long-term study and treatment of children and adults with Laron syndrome. *The Journal of Clinical Endocrinology & Metabolism*, *84*, 4397–4404.

Lipton, R. B., Hirsch, J., Katz, M. J., Wang, C., Sanders, A. E., Verghese, J., . . . Derby, C. A. (2010). Exceptional parental longevity associated with lower risk of Alzheimer's disease and memory decline. *Journal of the American Geriatrics Society*, *58*, 1043–1049. http://dx.doi.org/10.1111/j.1532-5415.2010.02868.x

Lucchi, T., Arosio, B., Caloni, M., Ceconi, I., Calabresi, C., Scurati, S., & Vergani, C. (2005). [I405V polymorphism of the cholesteryl ester transfer protein gene in young and very old individuals]. *Annali Italiani di Medicina Interna*, *20*, 45–50.

Marcus, R., Butterfield, G., Holloway, L., Gilliland, L., Baylink, D. J., Hintz, R. L., & Sherman, B. M. (1990). Effects of short term administration of recombinant human growth hormone to elderly people. *The Journal of Clinical Endocrinology & Metabolism*, *70*, 519–527.

McGue, M., Vaupel, J. W., Holm, N., & Harvald, B. (1993). Longevity is moderately heritable in a sample of Danish twins born 1870–1880. *The Journals of Gerontology*, *48*, B237–B244.

Mor, V. (2005). The compression of morbidity hypothesis: A review of research and prospects for the future. *Journal of the American Geriatrics Society*, *53*, S308–S309. http://dx.doi.org/10.1111/j.1532-5415.2005.53496.x

Orme, S. M., McNally, R. J., Cartwright, R. A., & Belchetz, P. E. (1998). Mortality and cancer incidence in acromegaly: A retrospective cohort study. United Kingdom Acromegaly Study Group. *The Journal of Clinical Endocrinology & Metabolism*, *83*, 2730–2734.

Perls, T., Kunkel, L., & Puca, A. (2002). The genetics of aging. *Current Opinion in Genetics & Development*, *12*, 362–369.

Perls, T., & Puca, A. (2002). The genetics of aging—Implications for pharmacogenomics. *Pharmacogenomics*, *3*, 469–484.

Perls, T. T., Wilmoth, J., Levenson, R., Drinkwater, M., Cohen, M., Bogan, H., . . . Puca, A. (2002). Life-long sustained mortality advantage of siblings of centenarians.

Proceedings of the National Academy of Sciences of the United States of America, *99*, 8442–8447.

Pollin, T. I., Damcott, C. M., Shen, H., Ott, S. H., Shelton, J., Horenstein, R. B., . . . Shuldiner, A. R. (2008). A null mutation in human APOC3 confers a favorable plasma lipid profile and apparent cardioprotection. *Science*, *322*, 1702–1705. http://dx.doi.org/10.1126/science.1161524

Rajpathak, S. N., Liu, Y., Ben-David, O., Reddy, S., Atzmon, G., Crandall, J., & Barzilai, N. (2011). Lifestyle factors of people with exceptional longevity. *Journal of the American Geriatrics Society*, *59*, 1509–1512. http://dx.doi.org/10.1111/j.1532-5415.2011.03498.x

Rozing, M. P., Houwing–Duistermaat, J. J., Slagboom, P. E., Beekman, M., Frolich, M., de Craen, A. J., . . . van Heemst, D. (2010). Familial longevity is associated with decreased thyroid function. *The Journal of Clinical Endocrinology & Metabolism*, *95*, 4979–4984.

Rudman, D., Kutner, M. H., Rogers, C. M., Lubin, M. F., Fleming, G. A., & Bain, R. P. (1981). Impaired growth hormone secretion in the adult population: Relation to age and adiposity. *Journal of Clinical Investigation*, *67*, 1361–1369.

Sanders, A. E., Wang, C., Katz, M., Derby, C. A., Barzilai, N., Ozelius, L., & Lipton, R. B. (2010). Association of a functional polymorphism in the cholesteryl ester transfer protein (CETP) gene with memory decline and incidence of dementia. *JAMA: The Journal of the American Medical Association*, *303*, 150–158. http://dx.doi.org/10.1001/jama.2009.1988

Serna, E., Gambini, J., Borras, C., Abdelaziz, K. M., Belenguer, A., Sanchis, P., . . . Vina, J. (2012). Centenarians, but not octogenarians, up-regulate the expression of microRNAs. *Scientific Reports*, 2, 961. http://dx.doi.org/10.1038/srep00961

Suh, Y., Atzmon, G., Cho, M. O., Hwang, D., Liu, B., Leahy, D. J., . . . Cohen, P. (2008). Functionally significant insulin-like growth factor I receptor mutations in centenarians. *Proceedings of the National Academy of Sciences of the United States of America*, *105*, 3438–3442. http://dx.doi.org/10.1073/pnas.0705467105

Tazearslan, C., Huang, J., Barzilai, N., & Suh, Y. (2011). Impaired IGF-IR signaling in cells expressing longevity-associated human IGF-IR alleles. *Aging Cell*, *10*, 551–554. http://dx.doi.org/10.1111/j.1474-9726.2011.00697.x

Vance, M. L., & Mauras, N. (1999). Growth hormone therapy in adults and children. *The New England Journal of Medicine*, *341*, 1206–1216. http://dx.doi.org/10.1056/NEJM199910143411607

Volkova, M., Garg, R., Dick, S., & Boheler, K. R. (2005). Aging-associated changes in cardiac gene expression. *Cardiovascular Research*, *66*, 194–204. http://dx.doi.org/10.1016/j.cardiores.2004.11.016

Yashin, A. I., De Benedictis, G., Vaupel, J. W., Tan, Q., Andreev, K. F., Iachine, I. A., . . . Franceschi, C. (2000). Genes and longevity: Lessons from studies of centenarians. *The Journals of Gerontology Series A: Biological Sciences and Medical Sciences*, *55*, B319–B328.

CHAPTER 7

Etiology of Individual Differences in Human Health and Longevity

Deborah Finkel, Lotte Gerritsen, Chandra A. Reynolds, Anna K. Dahl, and Nancy L. Pedersen

ABSTRACT

In this chapter, we review of the field of gerontological genetics with respect to subjective and objective health, the role of stress on health, and finally frailty and longevity. For most indices of subjective and objective health, frailty, and longevity, genetic influences contribute only modestly to individual differences, wherein heritabilities are typically on the order of 35%–40%. Notable exceptions are the moderate to strong heritabilities for lipid measures and brain structure and function, with a remarkably increasing role of genetic influences for longevity with advancing age. Although candidate gene and genome-wide association studies (GWAS) studies have identified gene variants associated with many subjective and objective health traits, their effect sizes are typically relatively small, as expected for complex traits. There is some evidence for gene–environment interactions, and stress may be an important moderator of genetic variance for health. For example, carrying a risk genotype for cardiovascular disease (CVD) in the angiotensin converting enzyme gene (*ACE*) may predict stress responsivity and risk of cardiovascular-related diagnoses. Moreover, the gene coding for apolipoprotein E (*APOE*) may moderate responsiveness to stress evoking experiences, impact of physical exercise, and associate with sleep characteristics in those who develop cognitive impairments. For metabolic syndrome (MetS), encompassing the co-occurrence of obesity, hypertension, hypertriglyceridemia,

http://dx.doi.org/10.1891/0198-8794.34.189

and hyperinsulinemia, promising associations exist although no single genotype or any gene clusters have been consistently associated with MetS across populations, suggesting that complex gene–environment interactions must be understood before the use of genetic markers can be realized in clinical practice. Future investigations of subjective and objective health, frailty, and longevity are needed to further identify sources of genetic and environmental contributions—and their dynamics across adulthood—to advance understanding of aging processes, prevention, and intervention avenues, and ultimately successful aging.

INTRODUCTION

During the last 30 years, several longitudinal studies of aging have begun to focus not only on normative behaviors and health but also on the etiology of individual differences and the role that genes have in phenotypic variation. Several twin studies of aging have matured and provided a wealth of information on heritability, whereas other studies of aging have increasingly taken a candidate gene approach or even applied genome-wide association studies (GWAS) to understand the magnitude and role of genetic influences on individual differences. Because human health and behavior is so complex, a review of the field of gerontological genetics could encompass a multitude of areas, spanning all aspects of behavior, such as cognitive aging, well-being, and adjustment to all aspects of health and longevity. In the following sections, we will focus on subjective and objective health, the role of stress on health, and finally frailty and longevity.

SUBJECTIVE HEALTH

Although most research investigating facets of the aging process that promote longevity focuses on biological and physical factors, subjective measures of functioning can provide insight into the functioning of the system as a whole. In a sense, measures of subjective health serve to put the person back into the stimulus-outcome equation. The physiological impact of environmental and psychological stressors, for example, will be mediated by the coping mechanisms of the individual. Assessing self-rated health (SRH) taps an individual's holistic perception of their functioning, over and above the data provided by objective measures of health. In this section, we review genetic investigations of measures subjective health and aging.

Psychosocial Stress and Health

It is commonly accepted that psychosocial stress is a risk factor for several severe illnesses, including cardiovascular disease (CVD; Steptoe & Kivimaki, 2012), immune disorders (Miller, Chen, & Parker, 2011), and dementia (Magri et al., 2006). Particularly, old age encompasses powerful stressors because of important life changes such as retirement and frequent occurrence of negative events such as loss of loved ones and new diseases. Chronic or repeated exposure to psychosocial stressors can induce alterations in the nervous system, the endocrine system, and the immune system (Juster, McEwen, & Lupien, 2010). In the nervous system, the experience of psychosocial stressors leads to structural and functional abnormalities in stress-sensitive regions such as the prefrontal cortex, the amygdala, and the hippocampus. In the endocrine system, exposure to psychosocial stressors is associated with chronic activation of the hypothalamic pituitary adrenal (HPA) axis, resulting in increased corticotropin-releasing factor (CRH) levels. Chronic stress is also associated with lower morning cortisol levels and elevated afternoon cortisol levels, resulting in flatter circadian variation and greater daily output of cortisol. HPA axis hyperactivity may not only be caused by alterations in the brain but can also be stimulated by elevated inflammation levels. In the immune system, chronic exposure to psychosocial stressors leads to long-lasting elevated levels of inflammatory markers and impaired cell-mediated acquired immunity. It has also been hypothesized that chronic exposure to stress may lead to accelerated cell aging (Wolkowitz, Epel, & Mellon, 2008) through dysregulation of the HPA axis, which can lead to a detrimental cascade of events, including intracellular glucose deficiency, glutamatergic hyperactivity, increased cellular calcium concentrations, mitochondrial damage, free radical generation, and increased oxidative stress. This cascade of events, coupled with increased levels of inflammatory markers, may lead to accelerated cellular aging via effects on the telomere/telomerase maintenance system, eventually leading to onset of age-related diseases (Tomiyama et al., 2012). Because aging itself is related to an increased basal activity and flattened diurnal amplitude of the HPA axis (Deuschle et al., 1997) and decreased telomere length (Njajou et al., 2009), chronic stress in old age may be particularly harmful (Bauer, Jeckel, & Luz, 2009).

The extent to which psychosocial stress will be harmful greatly depends on individual factors, including personality, coping style, preceding experiences, and genetic makeup (Hammen, 2006). Heritability for the experience of stressful events has been estimated between 5% and 45% (Bemmels, Burt, Legrand, Iacono, & McGue, 2008) depending on the type of stressor, where events dependent on the individual (e.g., getting laid off from job) are more heritable than familial (divorce of parents) or independent events (e.g., natural disasters; Bolinskey, Neale, Jacobson, Prescott, & Kendler, 2004; Plomin, Lichtenstein, Pedersen, McClearn, & Nesselroade, 1990). Furthermore, a twin study on HPA axis regulation found that genetics accounted for 40% of the variation of the mean increase in cortisol after awakening, and 48% of the variation of the of the overall area under the curve of the cortisol awakening response (Wust, Federenko,

Hellhammer, & Kirschbaum, 2000). Moreover, research has shown that whether a person develops an illness in response to stressful events is not explained by the same genetic risks as the sole experience of stressful events, suggesting that there are specific genetic factors that play a role in susceptibility for stress-related illnesses and not the experience of stress per se. The genetic factors that confer risk for trauma do not overlap completely with those that confer risk for stress-related disease (Amstadter, Aggen, Knudsen, Reichborn-Kjennerud, & Kendler, 2012). Because most people show resilience to stress, there is probably a vulnerable group of people who are more susceptible to the effects of stress (Feder, Nestler, & Charney, 2009).

Numerous studies have examined gene-by-stress interactions on the onset of neuropsychiatric diseases and cardiovascular outcomes. Genetic variations that consistently have shown to increase the risk for depression after the experience of stress are the short allele of the serotonin transporter promotor gene, 5-HTTLPR (Caspi, Hariri, Holmes, Uher, & Moffitt, 2010; Karg, Burmeister, Shedden, & Sen, 2011) and the met-allele of the gene coding for brain-derived neurotrophic factor(BDNF; Drachmann et al., 2009; Duman, 2009). With regard to dementia and cognitive aging, carriers of the *APOE*-e4 allele were found to be at higher risk for cognitive decline and mild cognitive impairment when they also had experienced stress compared to noncarriers (Gerritsen, Comijs, Deeg, Penninx, & Geerlings, 2011; Peavy, 2008), whereas another study found that genes involved in serotonin, estrogen, and cholesterol pathways can interact with stress on memory decline and depressive symptoms in elderly (Reynolds, Gatz, Berg, & Pedersen, 2007). Stress by gene interactions may also play a role in cardiovascular disorders because a recent study showed that the angiotensin converting enzyme (*ACE*) rs4291 TT genotype, which has been associated with HPA axis hyperactivity and higher levels of serum ACE, predicted acute stress response and more cardiovascular-related diagnoses after the experience of collective stress (e.g., 9/11; Holman, 2012).

Self-Rated Health

SRH is a complex variable that assesses personality and cognitive status as well as general physical health (e.g., Svedberg, Bardage, Sandin, & Pedersen, 2006). For example, in a factor analysis that included measures of cognition, objective health, lifestyle factors, and personality, SRH combined with neuroticism and physical exercise to form a single factor that was labeled "well-being" (Finkel, Pedersen, Berg, & Johansson, 2000). In a meta-analysis, Pinquart (2001) found that SRH was associated with functional, physical, and mental health. In spite of, or perhaps because of, this complex pedigree, SRH can predict longevity independent of objective health measures (Idler & Benyamini, 1997; Luszcz,

1996; McCallum, Shadbolt, & Wang, 1994). Behavior genetic investigations of SRH in older adults indicate that approximately 25%–40% of the individual differences results from genetic factors (Christensen, Holm, McGue, Corder, & Vaupel, 1999; Svedberg, Lichtenstein, & Pedersen, 2001). However, multivariate analyses demonstrate that much of the genetic variance for SRH is shared with genetic variance for associated phenotypes such as depression (Mosing, Pedersen, Martin, & Wright, 2010), cognitive function (Svedberg, Gatz, & Pedersen, 2009), and disease severity (Leinonen et al., 2005). In other words, the complex pedigree of SRH is reflected in its genetic architecture. In support of this conclusion, a recent GWAS reported that no genome-wide single nucleotide polymorphisms (SNPs) could be identified, indicating that SRH is likely influenced by a large number of genes with very small effect (Mosing, Verweij, et al., 2010). Indeed, these genes are as likely to reflect personality or cognitive traits as they are to impact SRH directly. For example, F. Zhang and colleagues (2008) reported an interaction between *APOE* allele status, physical exercise, and SRH. Their results suggested that the beneficial effects of physical exercise were attenuated among carriers of the *APOE*-e4 allele. Thus, attempts to identify genetic and environmental contributions to longevity will need to consider holistic measures such as SRH and stress as well as measures of objective health discussed in the following sections.

OBJECTIVE HEALTH

It can be difficult to discuss components of objective health as separate entities because functioning one area often overlaps or contributes to functioning in other areas. We begin our discussion of the etiology of individual differences in components of objective health associated with the aging process by focusing on physiological and biological phenotypes, leading up to the concept of metabolic syndrome, which incorporates many of those phenotypes. Then we discuss functional and behavioral phenotypes that typically engage multiple systems, leading up to investigations of the overarching construct of frailty. Finally, we examine the etiology of individual differences in the aging brain.

Obesity

The prevalence of obesity, usually defined as a body mass index (BMI) $\geq$ 30 kg/m^2, has increased dramatically across the world during the last century. The increase in obesity is mainly considered to originate from behavioral and environmental changes, such as high caloric intake and a sedentary lifestyle (Kopelman, 2000). Nevertheless, a large proportion of the variation in BMI is estimated to be influenced by genetic variants, as witnessed by a reported heritability of ~70%

(Silventoinen & Kaprio, 2009). Recent large-scale meta-analyses of GWAS have identified numerous genetic variants associated with BMI (Speliotes et al., 2010). The most well researched obesity gene is the fat mass and obesity associated (*FTO*) gene. *FTO* has been associated with variations in BMI in the population and has also been shown to be associated with weight gain in childhood and middle age (Haworth et al., 2008).

Although it is well-known that persons with normal weight (BMI of 18.5–24.9 kg/m^2) in midlife have a better prognosis of health and survival than obese persons in midlife, the association between BMI, health, and survival in late life is poorly understood (Ferrucci, Studenski, Alley, Barbagallo, & Harris, 2010). In late life, low BMI (often including normal weight) is often associated with negative health outcomes, such as an increased risk of dementia and mortality, whereas overweight (BMI of 25.0–29.9 kg/m^2) and sometimes even obesity is associated with a better health prognosis and survival (Dahl, Lopponen, Isoaho, Berg, & Kivela, 2008; Romero-Corral et al., 2006). This shift in association is often referred to as the obesity paradox and is hypothesized to be driven by weight loss primarily caused by disease processes. Therefore, the underlying causes as well as the implications of BMI and changes in BMI may differ across the life course.

So far, few twin studies and/or genetic studies have focused on unraveling the underlying causes of weight change in late life. Cross-sectional twin studies indicate that the heritability of BMI remains high in late life, that the nonshared environmental influences on BMI increase in late life, and that common environmental influences are negligible in late life (Nan et al., 2012). Extending these findings, longitudinal Swedish twin data indicate that both the nonshared environmental and genetic influence on change in BMI increase across the lifespan (Dahl & Reynolds, 2012). This raises the question whether there is amplification of genetic influences or perhaps new genetic influences emerging in late life. The influence of a genetic risk score, based on 32 SNPs (Speliotes et al., 2010), on BMI and change in BMI across the lifespan has been evaluated in two large Swedish population-based twin studies: the Swedish Adoption Twin Study of Aging (SATSA) and TwinGene. The obesity genetic risk score was associated with mean level BMI at age 65 years, and change in BMI up to the age of 65 years, but not with weight change after the age of 65 years (Dahl, Reynolds, Fall, Magnusson, & Pedersen, 2013). These initial findings emphasize the need for studies with a specific focus on BMI and changes BMI in late life because findings based on young or middle-aged adults likely do not apply to old persons.

Serum Lipids

Serum lipid traits—primarily total cholesterol (TC), LDL, HDL, and triglycerides (TG)—have been of enduring interest with respect to aging outcomes, including cardiovascular and cognitive health. Heritable variance across traits is moderate to strong, from 37% to 79% (Beekman et al., 2002; Cai, Hayakawa, Nishihara, & Kato, 2009; Goode, Cherny, Christian, Jarvik, & de Andrade, 2007, Middelberg, Spector, Swaminathan, & Snieder, 2002; Nilsson, Read, Berg, & Johansson, 2009; Pietiläinen et al., 2009; Pilia et al., 2006). Shared environmental contributions vary across studies but may contribute to HDL although such effects may wane with age (Dahlen, Ericson, de Faire, Iselius, & Lundman, 1983; Goode et al., 2007; Knoblauch et al., 1997; Middelberg, Martin, & Whitfield, 2006; Middelberg et al., 2002; Nilsson et al., 2009; S. Zhang et al., 2009). Longitudinal work suggests genes contribute to continuity of lipid levels across time (Friedlander et al., 1997; Middelberg et al., 2006). That said, partly unique genetic factors contribute to early adulthood lipid levels for HDL, LDL, and TG (age 18–35 years) but not in mid-adulthood (Friedlander et al., 1997; Middelberg et al., 2006), whereas new genetic factors emerge for LDL by midlife not present earlier (Middelberg et al., 2006). After age 50 years, heritable factors may decrease with age for TGs and apolipoprotein B (ApoB), the primary constituent of LDL (Heller, de Faire, Pedersen, Dahlen, & McClearn, 1993). Longitudinal analyses of aging male twins reported stable longitudinal genetic factors for TC, LDL, HD, and TG and modest amplification in heritability across nearly two decades (Goode et al., 2007). Gender differences in heritability and environmentality appear negligible (Heller et al., 1993; Middelberg et al., 2006), apart from ApoB with greater shared rearing environment influences for women than men (Heller et al., 1993).

Gene Candidates for Lipids. APOE encodes the primary cholesterol transporter in the brain, apolipoprotein E (ApoE), and is the most widely confirmed Alzheimer's disease candidate. Moreover, the *APOE* gene has evidenced the strongest signal in a recent GWAS of longevity (Deelen et al., 2011). The heritability of ApoE levels varies from .48 to .87 in middle-aged and older twins (Beekman et al., 2002; Cai et al., 2009). *APOE* genotype is associated with various serum lipid traits (Bennet et al., 2007; Bennet et al., 2010). Those carrying the e4 risk allele have poorer lipid profiles than e2 carriers or those with the e3/e3 genotype (Bennet et al., 2007).

Altogether, more than 95 genes reached genome-wide significance in a meta GWAS for lipid traits and explain as much as 25%–30% of the genetic variance (Teslovich et al., 2010). Four of the 95 candidates show heterogeneous impacts to lipid levels for men versus women and 5 candidates showed sex-specific associations; for example, the *KLF14* rs1562398 variant predicted TG levels in women ($p = 2 \times 10^{-12}$) but not men ($p = .05$). Eighteen of the identified genes were located near regions in which lipid-related Mendelian disorders had already been observed (Teslovich et al., 2010). Genetic risk scores from GWAS-identified lipid genes have been associated with clinically relevant outcomes such as coronary artery disease (CAD; Aulchenko et al., 2009).

A recent gene association study targeted variability in lipid and lipoprotein levels using a monozygotic (MZ) twin within-pair approach (Surakka et al., 2012). Indeed, a variant in the *APOE/APOC1* region on chromosome (chr) 19 as well as in the *DOCK1* gene on chr 10 (involved in cell surface restructuring and apoptosis) were associated with variability in both ApoE and ApoB levels in primary and replication sample sets. Overall, this work suggests that differential sensitivity to environmental factors based on genotype may be fruitful to pursue with measured environmental factors.

Diet and lifestyle factors, including smoking, alcohol consumption, obesity, and physically demanding occupations contribute to differences in lipid levels even amongst identical twin pairs (Hayakawa, Shimizu, Ohba, & Tomioka, 1987; Pietiläinen et al., 2009; Surakka et al., 2012). Moreover, rearing environments may be of lasting importance to total cholesterol even after the age of 50 years, as well as ApoA1 and ApoB levels in those 65 years and older suggesting cohort factors such as dietary habits may be important (Heller et al., 1993).

Blood Pressure

Blood pressure (BP) components, primarily systolic BP (SBP) and diastolic BP (DBP), generally evidence small to moderate heritability estimates about 19%–42% in population-based twin registry or family samples (Albarwani et al., 2012; Fagard, Loos, Beunen, Derom, & Vlietinck, 2003; Hottenga et al., 2005; Hottenga, Whitfield, de Geus, Boomsma, & Martin, 2006; Kupper et al., 2005; Pilia et al., 2006; Tarnoki et al., 2012; S. Zhang et al., 2009). Moreover, heritability for BP may increase with age (Colletto, Cardon, & Fulker, 1993; Friedlander et al., 1997; Pilia et al., 2006). Profile analysis of multiple gene loci supports this as well, suggesting overlapping polygenic contributions to blood pressure that increase in effect from childhood to adulthood (Taal et al., 2012). Effects of shared environmental contributions appear to be small at best (Elder et al., 2009), including no effect of chorionicity (Fagard et al., 2003). A higher heritability of BP traits has been reported in females than males, albeit it appears the same genetic factors are at work (Zeegers et al., 2004). Nevertheless, sex differences in relative magnitudes are not routinely observed (Hottenga et al., 2005; Pilia et al., 2006). The heritability of hypertension is strongly heritable at about 46%–63% (Kupper et al., 2005; McCaffery, Papandonatos, Lyons, & Niaura, 2008).

GWAS have identified several genes involved in blood pressure (SBP and DBP) and the risk of hypertension, although replications have not been consistent across efforts (Adeyemo et al., 2009; Ehret et al., 2008; Ganesh et al., 2013;

Kidambi et al., 2012; Levy et al., 2009; Newton-Cheh et al., 2009; Padmanabhan et al., 2010). Moreover, previously identified candidate genes such as that encoding *ACE* have not been replicated in GWAS using stringent *p* values, although meta-analysis suggests an association (Takeuchi et al., 2012). Altogether, several loci may be relevant across populations (e.g., *ATP2B1*, *CNNM2-NT5C2*, *FGF5*, *CASZ1*, *CSK-ULK3*, *MTHFR*). Select loci may be population specific: for example, amongst populations of East Asia, a variant in the *RPN6-PTPN11* gene (rs11066280) may derive its effect from the nearby *ALDH2* gene involved in alcohol metabolism (Kato et al., 2011).

Identified environmental influences include demographic (education, socioeconomic status [SES]), diet (e.g., salt intake, alcohol consumption), and lifestyle factors (e.g., physical exercise, obesity; Krieger, Chen, Coull, & Selby, 2005; Rebholz et al., 2012; Waller, Kujala, Kaprio, Koskenvuo, & Rantanen, 2010). For example, physical activity or weight loss interventions may be beneficial in those whose high BP is a result of salt or weight sensitivity, suggesting that those predisposed to higher BP via such pathways may particularly benefit from environmental treatments (Gu et al., 2013; Kostis et al., 2013; Rebholz et al., 2012). Lastly, educational attainment, which may be correlated with several health and lifestyle factors of relevance, appears to moderate heritability of hypertension in male twins, such that heritability was lower among twin pairs with 14 years or less of education (46%) and higher among twin pairs with 15 years or more (63%; McCaffery et al., 2008).

Heart Rate Variability

Heart period (HP), respiratory sinus arrhythmia (RSA), and other related indices from ECG that index heart rate variability (HRV), are predictive of cardiac events and mortality as well as associated with psychosocial stress and sleep problems among other health outcomes (Xhyheri, Manfrini, Mazzolini, Pizzi, & Bugiardini, 2012). Heart rate (HR), HP, and RSA are moderately to strongly heritable (De Geus, Boomsma, & Snieder, 2003; Kupper et al., 2004; Li et al., 2009; Singh et al., 1999; Snieder, van Doornen, Boomsma, & Thayer, 2007; Uusitalo et al., 2007), and estimates vary according to contexts such as at-rest and under experimentally induced stress conditions (De Geus, Kupper, Boomsma, & Snieder, 2007). Heritability estimates for RSA are similar in adolescent and middle-aged twins (31% and 32% at rest, 54% and 44% under stress, respectively; De Geus et al., 2007). Moreover, stress conditions appear to amplify existing genetic effects and engage added genes (De Geus et al., 2007). Lastly, resting RSA and a related measure, approximate entropy (ApEn), are similarly heritable in middle-aged men and women (30%–40%), despite the fact that women have higher HRV (Snieder et al., 2007). Little effect of shared environmental factors have been reported, with the remaining variation caused by person-specific environmental influences (Kupper et al., 2004).

Several gene candidates have been identified across several GWAS (Deo et al., 2013; Eijgelsheim et al., 2010; Holm et al., 2010; Newton-Cheh et al., 2007). We highlight two genes with variants confirmed for resting HR across populations that are of African, Asian, or European origins: (a) *GJA1* that encodes connexin 43, the major protein constituent of the human myocardial gap junction, and (b) *MYH6* (myosin, heavy chain 6, cardiac muscle, alpha) that encodes for a heavy chain subunit of cardiac muscle myosin (Deo et al., 2013).

Several health and lifestyle factors are associated with HRV, including caffeine, smoking, BMI, medication use, and chronic illness load. In a study of middle-aged twins, physical load of occupations emerged as explaining about 4% of individual differences among healthy middle-aged twins while BMI and coffee consumption explained about 2% each (Uusitalo et al., 2007); among a subset of twins who were ill, BMI and smoking explained a small amount of variation (Uusitalo et al., 2007). However, by and large, heritability estimates for most HRV measures were rather similar in healthy and unhealthy twins.

Self-reported exercise behaviors correlate with HP and RSA more strongly in adolescence than in middle age but appear to predominantly covary because of shared genetic etiologies when correlations are observed (De Geus et al., 2003). It is possible that although the benefits of exercise on HRV may be understood, individual choice to participate in exercise in adulthood (or not) is an example of gene–environment correlation or a selection process (Stubbe, Boomsma, & De Geus, 2005). Environmental selection factors notwithstanding, exercise interventions have shown benefits to HRV, for example, among postmenopausal women who have a confluence of risk factors for poor cardiovascular health (e.g., overweight, hypertension; Earnest, Blair, & Church, 2012).

Lastly, a body of literature has emerged on the impact of air pollution on HRV measures, with support for an inverse relationship in a recent meta-analysis (Pieters et al., 2012). Emerging small sample work suggests potential gene–environment interactions on the extent of pollutant effects. For example, individuals who are health compromised may be more vulnerable to the effects of air pollution on HRV given increased genetic risk for several gene variants associated with circadian rhythm (Hampel et al., 2012).

Metabolic Syndrome

Although obesity, hypertension, and hypertriglyceridemia have been discussed separately in this chapter thus far, these health states often co-occur, in conjunction with hyperinsulinemia, in a syndrome that has been referred to with various names such as insulin-resistance syndrome, syndrome X, and so forth but is most commonly referred to as the metabolic syndrome (MetS). Insulin-resistance and obesity (especially abdominal obesity) are key components of the syndrome, and one of the components might trigger the onset of the other components (Eckel, Grundy, & Zimmet, 2005). The prevalence is high in adults (about 24%) and increases with advancing age (Ford, Giles, & Dietz, 2002).

Given that high caloric diet and physical inactivity are risk factors for all the components, not the least obesity and insulin-resistance, lifestyle factors play an important role in the development of MetS. Other risk factors include inflammatory processes and genetic causes that will be discussed in the following sections.

Twin research indicated long before the GWAS era that there are genetic variants shared by the components of MetS (Hong, Pedersen, Brismar, & de Faire, 1997). In particular, obesity and insulin-resistance share the same genetic effects, and these genetic effects are also associated albeit to a lesser degree with the other components, HDL, TGs, and SBP.

Genes that have been associated with the individual components of MetS have also been associated with the syndrome as a whole, such as *FTO* (Al-Attar et al., 2008) and lipid variants residing in *APOC1* (Avery et al., 2011) and the *APOA1/C3/A4/A5* gene cluster (Kristiansson et al., 2012). Moreover, other pleiotropic genes may include *BRAP*, *IRS1*, and the immune-related *PLCG1* (Avery et al., 2011; Fall & Ingelsson, 2012). Although these findings are promising, no single genotype or cluster of genotypes has been identified that is consistently associated with MetS across populations (Joy, Lahiry, Pollex, & Hegele, 2008), as for many other complex traits. It is likely that there are complex gene–environment interactions that need to be understood before genomic DNA markers can be of use in clinical practice.

Muscle Strength

Grip strength is often considered a cost-effective proxy for general biological vitality (Frederiksen et al., 2002). A recent review of biomarkers assessed in the Health and Retirement Study verifies that measures of physical function including walking speed and grip strength are associated with longevity (Ailshire & Crimmins, 2013). In fact, physical function (including grip strength) has been shown to predict longevity even when age, BMI, smoking status, education, physical activity, and cognitive status are taken into account (De Buyser et al., 2013). Studies of older twins in Denmark, Finland, and Sweden indicate heritability estimates for both upper-body strength (e.g., hand grip) and lower-body strength (e.g., knee extension) range from 30% to 60% (Finkel et al., 2003; Frederiksen et al., 2002; Tiainen et al., 2004, 2005). McGue and Christensen (2013) recently confirmed that genetic contributions to grip strength are stable across the second half of the lifespan. Attempts to identify specific gene variants associated with muscle strength have met with limited success (e.g., Alfred et al., 2013; Vasunilashorn, Glei, Lin, & Goldman, 2013), although Charbonneau and colleagues (2008) reported a relationship between a polymorphism in the *ACE* gene, typically associated with cardiovascular health, and genetic variance in muscle strength.

Functional Ability

Disability is often assessed via self-report of activities of daily living (ADL); whereas functional ability is typically assessed via objective measures of functional tasks, such as walking, balance, and chair stands. Correlations between the two types of measures tend to be significant but modest, ranging from .30 to .54 (Ernsth-Bravel, Zarit, Johansson, 2011), and evidence suggests that self-reported ADL can reflect affect and personality as well as functional ability (Jagger et al., 2010; Kempen, Steverink, Ormel, & Deeg, 1996). Both ADL and function ability have been shown to predict longevity (Ailshire & Crimmins, 2013; Stineman et al., 2012; Taekema, Gussekloo, Westendorp, de Craen, & Maier, 2012; Tiainen, Luukkaala, Hervonen, & Jylha, 2013); moreover, slower rates of change over time in measures of functional performance predict longer survival (Hirsch, Buzkova, Robbins, Patel, & Newman, 2012; White et al., 2013). Behavior genetic investigations of functional ability have produced mixed results (Christensen, Frederiksen, Vaupel, & McGue, 2003; Finkel et al., 2000; Finkel et al., 2003; Finkel, Reynolds, Emery, & Pedersen, 2013). Evidence suggests, however, gender and age differences in genetic influences on physical functioning. Individual differences in physical functioning tend to be minimal before ages 65 or 70 years and to increase dramatically afterward; increases in variance reflect both genetic and environmental factors (Finkel et al., 2003; Finkel et al., 2013). In general, heritability estimates for measures of physical ability tend to be higher for women than for men, particularly for measures that tap gross motor movement such as walking and balance (Christensen et al., 2003; Finkel et al., 2013). The gender difference in heritability likely reflects the higher prevalence of genetically influenced chronic disabling diseases in women compared to men's more compressed history of disability prior to death (Sainio et al., 2006). In addition, differences in environmental exposures related to both work and leisure time activity (e.g., Gardner & Montgomery, 2008) could result in greater environmental variance for physical ability in men in older cohorts.

Lung Function

Lung function not only predicts mortality (Strachan, 1992; Young, Hopkins, & Eaton, 2007), but it is associated with general functional status of older adults in several domains, including walking speed, cognitive function, and self-rated health (e.g., Emery, Finkel, & Pedersen, 2012; Singh-Manoux et al., 2011). Recent work indicates that genetic variance for lung function drives subsequent genetic variance for cognitive aging (Finkel et al., 2013). In addition, research suggests that the link between lung function and mortality reflects both health and lifestyle factors (Sabia et al., 2010). Thus, it can be argued that lung function serves as a fairly good proxy for overall functioning in old age (Singh-Manoux et al., 2011). At the very least, lung function plays a fundamental role in the aging process. Quantitative genetic analyses indicate that the heritability of lung function ranges from 30% to 50%, depending on the spirometric measure used (Hukkinen et al., 2011; McClearn, Svartengren, Pedersen, Heller, & Plomin, 1994; Vasilopoulos et al., 2010; Whitfield, Wiggins, Belue, & Brandon, 2004). Moreover, multivariate analysis of several spirometric measures indicated only modest overlap in genetic variance, with significant genetic variance unique to each measure of lung function (Vasilopoulos et al., 2013). The complex etiology of lung function is reflected in the mixed results from attempts to identify specific genes associated with spirometric measures (Hancock et al., 2010; Repapi et al., 2010; Wilk et al., 2000). For example, a recent analysis had little success in replicating gene loci identified in previous studies (Obeidat et al., 2011). However, the researchers did identify possible gene by environment interactions—two loci (*SERPINA1* and *PDE4D*) demonstrated associations with lung function only in smokers. In a meta-analysis of GWAS studies that incorporated more than 48,000 individuals, 16 different gene loci were associated with lung function, however, neither *SERPINA1* nor *PDE4D* were on the list and no interactions with smoking were identified (Soler Artigas et al., 2011).

Sleep

Older age is associated with changes in sleep patterns, sleep quality, and several severe sleep problems including insomnia, parasomnia, and apnea (Dijk, Duffy, & Czeisler, 2000). In general, deep non-rapid eye movement (NREM) sleep is reduced, older persons have more awakenings from sleep, and their time spent awake in bed trying to sleep is increased. Age-related diseases such as CVD (Prinz, 1995), cancer (Asplund, 1999), nocturia (Asplund, 2005), pain (Prinz, 1995), diabetes (Foley, Ancoli-Israel, Britz, & Walsh, 2004), and dementia (Vitiello & Borson, 2001) can worsen these sleep disturbances. It is estimated that 40%–70% of older adults experience chronic sleep problems (Prinz, Vitiello, Raskind, & Thorpy, 1990). Aging is also associated with changes in the physiology of the internal circadian system that regulates the 24-hr rhythms in human physiology and behavior; these age-related changes in circadian physiology are thought to contribute to sleep problems (Dijk et al., 2000).

Twin studies on sleep report heritability estimates for sleep quality and duration between 33% and 53% for men and women, respectively (Paunio et al., 2009), whereas heritabilities for sleeping problems including insomnia are as high as 58% (Wing et al., 2012). Only one study looked into heritability in old age; in older men, heritability for sleep quality was around 20% and sleep duration was around 29% (Genderson et al., 2013). Given that sex differences in heritability have been reported in younger adults (age <65 years), it is unclear to what extent these results can be generalized to women.

Several genes, including adenosine deaminase (*ADA*), PERIOD3 (*PER3*), Circadian Locomotor Output Cycles Kaput (*CLOCK*), and Basic Helix-Loop-Helix Family, member e41 (*BHLHE41*) have been identified as contributing to sleep characteristics (Barclay & Gregory, 2013). Recently, a few genome-wide studies showed that genetic variation in the *CACNA1C* gene was associated with sleep quality and latency (Allebrandt et al., 2013; Parsons et al., 2013). The *CACNA1C* gene is an L-type voltage-dependent calcium channel previously associated with psychiatric disorders and is associated with sleep latency and sleep quality (Kalkman, 2012; Shimada et al., 2010). Another GWAS on sleep quality found that variation in the *ABCC9* gene, an ATP-sensitive potassium channel, was associated with sleep duration and accounted for 5% of the variance of this trait. Most genetic studies on sleep so far were conducted without consideration of age. In a study among patients with mild cognitive impairment (MCI), however, *APOE*-e4 carriers with MCI showed a larger reduction in REM sleep than noncarriers (Hita-Yañez, Atienza, Gil-Neciga, & Cantero, 2012), suggesting that there is an interaction between *APOE* genotype and MCI status on sleep characteristics.

Brain Morphology and Activity

The brain undergoes structural changes with aging and already early in adulthood, the brain begins decreasing in volume (Fotenos, Snyder, Girton, Morris, & Buckner, 2005). The loss in volume seems to be accelerated in those with cognitive impairment (den Heijer et al., 2012), and demented individuals have smaller brain volumes than clinically normal persons (Ikram et al., 2010). In a recent study using voxel-based morphometry to measure gray matter changes over the lifespan, age-related gray matter decline in nearly all parts of the brain were found, with particularly rapid decline in inferior regions of the frontal cortex (e.g., insula and left inferior frontal gyrus) and the central sulcus (Peelle, Cusack, & Henson, 2012). The healthy adult brain undergoes continual changes in white matter driven by development and repair processes devoted to creating and maintaining neural networks (Bartzokis et al., 2012). Besides structural brain changes, functional changes are also frequent in normal aging;

resting-state functional magnetic resonance imaging (fMRI) studies have found that age-related changes in functional connections tended to linearly increase in parts of the brain that play a role in processing of emotion, whereas decreasing connectivity was found in parts that play a role in sensorimotor functions (Wang, Su, Shen, & Hu, 2012). Vascular factors (e.g., atherosclerosis and dyslipidemia) also contribute to age-related brain changes, leading to white matter hyperintensities (WMH; Launer et al., 2000) and lacunar infarcts (Geerlings, Appelman, Vincken, Mali, & van der Graaf, 2009). WMHs in the brain increase with age (DeCarli et al., 2005) and have been implicated in cognitive decline and dementia (Stewart, 2012).

Normal aging is also associated with neuropathological changes in the brain, such as tau neurofibrillary tangles and amyloid plaques, and these neuropathological changes occur well before the start of cognitive changes, which may eventually lead to dementia (Braak & Braak, 1995). Nowadays, these neuropathological changes can be examined in vivo (Klunk et al., 2004; Small et al., 2006). In healthy elderly, changes in positron-emission tomography (PET) signals are also highly correlated with cognitive performance (Braskie et al., 2010).

Several twin studies examining the heritability of brain structure and function have been conducted. Among young adults, the heritabilities for gray and white matter volumes were estimated at 73% and 90%, respectively (Smit, Boomsma, Schnack, Hulshoff Pol, & de Geus, 2012). Although in a study among older male twins, the heritability of total brain volume was more than 70%, changes over time in total brain volume were not affected by genetic influences. Thus, variation in longitudinal change may have different underlying genetic and environmental pathways than variation seen cross-sectionally (Lessov-Schlaggar et al., 2012). In the same group of older male twins, heritability of white matter hyperintensities was 74% (Carmelli, Reed, & DeCarli, 2002). Moreover, they found that the associations between WMHs and poor cognitive and physical function in the elderly were to a great extent explained by genetic influences in common to the traits. In another large study among elderly male twins, heritabilities for subcortical volumes were between 60% and 80% (Kremen et al., 2010), whereas heritabilities for cortical thickness were around 40%–70% (Eyler et al., 2012).

Using young adult twins, Koten and colleagues (2009) investigated the heritability of brain activity and found that a substantial portion of response time and brain activity during working memory tasks proved to be under genetic influence (heritabilities up to 80%). Genetic effects were found bilaterally and included visual cortex, angular gyrus, intraparietal sulcus, temporoparietal junction, motor and premotor cortex, frontal eye field, inferior frontal gyrus, cuneus, and anterior cingulate cortex: all of which are regions that have been related to working memory functions (Koten et al., 2009).

Recently, several attempts have been made to identify genetic influences on brain imaging phenotypes. Two large GWAS have been conducted, combining neuroimaging data from several studies. No significant findings were found for total brain volume, but for intracranial volume, two loci were found: a known height-associated locus on chr 6q22 and a locus on chr 17q21 (Ikram et al., 2012). These findings need to be replicated in a study population of all ages.

In another GWAS, another locus located within the *HMGA2* gene at 12q14.3, was associated with intracranial volume (ICV; Stein et al., 2012). As the hippocampus is one of the brain regions that is most sensitive to age-related pathology (Scheltens, 2001), two GWAS have been conducted searching for genes that explain variation in hippocampal volume; one of these found that an intergenic variant in locus 12q24.22 (Stein et al., 2012) was associated with hippocampal volume, whereas the other study found one SNP at 2q24 within the *DPP4* gene and nine SNPs at 9p33 within the *ASTN2* gene (Bis et al., 2012). These associations implicate genes related to apoptosis (*HRK*), development (*WIF1*), oxidative stress (*MSR3B*), ubiquitination (*FBXW8*), and neuronal migration (*ASTN2*) as well as enzymes targeted by new diabetes medications (*DPP4*) indicating new genetic influences on hippocampal size and possibly the risk of cognitive decline and dementia.

The major genetic candidate for brain aging is of course the *APOE*-e4 allele. Compared to *APOE*-e4 noncarriers, it was found that *APOE*-e4 carriers show more white matter hyperintensities, increased total brain atrophy, smaller hippocampal volume and smaller entorhinal cortex volume, and altered cerebral blood flow and glucose metabolism patterns (Cherbuin, Leach, Christensen, & Anstey, 2007). By combining all genetic risks that previously were identified in a GWAS on Alzheimer's disease, Biffi and colleagues (2010) found that the GWAS-validated variants at the *CR1* and *PICALM* loci were also associated with decreased hippocampal and entorhinal cortex volume and decreased temporal pole cortical thickness.

Frailty

Frailty has been conceptualized in several ways. It has been used by demographers to describe susceptibility to morbidity or mortality (Vaupel, Manton, & Stallard, 1997), and implemented in correlated gamma-frailty models to evaluate the heritability of all-cause mortality (Iachine et al., 1998) and cause-specific mortality (e.g., coronary heart disease [CHD] mortality; Zdravkovic et al., 2004). Another conceptualization of frailty that combines many of objective health measures reviewed here was defined as a clinical syndrome in which three or more of the following criteria were present: unintentional weight loss (10 lb in the past year), self-reported exhaustion, weakness (grip strength), slow walking speed, and low physical activity (Fried et al., 2001). There are few studies that have estimated the heritability of various indices of frailty, and those that have focused on predictors of exceptional lifespan. In the Long Life Family Study, Matteini et al. (2010) computed principal components from 28 measurements in five domains (cardiovascular, cognition, physical function, pulmonary, and metabolic) and found heritabilities ranging from 16%–39%, the highest being for the principal component represented by poor lung and physical functioning. Another frailty index based on 34 health-related variables had a heritability of 39% in 86 full-sib pairs who were offspring of long-lived parents (Kim, Welsh, Cherry, Myers, & Jazwinski, 2013). Thus far, there are no reports of associations between candidate genes or genome-wide associations with indices of frailty.

LIFESPAN AND LONGEVITY

The search for longevity, and thereby its causes, is an enduring element of human nature. Although philosophers and scientists have speculated about the familial nature of longevity for centuries, there are few records of attempts to quantify the relative importance of genetic variance in lifespan and longevity prior to the 1990s. One approach has been to study exceptionally long-lived families. Hawkins et al. (1965) and Abbott et al. (1974) examined the familial component of longevity by studying the offspring of nonagenarians. Four decades later, several studies are using the same approach, such as the Leiden Longevity Study (Slagboom et al., 2011) and the study described in Chapter 6 of this volume.

Perhaps the best estimates of the heritability of human lifespan have come from twin studies. Population-based estimates of the heritability of lifespan based on Danish twins, first reported by McGue et al. (1993) and then expanded by Herskind et al. (1996), suggested a heritability of approximately 25%. Ljungqvist et al. (1998) applied the same liability threshold analyses to Swedish twins and reported that the heritability was approximately 30%. Using another technique, the correlated gamma-frailty model, Iachine et al. (1998) estimated the narrow sense heritability of survival in combined analyses of the Swedish, Danish, and Finnish twin cohorts at 50%. More recent combined analyses of these Nordic twin registries (Hjelmborg et al, 2006) indicate that before 60 years of age, there is no evidence of genetic variance for lifespan, whereas after 60 years, genetic influences increase in importance with increasing age.

There are several challenges in identifying genes for a complex phenotype such as longevity (or survival), not the least of which is finding suitable cases and controls (for association studies) or pedigrees with DNA (for linkage analyses). Only a few linkage studies have been carried out, mostly with conflicting findings. Nevertheless, recent analyses of 2,118 nonagenarian sibling pairs in the Genetics of Healthy Aging study (GEHA) suggested linkage at four regions: chr 14q11.2, chr 17q12-q22, chr 19p13-3-p18.11, and chr 19q13.11-q13.32 (Beekman et al., 2013). These regions were subsequently fine-mapped and the linkage at 19q133.11-q13-32 was attributed to *APOE* ε4 (risk) and ε2 (protective) alleles. Rare variants are likely to be the source of the peaks at the other three loci.

Early candidate gene studies typically compared centenarians with younger controls. Although numerous associations have been reported, only three genes have been well replicated across populations: *APOE*, *FOXO3A*, and *AKT1* in the insulin-IGF1 signaling pathway. The *APOE* finding most likely reflects the negative influence of the ε4 allele on cardiovascular health and age-related diseases such as Alzheimer's disease. Lack of ability to obtain replicated findings for other gene candidates most likely is a result of poorly chosen gene candidates, lack of appropriate controls, and publication bias (Christensen, Johnson, & Vaupel, 2006).

More recently, there have been several GWAS of longevity listed in the National Human Genome Research Institute (NHGRI) GWAS catalog (Hindorff et al., 2013; Table 7.1). In addition to the *APOE* and nearby *TOMM40* (Deelen et al., 2011), associations have been replicated for *MINPP1*, a highly conserved gene involved in cellular proliferation (Newman et al., 2010) *CAMKIV*, which activates proteins in longevity candidates *AKT1* and *FOXO3A* (Malovini et al., 2011); and *APOC1*, although this finding is attributable to linkage disequilibrium with *APOE* (Nebel et al., 2011).

SUMMARY

For most of the measures of subjective and objective health, frailty, and longevity, genetic variants contribute to only a modest proportion of individual differences; heritabilities are typically on the order of 35%–40%. Notable exceptions are some lipid measures, brain structure and function, and an increase in the role of genetic variance in longevity with increasing age. Candidate gene and GWAS studies are able to identify more and more SNPs associated with these traits, but their effect sizes are typically relatively small, as can be expected for complex traits. There is some evidence for gene–environment interactions, and stress may be an important moderator of genetic variance for health. Clearly, extensive investigations of genetic and environmental contributions and interactions are necessary to develop an understanding of the aging process that in turn may lead to adequate preventive measures, support effective interventions, and ultimately promote successful aging.

TABLE 7.1
Summary of GWAS Studies of Longevity in the NHGRI GWAS Catalog

First Author/ Year/Study	Initial Sample Size	Replication Sample Size	Region	Reported Gene(s)	Strongest SNP-Risk Allele	Context	Risk Allele Frequency in Controls	*p* Value	*OR* or Beta-Coefficient and [95% CI]
Sebastiani, P. 2012 Genetic signatures of exceptional longevity in humans.	801 European ancestry long-living individuals, 914 European ancestry controls	292 European ancestry long-living individuals, 21 long-living individuals, 867 controls	NS	*NS*	NS	NS	NS	NS	NS
Nebel, A. 2011 A genome-wide association study confirms APOE as the major gene influencing survival in long-lived individuals.	763 European ancestry individuals, 1,058 European ancestry individuals	754 European ancestry individuals, 860 European ancestry individuals	19q13.3	*APOC1*	rs4420638-?	nearGene-3	0.81	2×10^{-16}	NR

(Continued)

TABLE 7.1

Summary of GWAS Studies of Longevity in the NHGRI GWAS Catalog (Continued)

First Author/ Year/Study	Initial Sample Size	Replication Sample Size	Region	Reported Gene(s)	Strongest SNP-Risk Allele	Context	Risk Allele Frequency in Controls	p Value	*OR* or Beta-Coefficient and [95% CI]
Malovini, A. 2011 Association study on long-living individuals from Southern Italy identifies rs10491334 in the CAMKIV gene that regulates survival proteins.	410 long-living individuals, 553 young individuals	116 long-living individuals, 160 young individuals	5q22	*CAMKIV*	rs10491334-C		0.82	2×10^{-6}	1.82 [1.43–2.33]
Deelen, J. 2011 Genome-wide association study identifies a single major locus contributing to survival into old age; the APOE locus revisited.	403 European ancestry cases, 1,670 European ancestry controls	3,746 European ancestry cases, 5,912 European ancestry controls	19q13.3	*TOMM40*, *APOE*	rs2075650-?	intron	0.855	3×10^{-17}	1.41 [1.30–1.54]

Yashin, A. I. 2010 Joint influence of small-effect genetic variants on human longevity.	1,173 individuals	NR		16p13.3	*NTHL1*	rs2516739-?	intron;near-Gene-5	NR		1×10^{-6} (less than or equal to)	NR
				7p22	*C7orf50*	rs10256972-?	intron	NR		1×10^{-6} (less than or equal to)	NR
				4q21.1	*SDAD1*	rs2273-?	intron	NR		1×10^{-6} (less than or equal to)	NR
				17q25	*SLC38A10*	rs10445407-?	intron	NR		1×10^{-6} (less than or equal to)	NR

(Continued)

TABLE 7.1

Summary of GWAS Studies of Longevity in the NHGRI GWAS Catalog (Continued)

First Author/ Year/Study	Initial Sample Size	Replication Sample Size	Region	Reported Gene(s)	Strongest SNP-Risk Allele	Context	Risk Allele Frequency in Controls	*p* Value	*OR* or Beta-Coefficient and [95% CI]
			15q12	*GABRB3*	rs3212335-?	intron	NR	1×10^{-6} (less than or equal to)	NR
			13q31	*RP11-388D4.1*	rs2882281-?		NR	1×10^{-6} (less than or equal to)	NR
			3p21.3	*RP11-24C3.2*	rs9876781-?	nearGene-5	NR	1×10^{-6} (less than or equal to)	NR
			13q32	*STK24*	rs9517320-?	intron	NR	1×10^{-6} (less than or equal to)	NR
			13q32	*ABCC4*	rs4148546-?	intron	NR	1×10^{-6} (less than or equal to)	NR

			11p15.4	*CARS*	rs739401-?	intron	NR	1×10^{-6} (less than or equal to)	NR
Newman, A. B. 2010 A meta-analysis of four genome-wide association studies of survival to age 90 years or older: the Cohorts for Heart and Aging Research in Genomic Epidemiology Consortium.	1,836 long-lived Caucasian individuals, 1,955 Caucasian controls	2,594 long-lived Caucasian individuals, 3,431 Caucasian controls	10q23.2	*MINPP1*	rs9664222-C		0.79	7×10^{-7}	1.22 [NR]

Note. GWAS = genome-wide association studies; NHGRI = National Human Genome Research Institute; SNP = single nucleotide polymorphism.

REFERENCES

Abbott, M. H., Murphy, E. A., Bolling, D. R., Abbey, H. (1974). The familial component in longevity. A study of the offspring of nonagenerians. II. Preliminary analysis of the completed study. *Johns Hopkins Medical Journal, 134,* 1–16.

Adeyemo, A., Gerry, N., Chen, G., Herbert, A., Doumatey, A., Huang, H., . . . Rotimi, C. (2009). A genome-wide association study of hypertension and blood pressure in African Americans. *PLoS Genetics*, *5*(7), e1000564.

Ailshire, J., & Crimmins, E. (2013). Physical and biological indicators of health and functioning in U.S. oldest old. *Annual Review of Gerontology and Geriatrics*, *33*, 193–215.

Al-Attar, S. A., Pollex, R. L., Ban, M. R., Young, T. K., Bjerregaard, P., Anand, S. S., . . . Hegele R. A. (2008). Association between the FTO rs9939609 polymorphism and the metabolic syndrome in a non-Caucasian multi-ethnic sample. *Cardiovascular Diabetology*, *7*, 5.

Albarwani, S., Munoz, M. L., Voruganti, V. S., Jaju, D., Al-Yahyaee, V. S., Rizvi, S. G., . . . Hassan M. O. (2012). Heritability of ambulatory and beat-to-beat office blood pressure in large multigenerational Arab pedigrees: The "Oman Family study." *Twin Research and Human Genetics: The Official Journal of the International Society for Twin Studies*, *15*(6), 753–758.

Alfred, T., Ben-Shlomo, Y., Cooper, R., Hardy, R., Cooper, C., Deary, I. J., . . . Day, I. N.; HALCyon Study Team. (2013). Genetic markers of bone and joint health and physical capability in older adults: The HALCyon programme. *Bone*, *52*, 278–285.

Allebrandt, K. V., Amin, N., Muller-Myhsok, B., Esko, T., Teder-Laving, M., Azevedo, R. V., . . . Roenneberg, T. (2013). A K(ATP) channel gene effect on sleep duration: From genome-wide association studies to function in Drosophila. *Molecular Psychiatry*, *18*(1), 122–132.

Amstadter, A. B., Aggen, S. H., Knudsen, G. P., Reichborn-Kjennerud, T., & Kendler, K. S. (2012). A population-based study of familial and individual-specific environmental contributions to traumatic event exposure and posttraumatic stress disorder symptoms in a Norwegian twin sample. *Twin Research and Human Genetics*, *15*(5), 656–662.

Asplund, R. (1999). Sleep disorders in the elderly. *Drugs Aging*, *14*(2), 91–103.

Asplund, R. (2005). Nocturia in relation to sleep, health, and medical treatment in the elderly. *BJU International*, *96*(Suppl. 1), 15–21.

Aulchenko, Y. S., Ripatti, S., Lindqvist, I., Boomsma, D., Heid, I. M., Pramstaller, P. P., . . . Peltonen, L.; ENGAGE Consortium. (2009). Loci influencing lipid levels and coronary heart disease risk in 16 European population cohorts. *Nature Genetics*, *41*(1), 47–55.

Avery, C. L., He, Q., North, K. E., Ambite, J. L., Boerwinkle, E., Fornage, M., . . . Lin, D. Y. (2011). A phenomics-based strategy identifies loci on APOC1, BRAP, and PLCG1 associated with metabolic syndrome phenotype domains. *PLoS Genetics*, *7*(10), e1002322.

Barclay, N. L., & Gregory, A. M. (2013). Quantitative genetic research on sleep: A review of normal sleep, sleep disturbances and associated emotional, behavioural, and health-related difficulties. *Sleep Medicine Reviews*, *17*(1), 29–40.

Bartzokis, G., Lu, P. H., Heydari, P., Couvrette, A., Lee, G. J., Kalashyan, G., . . . Altshuler, L. L. (2012). Multimodal magnetic resonance imaging assessment of white matter aging trajectories over the lifespan of healthy individuals. *Biological Psychiatry*, *72*(12), 1026–1034.

Bauer, M. E., Jeckel, C. M., & Luz, C. (2009). The role of stress factors during aging of the immune system. *Annals of the New York Academy of Sciences*, *1153*, 139–152.

Beekman, M., Heijmans, B. T., Martin, N. G., Pedersen, N. L., Whitfield, J. B., DeFaire, U., . . . Boomsma, D. I. (2002). Heritabilities of apolipoprotein and lipid levels in three countries. *Twin Research*, *5*(2), 87–97.

Beekman, M., Blanché, H., Perola, M., Hervonen, A., Bezrukov, V., Sikora, E., . . . Sørensen, T. I. A. (2013). Genome-wide linkage analysis for human longevity: Genetics of Healthy Aging study. *Aging Cell, 12,* 184–193.

Bemmels, H. R., Burt, S. A., Legrand, L. N., Iacono, W. G., & McGue, M. (2008). The heritability of life events: An adolescent twin and adoption study. *Twin Research and Human Genetics*, *11*(3), 257–265.

Bennet, A. M., Di Angelantonio, E., Ye, Z., Wensley, F., Dahlin, A., Ahlbom, A., . . . Danesh, J. (2007). Association of apolipoprotein E genotypes with lipid levels and coronary risk. *JAMA: The Journal of the American Medical Association*, *298*(11), 1300–1311.

Bennet, A. M., Reynolds, C. A., Gatz, M., Blennow, K., Pedersen, N. L., & Prince, J. A. (2010). Pleiotropy in the presence of allelic heterogeneity: Alternative genetic models for the influence of APOE on serum LDL, CSF amyloid-beta42, and dementia. *Journal of Alzheimer's Disease*, *22*(1), 129–134.

Biffi, A., Anderson, C. D., Desikan, R. S., Sabuncu, M., Cortellini, L., Schmansky, N., . . . Rosand, J.; Alzheimer's Disease Neuroimaging Initiative. (2010). Genetic variation and neuroimaging measures in Alzheimer disease. *Archives of Neurology*, *67*(6), 677–685.

Bis, J. C., DeCarli, C., Smith, A. V., van der Lijn, F., Crivello, F., Fornage, M., . . . Seshadri, S.; Cohorts for Heart and Aging Research in Genomic Epidemiology Consortium. (2012). Common variants at 12q14 and 12q24 are associated with hippocampal volume. *National Genetics*, *44*(5), 545–551.

Bolinskey, P. K., Neale, M. C., Jacobson, K. C., Prescott, C. A., & Kendler, K. S. (2004). Sources of individual differences in stressful life event exposure in male and female twins. *Twin Research*, *7*(1), 33–38.

Braak, H., & Braak, E. (1995). Staging of Alzheimer's disease-related neurofibrillary changes. *Neurobiological Aging*, *16*(3), 271–278.

Braskie, M. N., Klunder, A. D., Hayashi, K. M., Protas, H., Kepe, V., Miller, K. J., . . . Thompson, P. M. (2010). Plaque and tangle imaging and cognition in normal aging and Alzheimer's disease. *Neurobiological Aging*, *31*(10), 1669–1678.

Cai, Y. P., Hayakawa, K., Nishihara, R., & Kato, K. (2009). Heritability of serum apolipoprotein concentrations in middle-aged Japanese twins. *Journal of Epidemiology*, *19*(5), 260–265.

Carmelli, D., Reed, T., & DeCarli, C. (2002). A bivariate genetic analysis of cerebral white matter hyperintensities and cognitive performance in elderly male twins. *Neurobiological Aging*, *23*(3), 413–420.

Caspi, A., Hariri, A. R., Holmes, A., Uher, R., & Moffitt, T. E. (2010). Genetic sensitivity to the environment: The case of the serotonin transporter gene and its implications for studying complex diseases and traits. *American Journal of Psychiatry, 167*(5), 509–527.

Charbonneau, D. E., Hanson, E. D., Ludlow, A. T., Delmonico, M. J., Hurley, B. F., & Roth, S. M. (2008). ACE genotype and the muscle hypertrophic and strength responses to strength training. *Medicine and Science in Sports and Exercise, 40*(4), 677–683.

Cherbuin, N., Leach, L. S., Christensen, H., & Anstey, K. J. (2007). Neuroimaging and APOE genotype: A systematic qualitative review. *Dementia and Geriatric Cognitive Disorders, 24*(5), 348–362.

Christensen, K., Frederiksen, H., Vaupel, J. W., & McGue, M. (2003). Age trajectories of genetic variance in physical functioning: A longitudinal study of Danish twins aged 70 years and older. *Behavior Genetics, 33*(2), 125–136.

Christensen, K., Holm, N. V., McGue, M., Corder, L., & Vaupel, J. W. (1999). A Danish population-based twin study on general health in the elderly. *Journal of Aging and Health, 11*(1), 49–64.

Christensen, K., Johnson, T. E., Vaupel, J. W. (2006). The quest for genetic determinants of human longevity: Challenges and insights. *Nature Reviews Genetics, 7*, 436–448.

Colletto, G. M., Cardon, L. R., & Fulker, D. W. (1993). A genetic and environmental time series analysis of blood pressure in male twins. *Genetic Epidemiology, 10*(6), 533–538.

Dahl, A. K., Lopponen, M., Isoaho, R., Berg, S., & Kivela, S. L. (2008). Overweight and obesity in old age are not associated with greater dementia risk. *Journal of the American Geriatrics Society, 56*(12), 2261–2266.

Dahl, A. K., & Reynolds, C. A. (2012). Heritability of the trajectory of body mass index across the adult life span [Abstract]. *Behavior Genetics, 43*, 927.

Dahl, A. K., Reynolds, C. A., Fall, T., Magnusson, P., & Pedersen, N. L. (2013). Multifactorial analysis of changes in body mass index across the adult life course—A study with 65 years of follow-up. *International Journal of Obesity*. Advance online publication.

Dahlen, G., Ericson, C., de Faire, U., Iselius, L., & Lundman, T. (1983). Genetic and environmental determinants of cholesterol and HDL-cholesterol concentrations in blood. *International Journal of Epidemiology, 12*(1), 32–35.

De Buyser, S. L., Petrovic, M., Taes, Y. E., Toye, K. R. C., Kaufman, J.-M., & Goemaere, S. (2013). Physical function measurements predict mortality in ambulatory older men. *European Journal of Clinical Investigation, 43*(4), 379–386.

De Geus, E. J., Boomsma, D. I., & Snieder, H. (2003). Genetic correlation of exercise with heart rate and respiratory sinus arrhythmia. *Medicine and Science in Sports and Exercise, 35*(8), 1287–1295.

De Geus, E. J., Kupper, N., Boomsma, D. I., & Snieder, H. (2007). Bivariate genetic modeling of cardiovascular stress reactivity: Does stress uncover genetic variance? *Psychosomatic Medicine, 69*(4), 356–364.

DeCarli, C., Massaro, J., Harvey, D., Hald, J., Tullberg, M., Au, R., . . . Wolf, P. A. (2005). Measures of brain morphology and infarction in the framingham heart study: Establishing what is normal. *Neurobiol Aging, 26*(4), 491–510.

Deelen, J., Beekman, M., Uh, H.-W., Helmer, Q., Kuningas, M., Christiansen, L., . . . Slagboom, P. E. (2011). Genome-wide association study identifies a single major locus contributing to survival into old age; the APOE locus revisited. *Aging Cell*, *10*(4), 686 698.

den Heijer, T., van der Lijn, F., Ikram, A., Koudstaal, P. J., van der Lugt, A., Krestin, G. P., . . . Breteler M. M. (2012). Vascular risk factors, apolipoprotein E, and hippocampal decline on magnetic resonance imaging over a 10-year follow-up. *Alzheimer's & Dementia*, *8*(5), 417–425.

Deo, R., Nalls, M. A., Avery, C. L., Smith, J. G., Evans, D. S., Keller, M. F., . . . Whitsel, E. A. (2013). Common genetic variation near the connexin-43 gene is associated with resting heart rate in African Americans: A genome-wide association study of 13,372 participants. *Heart Rhythm: The Official Journal of the Heart Rhythm Society*, *10*(3), 401–408.

Deuschle, M., Gotthardt, U., Schweiger, U., Weber, B., Korner, A., Schmider, J., . . . Heuser, I. (1997). With aging in humans the activity of the hypothalamus-pituitary-adrenal system increases and its diurnal amplitude flattens. *Life Sciences*, *61*(22), 2239–2246.

Dijk, D. J., Duffy, J. F., & Czeisler, C. A. (2000). Contribution of circadian physiology and sleep homeostasis to age-related changes in human sleep. *Chronobiology International*, *17*(3), 285–311.

Drachmann, B. J., Bock, C., Vinberg, M., Werge, T., Gether, U., & Vedel, K. L. (2009). Interaction between genetic polymorphisms and stressful life events in first episode depression. *Journal of Affective Disorders*, *119*(1–3), 107–115.

Duman, R. S. (2009). Neuronal damage and protection in the pathophysiology and treatment of psychiatric illness: Stress and depression. *Dialogues in Clinical Neuroscience*, *11*(3), 239–255.

Earnest, C. P., Blair, S. N., & Church, T. S. (2012). Heart rate variability and exercise in aging women. *Journal of Women's Health*, *21*(3), 334–339.

Eckel, R. H., Grundy, S. M., & Zimmet, P. Z. (2005). The metabolic syndrome. *Lancet*, *365*(9468), 1415–1428.

Ehret, G. B., Morrison, A. C., O'Connor, A. A., Grove, M. L., Baird, L., Schwander, K., . . . Chakravarti, A. (2008). Replication of the Wellcome Trust genome-wide association study of essential hypertension: The Family Blood Pressure Program. *European Journal of Human Genetics: EJHG*, *16*(12), 1507–1511.

Eijgelsheim, M., Newton-Cheh, C., Sotoodehnia, N., de Bakker, P. I., Muller, M., Morrison, A. C., . . . O'Donnell, C. J. (2010). Genome-wide association analysis identifies multiple loci related to resting heart rate. *Human Molecular Genetics*, *19*(19), 3885–3894.

Elder, S. J., Lichtenstein, A. H., Pittas, A. G., Roberts, S. B., Fuss, P. J., Greenberg, A. S., . . . Neale, M. C. (2009). Genetic and environmental influences on factors associated with cardiovascular disease and the metabolic syndrome. *Journal of Lipid Research*, *50*(9), 1917–1926.

Emery, C. F., Finkel, D., & Pedersen, N. L. (2012). Pulmonary function as a cause of cognitive aging. *Psychological Science*, *23*(9), 1024–1032.

Ernsth-Bravel, M., Zarit, S. H., & Johansson, B. (2011). Self-reported activities of daily living and performance-based functional ability: A study of congruence in the oldest-old. *European Journal of Ageing*, *8*, 199–209.

Eyler, L. T., Chen, C. H., Panizzon, M. S., Fennema-Notestine, C., Neale, M. C., Jak, A., . . . Kremen W. S. (2012). A comparison of heritability maps of cortical surface area and thickness and the influence of adjustment for whole brain measures: A magnetic resonance imaging twin study. *Twin Research and Human Genetics*, *15*(3), 304–314.

Fagard, R. H., Loos, R. J., Beunen, G., Derom, C., & Vlietinck, R. (2003). Influence of chorionicity on the heritability estimates of blood pressure: A study in twins. *Journal of Hypertension*, *21*(7), 1313–1318.

Fall, T., & Ingelsson, E. (2012). Genome-wide association studies of obesity and metabolic syndrome. *Molecular and Cellular Endocrinology*. Advance online publication.

Feder, A., Nestler, E. J., & Charney, D. S. (2009). Psychobiology and molecular genetics of resilience. *Nature Reviews Neuroscience*, *10*(6), 446–457.

Ferrucci, L., Studenski, S. A., Alley, D. E., Barbagallo, M., & Harris, T. B. (2010). Obesity in aging and art. *The Journals of Gerontology Series A: Biological Sciences and Medical Sciences*, *65*(1), 53–56.

Finkel, D., Pedersen, N. L., Berg, S., & Johansson, B. (2000). Quantitative genetic analysis of biobehavioral markers of aging in Swedish studies of aging twins. *Journal of Aging and Health*, *12*, 47–68.

Finkel, D., Pedersen, N. L., Reynolds, C. A., Berg, S., de Faire, U., & Svartengren, M. (2003). Genetic and environmental influences on decline in biobehavioral markers of aging. *Behavior Genetics*, *33*(2), 107–123.

Finkel, D., Reynolds, C. A., Emery, C. F., & Pedersen, N. L. (2013). Genetic and environmental variation in lung function drives subsequent variation in aging of fluid intelligence. *Behavior Genetics*, *43*(4), 274–285.

Foley, D., Ancoli-Israel, S., Britz, P., & Walsh, J. (2004). Sleep disturbances and chronic disease in older adults: Results of the 2003 National Sleep Foundation Sleep in America Survey. *Journal of Psychosomatic Research*, *56*(5), 497–502.

Ford, E. S., Giles, W. H., & Dietz, W. H. (2002). Prevalence of the metabolic syndrome among US adults: Findings from the third National Health and Nutrition Examination Survey. *JAMA: The Journal of the American Medical Association*, *287*(3), 356–359.

Fotenos, A. F., Snyder, A. Z., Girton, L. E., Morris, J. C., & Buckner, R. L. (2005). Normative estimates of cross-sectional and longitudinal brain volume decline in aging and AD. *Neurology*, *64*(6), 1032–1039.

Frederiksen, H., Gaist, D., Petersen, H. C., Hjelmborg, J., McGue, M., Vaupel, J. W., & Christensen K. (2002). Hand grip strength: A phenotype suitable for identifying genetic variants affecting mid- and late-life physical functioning. *Genetic Epidemiology*, *23*(2), 110–122.

Fried, L. P., Tangen, C. M., Walston, J., Newman, A. B., Hirsch, C., Gottdiener, J., . . . McBurnie, M. A.; Cardiovascular Health Study Collaborative Research Group.

(2001). Frailty in older adults: Evidence for a phenotype. *The Journals of Gerontology Series A: Biological Sciences and Medical Sciences*, *56*(3), M146–M156.

Friedlander, Y., Austin, M. A., Newman, B., Edwards, K., Mayer-Davis, E. I., & King, M. C. (1997). Heritability of longitudinal changes in coronary-heart-disease risk factors in women twins. *American Journal of Human Genetics*, *60*(6), 1502–1512.

Ganesh, S. K., Tragante, V., Guo, W., Guo, Y., Lanktree, M. B., Smith, E. N., . . . Asselbergs, F. W. (2013). Loci influencing blood pressure identified using a cardiovascular gene-centric array. *Human Molecular Genetics*, *22*(8), 1663–1678.

Gardner, A. W., & Montgomery, P. S. (2008). DIFFERENCES IN EXERCISE PERFORMANCE AND LEISURE-TIME PHYSICAL ACTIVITY IN OLDER CAUCASIANS AND AFRICAN-AMERICANS. *Clinical Medicine. Geriatrics*, *1*, 1–7.

Geerlings, M. I., Appelman, A. P., Vincken, K. L., Mali, W. P., & van der Graaf, Y.; SMART Study Group. (2009). Association of white matter lesions and lacunar infarcts with executive functioning: The SMART-MR study. *American Journal of Epidemiology*, *170*(9), 1147–1155.

Genderson, M. R., Rana, B. K., Panizzon, M. S., Grant, M. D., Toomey, R., Jacobson, K. C., . . . Lyons, M. J. (2013). Genetic and environmental influences on sleep quality in middle-aged men: A twin study. *Journal of Sleep Research*, *22*(5), 519–526.

Gerritsen, L., Comijs, H. C., Deeg, D. J., Penninx, B. W., & Geerlings, M. I. (2011). Salivary cortisol, APOE-epsilon4 allele and cognitive decline in a prospective study of older persons. *Neurobiological Aging*, *32*(9), 1615–1625.

Goode, E. L., Cherny, S. S., Christian, J. C., Jarvik, G. P., & de Andrade, M. (2007). Heritability of longitudinal measures of body mass index and lipid and lipoprotein levels in aging twins. *Twin Research and Human Genetics: The Official Journal of the International Society for Twin Studies*, *10*(5), 703–711.

Gu, D., Zhao, Q., Chen, J., Chen, J. C., Huang, J., Bazzano, L. A., . . . He, J. (2013). Reproducibility of blood pressure responses to dietary sodium and potassium interventions: The GenSalt Study. *Hypertension*, *62*(3), 499–505.

Hammen, C. (2006). Stress generation in depression: Reflections on origins, research, and future directions. *Journal of Clinical Psychology*, *62*(9), 1065–1082.

Hampel, R., Breitner, S., Schneider, A., Zareba, W., Kraus, U., Cyrys, J., . . . Peters, A.; Cooperative Health Research in the Region of Augsburg (KORA) Study Group. (2012). Acute air pollution effects on heart rate variability are modified by SNPs involved in cardiac rhythm in individuals with diabetes or impaired glucose tolerance. *Environmental Research*, *112*, 177–185.

Hancock, D. B., Eijgelsheim, M., Wilk, J. B., Gharib, S. A., Loehr, L. R., Marciante, K. D., . . . London, S. J. (2010). Meta-analyses of genome-wide association studies identify multiple loci associated with pulmonary function. *Nature Genetics*, *42*(1), 45–52.

Hawkins, M. R., & Murphy, E. A. (1965). The familial component in longevity. A study of the offspring of nonagenerians. I. Methods and preliminary report. *Bulletin of Johns Hopkins Hospital*, *117*, 24–36.

Haworth, C. M., Carnell, S., Meaburn, E. L., Davis, O. S., Plomin, R., & Wardle, J. (2008). Increasing heritability of BMI and stronger associations with the FTO gene over childhood. *Obesity (Silver Spring)*, *16*(12), 2663–2668.

Hayakawa, K., Shimizu, T., Ohba, Y., & Tomioka, S. (1987). Lifestyle factors affecting intrapair differences of serum apoproteins and cholesterol concentrations in adult identical twins. *Atherosclerosis*, *66*(1–2), 1–9.

Heller, D. A., de Faire, U., Pedersen, N. L., Dahlen, G., & McClearn, G. E. (1993). Genetic and environmental influences on serum lipid levels in twins. *New England Journal of Medicine*, *328*(16), 1150–1156.

Herskind, A. M., McGue, M., Holm, N. V., Sørensen, T. I., Harvald, B., & Vaupel, J. W. (1996). The heritability of human longevity: A population-based study of 2,872 Danish twin pairs born 1870-1900. *Human Genetics, 97,* 319–23.

Hindorff, L. A., MacArthur, J., Morales, J., Junkins, H. A., Hall, P. N., Klemm, A. K., & Manolio, T. A. (2013). A catalog of published genome-wide association studies. Retrieved from www.genome.gov/gwastudies

Hirsch, C. H., Buzkova, P., Robbins, J. A., Patel, K. V., & Newman, A. B. (2012). Predicting late-life disability and death by the rate of decline in physical performance measures. *Age Ageing*, *41*(2), 155–161.

Hita-Yañez, E., Atienza, M., Gil-Neciga, E., & Cantero, J. L. (2012). Disturbed sleep patterns in elders with mild cognitive impairment: The role of memory decline and ApoE epsilon4 genotype. *Current Alzheimer Research*, *9*(3), 290-297.

Hjelmborg, J. vB., Iachine, I., Skytthe, A., Vaupel, J. W., McGue, M., Koskenvuo, M., . . . Christensen, K. (2006). Genetic influences on human lifespan and longevity. *Human Genetics, 119,* 312–321.

Holm, H., Gudbjartsson, D. F., Arnar, D. O., Thorleifsson, G., Thorgeirsson, G., Stefansdottir, H., . . . Stefansson, K. (2010). Several common variants modulate heart rate, PR interval and QRS duration. *Nature Genetics*, *42*(2), 117–122.

Holman, E. A. (2012). Acute stress and cardiovascular health: Is there an ACE gene connection? *Journal of Traumatic Stress*, *25*(5), 592–597.

Hong, Y., Pedersen, N. L., Brismar, K., & de Faire, U. (1997). Genetic and environmental architecture of the features of the insulin-resistance syndrome. *The American Journal of Human Genetics*, *60*(1), 143–152.

Hottenga, J. J., Boomsma, D. I., Kupper, N., Posthuma, D., Snieder, H., Willemsen, G., & de Geus, E. J. (2005). Heritability and stability of resting blood pressure. *Twin Research and Human Genetics: The Official Journal of the International Society for Twin Studies*, *8*(5), 499–508.

Hottenga, J. J., Whitfield, J. B., de Geus, E. J., Boomsma, D. I., & Martin, N. G. (2006). Heritability and stability of resting blood pressure in Australian twins. *Twin Research and Human Genetics: The Official Journal of the International Society for Twin Studies*, *9*(2), 205–209.

Hukkinen, M., Kaprio, J., Broms, U., Viljanen, A., Kotz, D., Rantanen, T., & Korhonen, T. (2011). Heritability of lung function: A twin study among never-smoking elderly women. *Twin Research and Human Genetics*, *14*(5), 401–407.

Iachine, I. A., Holm, N. V., Harris, J. R., Begun, A. Z., Iachina, M. K., Laitinen, M., . . . Yashin, A. I. (1998). How heritable is individual susceptibility to death? The results of an analysis of survival data on Danish, Swedish and Finnish twins. *Twin Research, 1*(4), 196–203.

Idler, E. L., & Benyamini, Y. (1997). Self-rated health and mortality: A review of twenty-seven community studies. *Journal of Health and Social Behavior, 38*(1), 21–37.

Ikram, M. A., Fornage, M., Smith, A. V., Seshadri, S., Schmidt, R., Debette, S., . . . DeCarli, C.; Cohorts for Heart and Aging Research in Genomic Epidemiology Consortium. (2012). Common variants at 6q22 and 17q21 are associated with intracranial volume. *Nature Genetics, 44*(5), 539–544.

Ikram, M. A., Vrooman, H. A., Vernooij, M. W., den Heijer, T., Hofman, A., Niessen, W. J., . . . Breteler, M. M. (2010). Brain tissue volumes in relation to cognitive function and risk of dementia. *Neurobiological Aging, 31*(3), 378–386.

Jagger, C., Gillies, C., Cambois, E., Van Oyen, H., Nusselder, W., & Robine, J.-M. (2010). The Global Activity Limitation Index measured function and disability similarly across European countries. *Journal of Clinical Epidemiology, 63*(8), 892–899.

Joy, T., Lahiry, P., Pollex, R. L., & Hegele, R. A. (2008). Genetics of metabolic syndrome. *Current Diabetes Reports, 8*(2), 141–148.

Juster, R. P., McEwen, B. S., & Lupien, S. J. (2010). Allostatic load biomarkers of chronic stress and impact on health and cognition. *Neuroscience & Biobehavioral Reviews, 35*(1), 2–16.

Kalkman, H. O. (2012). Potential opposite roles of the extracellular signal-regulated kinase (ERK) pathway in autism spectrum and bipolar disorders. *Neuroscience & Biobehavioral Reviews, 36*(10), 2206–2213.

Karg, K., Burmeister, M., Shedden, K., & Sen, S. (2011). The serotonin transporter promoter variant (5-HTTLPR), stress, and depression meta-analysis revisited: Evidence of genetic moderation. *Archives of General Psychiatry, 68*(5), 444–454.

Kato, N., Takeuchi, F., Tabara, Y., Kelly, T. N., Go, M. J., Sim, X., . . . He, J. (2011). Meta-analysis of genome-wide association studies identifies common variants associated with blood pressure variation in east Asians. *Nature Genetics, 43*(6), 531–538.

Kempen, G. I., Steverink, N., Ormel, J., & Deeg, D. J. (1996). The assessment of ADL among frail elderly in an interview survey: Self-report versus performance-based tests and determinants of discrepancies. *The Journals of Gerontology Series B: Psychological Sciences and Social Sciences, 51*, 254–260.

Kidambi, S., Ghosh, S., Kotchen, J. M., Grim, C. E., Krishnaswami, S., Kaldunski, M. L., . . . Kotchen, T. A. (2012). Non-replication study of a genome-wide association study for hypertension and blood pressure in African Americans. *BMC Medical Genetics, 13*, 27.

Kim, S., Welsh, D. A., Cherry, K. E., Myers, L., & Jazwinski, S. M. (2013). Association of healthy aging with parental longevity. *Age, 35*, 1975–1982.

Klunk, W. F., Engler, H., Nordberg, A., Wang, Y., Blomqvist, G., Holt, D. P., . . . Långström, B. (2004). Imaging brain amyloid in Alzheimer's disease with Pittsburgh Compound-B. *Annals of Neurology, 55*(3), 306–319.

Knoblauch, H., Busjahn, A., Münter, S., Nagy, Z., Faulhaber, H.-D., Schuster, H., & Luft, F. C. (1997). Heritability analysis of lipids and three gene loci in twins link the macrophage scavenger receptor to HDL cholesterol concentrations. *Arteriosclerosis, Thrombosis, and Vascular Biology*, *17*(10), 2054–2060.

Kopelman, P. G. (2000). Obesity as a medical problem. *Nature*, *404*(6778), 635–643.

Kostis, W. J., Cabrera, J., Hooper, W. C., Whelton, P. K., Espeland, M. A., Cosgrove, N. M., . . . Kostis, J. B. (2013). Relationships between selected gene polymorphisms and blood pressure sensitivity to weight loss in elderly persons with hypertension. *Hypertension*, *61*(4), 857–863.

Koten, J. W., Jr., Wood, G., Hagoort, P., Goebel, R., Propping, P., Willmes, K., & Boomsma, D. I. (2009). Genetic contribution to variation in cognitive function: An FMRI study in twins. *Science*, *323*(5922), 1737–1740.

Kremen, W. S., Prom-Wormley, E., Panizzon, M. S., Eyler, L. T., Fischl, B., Neale, M. C., . . . Fennema-Notestine, C. (2010). Genetic and environmental influences on the size of specific brain regions in midlife: The VETSA MRI study. *Neuroimage*, *49*(2), 1213–1223.

Krieger, N., Chen, J. T., Coull, B. A., & Selby, J. V. (2005). Lifetime socioeconomic position and twins' health: An analysis of 308 pairs of United States women twins. *PLoS Medicine*, *2*(7), e162.

Kristiansson, K., Perola, M., Tikkanen, E., Kettunen, J., Surakka, I., Havulinna, A. S., . . . Salomaa, V. (2012). Genome-wide screen for metabolic syndrome susceptibility loci reveals strong lipid gene contribution but no evidence for common genetic basis for clustering of metabolic syndrome traits. *Circulation: Cardiovascular Genetics*, *5*(2), 242–249.

Kupper, N., Willemsen, G., Riese, H., Posthuma, D., Boomsma, D. I., & de Geus, E. J. (2005). Heritability of daytime ambulatory blood pressure in an extended twin design. *Hypertension*, *45*(1), 80–85.

Kupper, N. H., Willemsen, G., van den Berg, M., de Boer, D., Posthuma, D., Boomsma, D. I., & de Geus, E. J. (2004). Heritability of ambulatory heart rate variability. *Circulation*, *110*(18), 2792–2796.

Launer, L. J., Oudkerk, M., Nilsson, L. G., Alperovitch, A., Berger, K., Breteler, M. M., . . . Hofman, A. (2000). CASCADE: A European collaborative study on vascular determinants of brain lesions. Study design and objectives. *Neuroepidemiology*, *19*(3), 113–120.

Leinonen, R., Kaprio, J., Jylha, M., Tolvanen, A., Koskenvuo, M., Heikkinen, E., & Rantanen, T. (2005). Genetic influences underlying self-rated health in older female twins. *Journal of the American Geriatrics Society*, *53*(6), 1002–1007.

Lessov-Schlaggar, C. N., Hardin, J., DeCarli, C., Krasnow, R. E., Reed, T., Wolf, P. A., & Carmelli, D. (2012). Longitudinal genetic analysis of brain volumes in normal elderly male twins. *Neurobiological Aging*, *33*(4), 636–644.

Levy, D., Ehret, G. B., Rice, K., Verwoert, G. C., Launer, L. J., Dehghan, A., . . . van Duijn, C. M. (2009). Genome-wide association study of blood pressure and hypertension. *Nature Genetics*, *41*(6), 677–687.

Li, J., Huo, Y., Zhang, Y., Fang, Z., Yang, J., Zang, T., . . . Xu, X. (2009). Familial aggregation and heritability of electrocardiographic intervals and heart rate in a rural Chinese population. *Annals of Noninvasive Electrocardiology: The Official Journal of the International Society for Holter and Noninvasive Electrocardiology, Inc.*, *14*(2), 147–152.

Ljungquist, B., Berg, S., Lanke, J., McClearn, G. E., & Pedersen, N. L. (1998). The effect of genetic factors for longevity: A comparison of identical and fraternal twins in the Swedish Twin Registry. *Journal of Gerontology Series A: Biological Sciences and Medical Sciences*, *53*(6), M441–M446.

Luszcz, M. A. (1996). Beliefs about control in later life: Implications of perceptions of health, memory and global control. *Hong Kong Journal of Gerontology*, *10*, 502–506.

Magri, F., Cravello, L., Barili, L., Sarra, S., Cinchetti, W., Salmoiraghi, F., . . . Ferrari E. (2006). Stress and dementia: The role of the hypothalamic pituitary-adrenal axis. *Aging Clinical and Experimental Research*, *18*(2), 167–170.

Malovini, A., Illario, M., Iaccarino, G., Villa, F., Ferrario, A., Roncarati, R., . . . Puca, A. A. (2011). Association study on long-living individuals from Southern Italy identifies rs10491334 in the CAMKIV gene that regulates survival proteins. *Rejuvenation Research*, *14*, 283–291.

Matteini, A. M., Fallin, M. D., Kammerer, C. M., Schupf, N., Yashin, A. I., Christensen, K., . . . Walston, J. D. (2010). Heritability estimates of endophenotypes of long and health life: The Long Life Family Study. *The Journals of Gerontology Series A: Biological Sciences and Medical Sciences*, *65*(12), 1375–1379.

McCaffery, J. M., Papandonatos, G. D., Lyons, M. J., & Niaura, R. (2008). Educational attainment and the heritability of self-reported hypertension among male Vietnam-era twins. *Psychosomatic Medicine*, *70*(7), 781–786.

McCallum, J., Shadbolt, B., & Wang, D. (1994). Self-rated health and survival: A 7-year follow-up study of Australian elderly. *American Journal of Public Health*, *84*(7), 1100–1105.

McClearn, G. E., Svartengren, M., Pedersen, N. L., Heller, D. A., & Plomin, R. (1994). Genetic and environmental influences on pulmonary function in aging Swedish twins. *The Journals of Gerontology*, *49*(6), 264–268.

McGue, M., Vaupel, J. W., Holm, N., & Harvald, B. (1993). Longevity is moderately heritable in a sample of Danish twins born 1870–1880. *Journal of Gerontology*, *48*, B237–B245.

McGue, M., & Christensen, K. (2013). Growing old but not growing apart: Twin similarity in the latter half of the lifespan. *Behavior Genetics*, *43*(1), 1–12.

Middelberg, R. P., Martin, N. G., & Whitfield, J. B. (2006). Longitudinal genetic analysis of plasma lipids. *Twin Research and Human Genetics: The Official Journal of the International Society for Twin Studies*, *9*(4), 550–557.

Middelberg, R. P., Spector, T. D., Swaminathan, R., & Snieder, H. (2002). Genetic and environmental influences on lipids, lipoproteins, and apolipoproteins: Effects of menopause. *Arteriosclerosis, Thrombosis, and Vascular Biology*, *22*(7), 1142–1147.

Miller, G. E., Chen, E., & Parker, K. J. (2011). Psychological stress in childhood and susceptibility to the chronic diseases of aging: Moving toward a model of behavioral and biological mechanisms. *Psychological Bulletin*, *137*(6), 959–997.

Mosing, M. A., Pedersen, N. L., Martin, N. G., & Wright, M. J. (2010). Sex differences in the genetic architecture of optimism and health and their interrelation: A study of Australian and Swedish twins. *Twin Research and Human Genetics*, *13*(4), 322–329.

Mosing, M. A., Verweij, K. J. H., Medland, S. E., Painter, J., Gordon, S. D., Heath, A. C., . . . Martin, N. G. (2010). A genome-wide association study of self-rated health. *Twin Research and Human Genetics*, *13*(4), 398–403.

Nan, C., Guo, B., Warner, C., Fowler, T., Barrett, T., Boomsma, D., . . . Zeegers, M. (2012). Heritability of body mass index in pre-adolescence, young adulthood and late adulthood. *European Journal of Epidemiology*, 27(4), 247–253.

Nebel, A., Kleindorp, R., Caliebe, A., Nothnagel, M., Blanche, H., Junge, O., . . . Schreiber, S. (2011). A genome-wide association study confirms APOE as the major gene influencing survival in long-lived individuals. *Mechanisms of Ageing & Development, 132,* 324–30.

Newman, A. B., Walter, S., Lunetta, K. L., Garcia, M. E., Slagboom, P. E., Christensen, K., . . . Murabito, J. M. (2010). A meta-analysis of four genome-wide association studies of survival to age 90 years or older: The cohorts for heart and aging research in genomic epidemiology consortium. *The Journals of Gerontology Series A: Biological Sciences and Medical Sciences, 65,* 478–87.

Newton-Cheh, C., Guo, C. Y., Wang, T. J., O'Donnell, C., J., Levy, D., & Larson, M. G. (2007). Genome-wide association study of electrocardiographic and heart rate variability traits: The Framingham Heart Study. *BMC Medical Genetics*, *8*(Suppl. 1), S7.

Newton-Cheh, C., Johnson, T., Gateva, V., Tobin, M. D., Bochud, M., Coin, L., . . . Munroe, P. B. (2009). Genome-wide association study identifies eight loci associated with blood pressure. *Nature Genetics*, *41*(6), 666–676.

Nilsson, S. E., Read, S., Berg, S., & Johansson, B. (2009). Heritabilities for fifteen routine biochemical values: Findings in 215 Swedish twin pairs 82 years of age or older. *Scandinavian Journal of Clinical and Laboratory Investigation*, *69*(5), 562–569.

Njajou, O. T., Hsueh, W. C., Blackburn, E. H., Newman, A. B., Wu, S. H., Li, R., . . . Cawthon, R. M.; Health ABC study. (2009). Association between telomere length, specific causes of death, and years of healthy life in health, aging, and body composition, a population-based cohort study. *The Journals of Gerontology Series A: Biological Sciences and Medical Sciences*, *64*(8), 860–864.

Obeidat, M., Wain, L. V., Shrine, N., Kalsheker, N., Soler Artigas, M., Repapi, E., . . . Hall, I. P.; SpiroMeta Consortium. (2011). A comprehensive evaluation of potential lung function associated genes in the SpiroMeta general population sample. *PLoS One*, 6(5), e19382.

Padmanabhan, S., Melander, O., Johnson, T., Di Blasio, A. M., Lee, W. K., Gentilini, D., . . . Dominiczak, A. F. (2010). Genome-wide association study of blood pressure extremes identifies variant near UMOD associated with hypertension. *PLoS Genetics*, 6(10), e1001177.

Parsons, M. J., Lester, K. J., Barclay, N. L., Nolan, P. M., Eley, T. C., & Gregory, A. M. (2013). Replication of Genome-Wide association Studies (GWAS) loci for sleep in the

British G1219 cohort. *American Journal of Medical Genetics Part B: Neuropsychiatric Genetics*, *162B*(5), 431–438.

Paunio, T., Korhonen, T., Hublin, C., Partinen, M., Kivimaki, M., Koskenvuo, M., & Kaprio, J. (2009). Longitudinal study on poor sleep and life dissatisfaction in a nationwide cohort of twins. *American Journal of Epidemiology*, *169*(2), 206–213.

Peavy, G. M. (2008). The effects of stress and APOE genotype on cognition in older adults. *American Journal of Psychiatry*, *165*(11), 1376–1378.

Peelle, J. E., Cusack, R., & Henson, R. N. (2012). Adjusting for global effects in voxel-based morphometry: Gray matter decline in normal aging. *Neuroimage*, *60*(2), 1503–1516.

Pieters, N., Plusquin, M., Cox, B., Kicinski, M., Vangronsveld, J., & Nawrot, T. S. (2012). An epidemiological appraisal of the association between heart rate variability and particulate air pollution: A meta-analysis. *Heart*, *98*(15), 1127–1135.

Pietiläinen, K. H., Söderlund, S., Rissanen, A., Nakanishi, S., Jauhiainen, M., Taskinen, M.-R., & Kaprio, J. (2009). HDL subspecies in young adult twins: Heritability and impact of overweight. *Obesity*, *17*(6), 1208–1214.

Pilia, G., Chen, W. M., Scuteri, A., Orru, M., Albai, G., Dei, M., . . . Schlessinger, D. (2006). Heritability of cardiovascular and personality traits in 6,148 Sardinians. *PLoS Genetics*, *2*(8), e132.

Pinquart, M. (2001). Correlates of subjective health in older adults: A meta-analysis. *Psychology and Aging*, *16*(3), 414–426.

Plomin, R., Lichtenstein, P., Pedersen, N. L., McClearn, G. E., & Nesselroade, J. R. (1990). Genetic influence on life events during the last half of the life span. *Psychology and Aging*, *5*(1), 25–30.

Prinz, P. N. (1995). Sleep and sleep disorders in older adults. *Journal of Clinical Neurophysiology*, *12*(2), 139–146.

Prinz, P. N., Vitiello, M. V., Raskind, M. A., & Thorpy, M. J. (1990). Geriatrics: Sleep disorders and aging. *The New England Journal of Medicine*, *323*(8), 520–526.

Rebholz, C. M., Gu, D., Chen, J., Huang, J. F., Cao, J., Chen, J. C., . . . He, J.; GenSalt Collaborative Research Group. (2012). Physical activity reduces salt sensitivity of blood pressure: The Genetic Epidemiology Network of Salt Sensitivity Study. *American Journal of Epidemiology*, *176*(Suppl. 7), S106–S113.

Repapi, E., Sayers, I., Wain, L. V., Burton, P. R., Johnson, T., Obeidat, M., . . . Tobin, M. D. (2010). Genome-wide association study identifies five loci associated with lung function. *Nature Genetics*, *42*(1), 36–44.

Reynolds, C. A., Gatz, M., Berg, S., & Pedersen, N. L. (2007). Genotype-environment interactions: Cognitive aging and social factors. *Twin Research and Human Genetics*, *10*(2), 241–254.

Romero-Corral, A., Montori, V. M., Somers, V. K., Korinek, J., Thomas, R. J., Allison, T. G., . . . Lopez-Jimenez, F. (2006). Association of bodyweight with total mortality and with cardiovascular events in coronary artery disease: A systematic review of cohort studies. *Lancet*, *368*(9536), 666–678.

Sabia, S., Shipley, M., Elbaz, A., Marmot, M., Kivimaki, M., Kauffmann, F., & Singh-Manoux, A. (2010). Why does lung function predict mortality? Results from the Whitehall II Cohort Study. *American Journal of Epidemiology*, *172*(12), 1415–1423.

Sainio, P., Koskinen, S., Heliovaara, M., Martelin, T., Harkanen, T., Hurri, H., . . . Aromaa, A. (2006). Self-reported and test-based mobility limitations in a representative sample of Finns aged 30+. *Scand J Public Health*, *34*(4), 378–386.

Scheltens, P. H. (2001). Structural neuroimaging of Alzheimer's disease and other dementias. *Aging (Milano)*, *13*(3), 203–209.

Shimada, M., Miyagawa, T., Kawashima, M., Tanaka, S., Honda, Y., Honda, M., & Tokunaga, K. (2010). An approach based on a genome-wide association study reveals candidate loci for narcolepsy. *Human Genetics*, *128*(4), 433–441.

Silventoinen, K., & Kaprio, J. (2009). Genetics of tracking of body mass index from birth to late middle age: Evidence from twin and family studies. *Obesity Facts*, *2*(3), 196–202.

Singh, J. P., Larson, M. G., O'Donnell, C. J., Tsuji, H., Evans, J. C., & Levy, D. (1999). Heritability of heart rate variability: The Framingham Heart Study. *Circulation*, *99*(17), 2251–2254.

Singh-Manoux, A., Dugravot, A., Kauffmann, F., Elbaz, A., Ankri, J., Nabi, H., . . . Sabia, S. (2011). Association of lung function with physical, mental and cognitive function in early old age. *Age (Dordr)*, *33*(3), 385–392.

Slagboom, P. E., Beekman, M., Passtoors, W. M., Deelen, J., Vaarhorst, A. A., Boer, J. M., . . . Westendorp, R. G. (2011). Genomics of human longevity. *Philosophical Transactions of the Royal Society B: Biological Sciences, 12*, 35–42.

Small, G. W., Kepe, V., Ercoli, L. M., Siddarth, P., Bookheimer, S. Y., Miller, K. J., . . . Barrio, J. R. (2006). PET of brain amyloid and tau in mild cognitive impairment. *The New England Journal of Medicine*, *355*(25), 2652–2663.

Smit, D. J., Boomsma, D. I., Schnack, H. G., Hulshoff Pol, H. E., & de Geus, E. J. (2012). Individual differences in EEG spectral power reflect genetic variance in gray and white matter volumes. *Twin Research and Human Genetics*, *15*(3), 384–392.

Snieder, H., van Doornen, L. J., Boomsma, D. I., & Thayer, J. F. (2007). Sex differences and heritability of two indices of heart rate dynamics: A twin study. *Twin Research and Human Genetics: The Official Journal of the International Society for Twin Studies*, *10*(2), 364–372.

Soler Artigas, M., Loth, D. W., Wain, L. V., Gharib, S. A., Obeidat, M., Tang, W., . . . Tobin, M. D. (2011). Genome-wide association and large-scale follow up identifies 16 new loci influencing lung function. *Nature Genetics*, *43*(11), 1082–1090.

Speliotes, E. K., Willer, C. J., Berndt, S. I., Monda, K. L., Thorleifsson, G., Jackson, A. U., . . . Loos, R. J. (2010). Association analyses of 249,796 individuals reveal 18 new loci associated with body mass index. *Nature Genetics*, *42*(11), 937–948.

Stein, J. L., Medland, S. E., Vasquez, A. A., Hibar, D. P., Senstad, R. E., Winkler, A. M., . . . Thompson, P. M.; Enhancing Neuro Imaging Genetics through Meta-Analysis Consortium. (2012). Identification of common variants associated with human hippocampal and intracranial volumes. *Nature Genetics*, *44*(5), 552–561.

Steptoe, A., & Kivimaki, M. (2012). Stress and cardiovascular disease. *Nature Reviews Cardiology*, *9*(6), 360–370.

Stewart, A. R. (2012). White matter hyperintensities: Age appropriate or risk indicator? *Journal of Insurance Medicine*, *43*(2), 84–91.

Stineman, M. G., Xie, D., Pan, Q., Kurichi, J. E., Zhang, Z., Saliba, D., . . . Streim, J. (2012). All-cause 1-, 5-, and 10-year mortality in elderly people according to activities of daily living stage. *Journal of the American Geriatrics Society*, *60*(3), 485–492.

Strachan, D. P. (1992). Causes and control of chronic respiratory disease: Looking beyond the smokescreen. *Journal of Epidemiology & Community Health*, *46*(3), 177–179.

Stubbe, J. H., Boomsma, D. I., & De Geus, E. J. (2005). Sports participation during adolescence: A shift from environmental to genetic factors. *Medicine and Science in Sports and Exercise*, *37*(4), 563–570.

Surakka, I., Whitfield, J. B., Perola, M., Visscher, P. M., Montgomery, G. W., Falchi, M., . . . Peltonen, L.; GenomEUtwin Project. (2012). A genome-wide association study of monozygotic twin-pairs suggests a locus related to variability of serum high-density lipoprotein cholesterol. *Twin Research and Human Genetics*, *15*(6), 691–699.

Svedberg, P., Bardage, C., Sandin, S., & Pedersen, N. L. (2006). A prospective study of health, life-style and psychosocial predictors of self-rated health. *European Journal of Epidemiology*, *21*(10), 767–776.

Svedberg, P., Gatz, M., & Pedersen, N. L. (2009). Genetic and environmental mediation of the associations between self-rated health and cognitive abilities. *Experimental Aging Research*, *35*(2), 178–201.

Svedberg, P., Lichtenstein, P., & Pedersen, N. L. (2001). Age and sex differences in genetic and environmental factors for self-rated health: A twin study. *The Journals of Gerontology Series B: Psychological Sciences and Social Sciences*, *56*, 171–178.

Taal, H. R., Verwoert, G. C., Demirkan, A., Janssens, A. C., Rice, K., Ehret, G., . . . van Duijn, C. M. (2012). Genome-wide profiling of blood pressure in adults and children. *Hypertension*, *59*(2), 241–247.

Taekema, D. G., Gussekloo, J., Westendorp, R. G. J., de Craen, A. J. M., & Maier, A. B. (2012). Predicting survival in oldest old people. *American Journal of Medicine*, *125*(12), 1188–1194.

Takeuchi, F., Yamamoto, K., Katsuya, T., Sugiyama, T., Nabika, T., Ohnaka, K., . . . Kato, N. (2012). Reevaluation of the association of seven candidate genes with blood pressure and hypertension: A replication study and meta-analysis with a larger sample size. *Hypertension Research: Official Journal of the Japanese Society of Hypertension*, *35*(8), 825–831.

Tarnoki, A. D., Tarnoki, D. L., Stazi, M. A., Medda, E., Cotichini, R., Nistico, L., . . . Schillaci, G. (2012). Heritability of central blood pressure and arterial stiffness: A twin study. *Journal of Hypertension*, *30*(8), 1564–1571.

Teslovich, T. M., Musunuru, K., Smith, A. V., Edmondson, A. C., Stylianou, I. M., Koseki, M., . . . Kathiresan, S. (2010). Biological, clinical and population relevance of 95 loci for blood lipids. *Nature*, *466*(7307), 707–713.

Tiainen, K., Luukkaala, T., Hervonen, A., & Jylha, M. (2013). Predictors of mortality in men and women aged 90 and older: A nine-year follow-up study in the Vitality 90+ study. *Age Ageing*, *42*(4), 468–475.

Tiainen, K., Sipilä, S., Alen, M., Heikkinen, E., Kaprio, J., Koskenvuo, M., . . . Rantanen, T. (2004). Heritability of maximal isometric muscle strength in older female twins. *Journal of Applied Physiology*, *96*(1), 173–180.

Tiainen, K., Sipilä, S., Alen, M., Heikkinen, E., Kaprio, J., Koskenvuo, M., . . . Rantanen, T. (2005). Shared genetic and environmental effects on strength and power in older female twins. *Medicine and Science in Sports and Exercise*, *37*(1), 72–78.

Tomiyama, A. J., O'Donovan, A., Lin, J., Puterman, E., Lazaro, A., Chan, J., . . . Epel, E. (2012). Does cellular aging relate to patterns of allostasis? An examination of basal and stress reactive HPA axis activity and telomere length. *Physiology & Behavior*, *106*(1), 40–45.

Uusitalo, A. L., Vanninen, E., Levalahti, E., Battie, M. C., Videman, T., & Kaprio, J. (2007). Role of genetic and environmental influences on heart rate variability in middle-aged men. *American Journal of Physiology. Heart and Circulatory Physiology*, *293*(2), H1013–H1022.

Vasilopoulos, T., Grant, M. D., Franz, C. E., Panizzon, M. S., Xian, H., Toomey, R., . . . Jacobson, K. C. (2013). Shared and distinct genetic influences among different measures of pulmonary function. *Behavior Genetics*, *43*(2), 141–150.

Vasilopoulos, T., Mack, H. A., McClearn, G. E., Berg, S., Johansson, B., & Vogler, G. P. (2010). Stability of genetic influences on pulmonary function in a longitudinal study of octogenarian twins. *American Journal of Human Biology*, *22*(3), 375–377.

Vasunilashorn, S., Glei, D. A., Lin, Y.-H., & Goldman, N. (2013). Apolipoprotein e and measured physical and pulmonary function in older Taiwanese adults. *Biodemography and Social Biology*, *59*(1), 57–67.

Vaupel, J. W., Manton, K. G., & Stallard, E. (1997). The impact of heterogeneity in individual frailty on the dynamics of mortality. *Demography*, *16*, 439.

Vitiello, M. V., & Borson, S. (2001). Sleep disturbances in patients with Alzheimer's disease: Epidemiology, pathophysiology and treatment. *CNS Drugs*, *15*(10), 777–796.

Waller, K., Kujala, U. M., Kaprio, J., Koskenvuo, M., & Rantanen, T. (2010). Effect of physical activity on health in twins: A 30-yr longitudinal study. *Medicine and Science in Sports and Exercise*, *42*(4), 658–664.

Wang, L., Su, L., Shen, H., & Hu, D. (2012). Decoding lifespan changes of the human brain using resting-state functional connectivity MRI. *PLoS One*, *7*(8), e44530.

White, D. K., Neogi, T., Nevitt, M. C., Peloquin, C. E., Zhu, Y., Boudreau, R. M., . . . Zhang, Y. (2013). Trajectories of gait speed predict mortality in well-functioning older adults: The Health, Aging and Body Composition study. *The Journals of Gerontology. Series A, Biological Sciences and Medical Sciences*, *68*(4), 456–464.

Whitfield, K. E., Wiggins, S. A., Belue, R., & Brandon, D. T. (2004). Genetic and environmental influences on forced expiratory volume in African Americans: The Carolina African-American Twin Study of Aging. *Ethnicity & Disease*, *14*(2), 206–211.

Wilk, J. B., Djousse, L., Arnett, D. K., Rich, S. S., Province, M. A., Hunt, S. C., . . . Myers, R. H. (2000). Evidence for major genes influencing pulmonary function in the NHLBI family heart study. *Genetic Epidemiology*, *19*(1), 81–94.

Wing, Y. K., Zhang, J., Lam, S. P., Li, S. X., Tang, N. L., Lai, K. Y., & Li, A. M. (2012). Familial aggregation and heritability of insomnia in a community-based study. *Sleep Medicine, 13*(8), 985–990.

Wolkowitz, O. M., Epel, E. S., & Mellon, S. (2008). When blue turns to grey: Do stress and depression accelerate cell aging? *The World Journal of Biological Psychiatry*, 9(1), 2–5.

Wust, S., Federenko, I., Hellhammer, D. H., & Kirschbaum, C. (2000). Genetic factors, perceived chronic stress, and the free cortisol response to awakening. *Psychoneuroendocrinology, 25*(7), 707–720.

Xhyheri, B., Manfrini, O., Mazzolini, M., Pizzi, C., & Bugiardini, R. (2012). Heart rate variability today. *Progress in Cardiovascular Diseases, 55*(3), 321–331.

Young, R. P., Hopkins, R., & Eaton, T. E. (2007). Forced expiratory volume in one second: Not just a lung function test but a marker of premature death from all causes. *European Respiratory Journal, 30*(4), 616–622.

Zdravkovic, S., Wienke, A., Pedersen, N. L., Marenberg, M. E., Yashin, A. I., & de Faire, U. (2004). Genetic influences on CHD-death and the impact of known risk factors: Comparison of two frailty models. *Behavior Genetics, 34*(6), 585–592.

Zeegers, M. P., Rijsdijk, F., Sham, P., Fagard, R., Gielen, M., De Leeuw, P. W., & Vlietinck, R. (2004). The contribution of risk factors to blood pressure heritability estimates in young adults: The East flanders prospective twin study. *Twin Research: The Official Journal of the International Society for Twin Studies, 7*(3), 245–253.

Zhang, F., Lewis, M., Yang, G., Iriondo-Perez, J., Zeng, Y., & Liu, J. (2008). Apolipoprotein E polymorphism, life stress and self-reported health among older adults. *Journal of Epidemiology and Community Health, 62*(4), e3.

Zhang, S., Liu, X., Yu, Y., Hong, X., Christoffel, K. K., Wang, B., . . . Wang, X. (2009). Genetic and environmental contributions to phenotypic components of metabolic syndrome: A population-based twin study. *Obesity, 17*(8), 1581–1587.

CHAPTER 8

Exploiting Causal Complexity in Aging

Gerald E. McClearn, David J. Vandenbergh, J. Tobias Stout, and Roger J. McCarter

ABSTRACT

Gerontological genetics is a paradigm case of complexity, with many genes affecting the biological processes of aging, many environmental features influencing the same processes, and conglomerates of interactions within and between each of these sources of variance. To address this complexity, researchers have available increasingly powerful and precise tools. The relative stability and uniformity of genotype of inbred strains, the precision of localization of base pairs in DNA, the standardization of biomarker measures, and the specific-pathogen-free environments—these features, among others, make possible the repeatability of experimental circumstance from laboratory to laboratory that is a defining characteristic of experimental science. However, it is increasingly apparent that the results obtained from such tightly controlled experimental features may be severely limited in their generalizability. In this work, we seek to illustrate the complexity associated even within a set of controlled studies in mice. In these studies, a relatively simple phenotype, end-of-life, was used as a main outcome measure, with predictions based on particular genetic configurations previously shown to be associated with either increased or decreased median length of life. In addition, several other phenotypes were assessed to provide possible mechanistic insights into causal pathways. The results obtained provide salutary warning of the many variables involved in determining length of life and the

http://dx.doi.org/10.1891/0198-8794.34.229

great difficulty of controlling for all possible sources of variance. This complexity may be regarded as a major nuisance in the search for the dynamics of aging. The argument can be made, however, that specific examples of interaction "hot-spots" are research targets whose study may be particularly fruitful.

INTRODUCTION

The search for mechanisms underlying aging processes has often focused on the importance of genetic inheritance (McClearn et al., 1997). In support of this focus, current studies in human beings and in animal models indicate strong association between length of life and the presence or absence of particular genes or alleles (Jiang, Kirchman, Zagulski, Hunt, & Jazwinski, 1998). Discovery of genes regulating lifespan in model organisms and genes associated with extreme longevity in men and women led to the concept of longevity assurance genes (LAG) and raised the possibility of "individualized" medical care or care directed at the genetic milieu of particular patients (Barzilai et al., 2012). Because extended longevity is often associated with the decreased presence of disease, or extended health span, a so-called "longevity dividend" has been postulated to accrue from the manipulation of human lifespan in response to the slowing down of aging processes in men and women of even a few years (Olshansky, Perry, Miller, & Butler, 2006). This dividend would involve increased duration of health and productivity over the lifespan but would also provide large financial benefits from reduced costs of medical care for the elderly. Such a slowdown in the rate of aging is theoretically possible because the current status of knowledge of molecular pathways associated with manipulated length of life in model organisms supports the possibility of slowing aging using pharmaceutical interventions (such as rapamycin, resveratrol, etc.) based on the actions of genes and transcription factors (such as sirtuins and FOXO) known to be involved in extended longevity. In short, there exists today much optimism concerning benefits associated with the manipulation of human longevity.

Such optimistic forecasts must however face the reality of the particularity of the experimental results on which these forecasts are based and of the large complexity of the aging phenotype. Genetic research over the past 50 years has increasingly demonstrated the variability of gene expression with advancing age in a given species and the dependence of gene expression at any given age on environmental and other factors. For example, epigenetic phenomena and the modulation of gene expression by small RNA molecules suggests that extrapolation of genetic identity to phenotypic outcome is hazardous at best and may be far more complicated than as suggested earlier. In particular, focus on epigenetic marks and small RNA function brings the possibility of a mechanism by which the genome can respond to life experiences, shutting down some genes and turning on others; however, this focus must address two issues. The first is that of a target tissue—changes in either domain in one tissue might be irrelevant to changes in another, more critical, tissue for aging outcomes, even if the changes are well correlated with lifespan. The second issue to consider is that changes in epigenetic patterns are themselves modulated by genotype. Thus, although there are many avenues to take in studies of aging, significant progress will most likely be made by well-focused studies that are replicable and generalizable and designed to be pieced together with other work to make sense of the "jigsaw puzzle" that is aging.

THE SEQUEL TO QTL NOMINATION

As part of the vast literature now accumulated that identifies QTLs affecting aging processes, several were previously nominated from data reported by Gelman, Watson, Bronson, and Yunis (1988) and by our group (Lang et al., 2010) as lifespan-influencing in female BXD (C57BL/6 X DBA/2) recombinant inbred (RI) strains of mice. Of particular interest was an epistatic relationship between a locus on Chromosome 2 and one on Chromosome 7 (labeled using the polymorphism closest to the center of the loci D2Mit9 and D7Mit178; hereafter abbreviated 2-9 and 7-178, respectively).

Briefly stated, presence of the lifespan-increasing allele of either QTL in homozygous state appeared to be sufficient to "rescue" the animals from the effects of a lifespan-decreasing genotype of the other locus. This study sought to confirm these initial results and to begin a probe into the mechanism(s) through which they occur.

STUDY DESIGN

In the current project, genotypic selective breeding from an F2 population derived from C57BL/6 and DBA/2 progenitor inbred strains generated four strains of mice with respect to 2-9 and 7-178. The four strains were homozygous at these loci in the configurations of lifespan-decreasing alleles at both loci (Strain 1); lifespan-increasing alleles at both loci (Strain 4); and increasing alleles at one locus and decreasing alleles at the other (Strains 2 and 3). (Further detail is given in Table 8.1.) In addition, two other QTLs identified as female-lifespan-affecting (D1Mit218 and D6Mit102; 1-218 and 6-102, respectively; Lang et al., 2010) were assessed in a subsample. Thus, the study design permits evaluation in homozygous genotype combinations of two loci fixed by selective breeding and,

TABLE 8.1

Sample Structure (Numbers of Mice, Females Only) of Selectively Bred Strains and of Test Group Membership

Strain	2-9 Locus	7-178 Locus	LIFESPAN	BEHAVIOR/ IGF1	BODYCOMP	Total N
1	DD	DD	54	30	30	114
2	DD	BB	47	25	23	95
3	BB	DD	46	18	19	83
4	BB	BB	49	29	30	108
Total Number			196	102	102	400

in two other loci, in segregating genotypes (including heterozygotes). In both situations, the loci under examination exist in a context of varying combinations of segregating genetic factors derived from the C57BL/6 and DBA/2 gene pools.

In addition to testing of generalizability of the lifespan-altering effects of specific loci, the project offered an opportunity to assess the influence of several biomarker domains and experimental design features, both as intrinsic predictors of longevity and as factors interacting with genetic influences.

Three test groups (all females) were established within each of the four selectively bred strains. All animals were housed four per cage and were maintained under specific-pathogen-free (SPF) barrier conditions until natural death (or meeting of moribundity criteria). The LIFESPAN group was undisturbed except for routine husbandry procedures and a one-time tail tip sampling for 1-218 and 6-102 assay. Two biomarker groups were measured at approximately 150, 450, and 750 days of age. One of these groups (BEHAVIOR/IGF1) was measured on behavioral variables putatively related to aging—including strength, agility, and exploratory behavior—and was also assessed for plasma levels of insulin-like growth factor (IGF). A third group (BODYCOMP) was assessed for body composition variables including body weight, body length, body fat, lean mass, and bone mineral density (BMD). Apart from the procedures necessary for their particular biomarker measurements, the BEHAVIOR/IGF1 and BODYCOMP animals were maintained under the same barrier conditions as were the LIFESPAN group. Litters were maintained together until weaning, when females and males were separated. Females for this study were maintained thereafter in sibship groups in conventional barrier caging until death.

The sample structure of the project and the numbers of each subgroup are shown in Table 8.1. The strains are identified by numerals, with a letter code (D or B) specifying their genotypes with respect to the two selected loci, 2-9 and 7-178, respectively. The initial nominating project had identified the D allele, from the DBA parentage, to be the decreasing allele at each locus; similarly, the B allele from the C57BL/6 parentage is the increasing allele. Thus, for example, DD/BB identifies Strain 2 as having been bred selectively to be homozygous for the decreasing allele at the Chromosome 2 locus and homozygous for the increasing allele at the Chromosome 7 locus, and so forth.

GENETIC EVALUATIONS

Response of Longevity to Genotypic Selective Breeding

The principal operational question of the selective breeding program was whether the differences in age at death that served to nominate 2-9 and 7-178 in the original RI strain context would be evident when these QTLs are organized in four homozygous relationships, each on a segregating genetic background derived from the C57BL/6 and DBA/2 gene pool. In general, results reported were obtained from nonparametric statistical procedures using SPSS version 20, so as to minimize reliance on interval scale assumptions. Briefly stated, the distributions of the initial RI strain *median* age-at-death values were such that the double-decreasing homozygotes (DDDD) did not overlap the medians of the other three distributions. Thus, the simplest and most direct confirmation of the original nomination would show Strain 4 animals to have a higher median longevity than those of Strain 1. The results for Strains 2 and 3 should be closer to Strain 4 than to Strain 1, and preferably, in keeping with the interaction theme, would not differ from each other.

Distributions of age of death (AOD: age at date of death measured in days) measures for the standard, "undisturbed" LIFESPAN Test Group are given in Figure 8.1. The Kruskal-Wallis test revealed no significant difference among the strains ($H = 1.0$, $n = 196$, $p < .80$).

Influence of QTL 1-218 and 6-102 on Genetically Heterogeneous Backgrounds

For determining the genotypes of the two nominated QTLs of interest on Chromosomes 1 and 6, tail tips were collected at weaning and the DNA purified from this tissue was genotyped at a pair of markers that flank the QTL regions of interest. Animals of this phase were maintained in the LIFESPAN mode. Table 8.2 gives the sample size for each genotype group.

No significant relationship was found between allelic state (0, 1, or 2 "increasing" alleles) and age at death for either locus (Kruskal-Wallis $H = .526$, $p < .77$ and $H = .106$, $p < .95$ for 1-218 and 6-102, respectively).

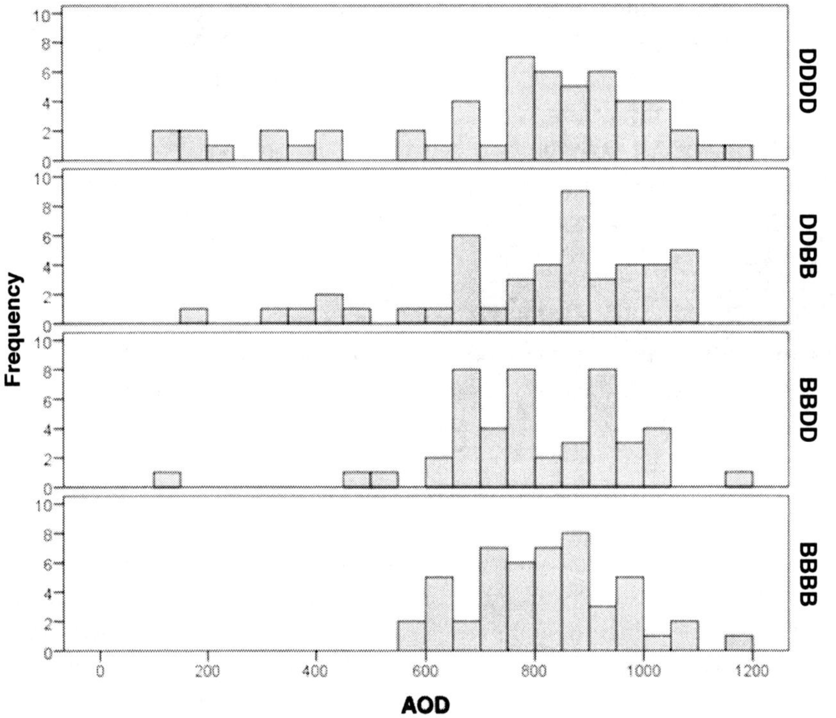

FIGURE 8.1 Distributions of ages at death of selectively bred strains maintained under LIFESPAN conditions.

Thus, so far as median lifespans of the selectively bred strains were concerned, there was failure to confirm the original nominations. However, differences among the strains in incidence of low values (see Figure 8.1) suggest the presence in this population of at least two subprocesses, one of which promotes early death. They also indicate that Strain 1 (DDDD), homozygous for the presumptive decreasing alleles at both selected loci, appears most susceptible to early death; Strain 4 (BBBB), homozygous for the increasing alleles,

TABLE 8.2
Numbers of Animals With Chromosome 1 and Chromosome 6 Genotypes

	Numbers of Increasing Alleles			
QTL	0	1	2	Total
1-218	16	40	32	88
6-102	20	33	26	79

may be most resistant, with other strains intermediate. Although not a direct confirmation of the QTLs' influence on the AOD phenotype for which it was nominated, these results are indicative of some process or processes and may identify a valuable research objective. Several analyses were directed toward this prospect.

GENES AND ENVIRONMENTS

A central consideration of complex causal fields in biological systems is the interaction of genes and environments. Relevant environmental factors may include those deliberately manipulated as a central focus of the research program as well as those that occur without systematic manipulation. In particular, features of the environment and husbandry in which the test animals are born, reared, nurtured, and measured may potentially exert considerable influence on the research outcomes.

A primary current issue was whether there was a detectable effect of rearing and maintenance in the different test groups on either AOD or early deaths.

For the present analysis, a threshold of AOD of 400 days (approximately two standard deviations lower than the mean of the total LIFESPAN group distribution) was chosen to differentiate "early" deaths from those in the "normal" range. Distribution of these deaths within strain and test groups is shown in Table 8.3.

Testing Regimens

The LIFESPAN group of this study was intended to provide a minimally disturbed group as a reference "control" for evaluating the possible effects on aging of the measurement processes involved in assessing the biomarker variables of the BEHAVIOR/IGF1 and BODYCOMP test groups.

In the total population, Kruskal-Wallis analyses demonstrated no significant difference among test groups in median ages at death. Furthermore, no

TABLE 8.3

Incidence of Early Deaths as Fractions of Strain and Test Groups

Testing Group	Strain 1 DDDD	Strain 2 DDBB	Strain 3 BBDD	Strain 4 BBBB	Total
LIFESPAN	8/54	3/47	1/46	0/49	12/196
BEHAVIOR/IGF1	0/30	0/25	1/18	1/29	2/102
BODYCOMP	2/30	3/23	0/19	0/30	5/102
Total	10/114	6/95	2/83	1/108	19/400

influence of test group was found *within* any of the strains. However, a more complex situation is revealed when strains are compared within test groups with respect to the distribution of AOD. The strain differences in incidence of early death shown in Figure 8.1 and Table 8.3 (with Strains 1 and 2 showing higher incidence of early death than Strains 3 or 4) are significant only within the LIFESPAN group. Strains 1 and 2 share the DD genotype for 2-9; Strains 3 and 4 share the BB allele. Crosstabs analysis indicates that the difference between these pairs is statistically significant (chi square $p < .004$). A parallel analysis revealed no significant influence of 7-178 in any test group.

The result suggests a vulnerability of individuals homozygous for the decreasing allele (DD) of the 2-9 QTL for early death and illustrates that influence of environmental features of experimental design on early deaths may depend on both the genotype of the organisms under study as well as the stressors. Thus, results based on a single strain or single environmental intervention may be seriously limited in range of applicability. That a detrimental effect for one strain in this study was obtained in the test group intended to be *least* disturbed by measurement stress invites further study. It may be that stress can have curvilinear effects on longevity, with some levels being beneficial, others harmful (Neafsey, 1990; Salmon et al., 2005).

Litter Birth Order

Other aspects of gestation and development may affect key experimental parameters. For example, programs requiring assignment of animals to several projects with diverse testing calendars are potentially subject to major logistical issues attendant upon litter birth order. In this study, test animals were assigned from 1st, 2nd, or 3rd litters. Kruskal-Wallis analyses of LIFESPAN animals revealed no significant difference in AOD among these groups. However, analysis of all test groups together yielded a significant effect ($H = 8.1$; $n = 391$, $p < .017$) with longer lives among animals from later litters. Furthermore, analysis separately by strain showed a significant effect of litter number, but only within the LIFESPAN group of Strain 2 ($H = 7.4$, $n = 92$, $p < .02$). By inspection of the distributions of Strain 2 animals (see Figure 8.2), and of Strain 2 LIFESPAN animals (see Figure 8.3), the beneficial effect appears to be caused principally by reduction (or elimination) of early mortality. This invites speculation about protective features of older, more experienced mothers or other (as yet unknown) variables.

BIOMARKERS

Body Composition

The five primary body composition variables examined were body length (LENGTH), body weight (WT), PerCent total lean (PERTLEAN), PerCent total

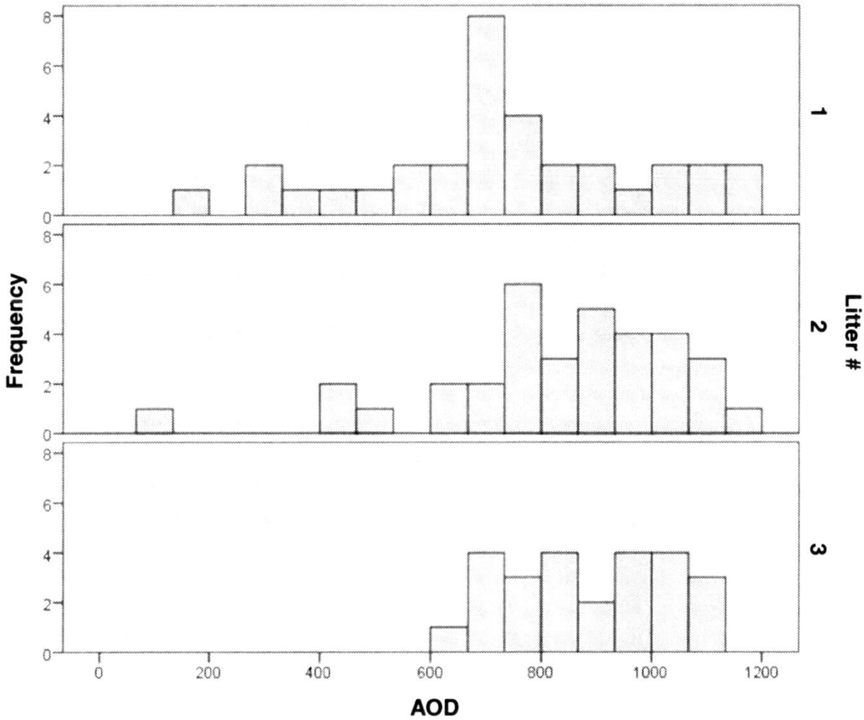

FIGURE 8.2 Distributions of ages at death of animals of three litters in Strain 2.

fat (PERTFAT), and BMD. All of these measures were substantially to highly intercorrelated, with absolute rho values ranging from .55 to .95 at all ages.

The initial assessment of the predictive value of these measures was made by simple correlations with AOD. None of the 150-day measures was predictive of total remaining lifetime; PERTLEAN and PERTFAT measured at 450 days produced modest predictive value, overall (rho = −.26, $n = 90$, $p < .01$ and .35, $n = 90$, $p < .002$).

Within Strains 1, 2, and 4, however, none of the relationships was significant. Within Strain 3 alone, rho = −.49, $n = 18$, $p < .04$ and .46, $p < .05$ (for PERTLEAN450 and PERTFAT450 respectively). For the 750-day assays, the stress of testing procedures (for example, anesthetizing animals for measurement of BMD) was judged to be sufficient to affect measures of remaining lifespan. Testing was therefore terminated after 19 observations had been made.

All of these 750-day measures excepting body length produced substantial predictive value (rho indices ranging from .50 to .64; p values from .003 to .031) for the life expectancy of this sample of tested 750-day survivors.

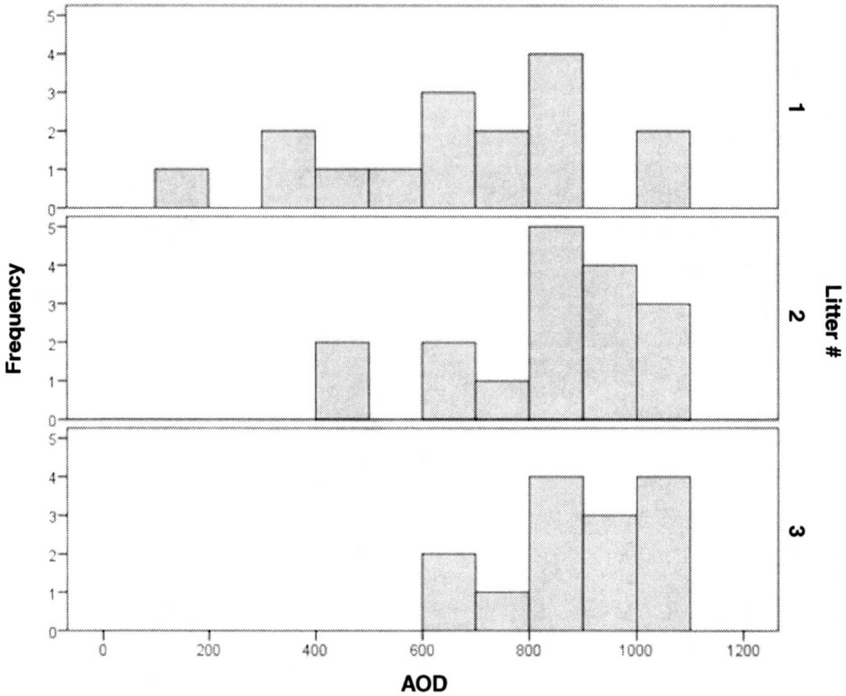

FIGURE 8.3 Distributions of ages at death of animals of three litter birth orders within Strain 2, maintained under LIFESPAN conditions.

Behavioral Biomarkers

Previous work on mice in our laboratory has examined batteries of behavioral variables for relationship to lifespan (e.g., Foreman et al., 2009; Heller, Ahern, Stout, & McClearn, 1998). This study offered a confirmation test for evaluating the generalizability of these previous results. The mice used in the previous studies were from the heterogeneous stock (HS) colony derived from eight inbred strains, including the C57BL and DBA/2. In particular, attention was directed to three tests, presumed measures of exploration/curiosity, when mice were placed singly in unfamiliar situations. Among the tests employed were the File apparatus (a small enclosed arena with floor marked in four equal squares, each with a centered small hole) and the CORD apparatus (a horizontal cord suspended tautly between supports). Specific measures found relevant to length of life (Heller et al., 1998) included file activity (number of floor-squares entered in a 3-min period), headpokes (number of thrusts of nose into the floor openings), and cord drop times (cling time after being placed on a cord before dropping to a foam mat. To summarize, in female mice, file acivity, headpokes, and longer cord drop times were significantly related to lifespans.

In the current data, no one of these particular behavioral measures from any of the three ages correlated significantly with age at death, either in the overall data or within any single strain.

Insulin-Like Growth Factor

Considerable research attention has been devoted to the inverse relation between longevity and plasma levels of IGF in several inbred strains of mice and in other species (Sonntag, Csiszar, deCabo, Ferrucci, & Ungvari, 2012). In this study, animals of the BEHAVIOR/IGF1 group were assayed for plasma levels at all three testing ages.

In overall analysis and separately in Strains 1, 3, and 4, there was no correlation between measured IGF1 and age at death. In Strain 2, however, significant relationships were obtained both for IGF1-150 (rho $= -.55$, $p < .005$) and IGF1-450 (rho $= -.45$, $p < .03$).

Thus, the efficacy of IGF1 as a predictor biomarker of lifespan (and, presumably as an agent in the causal field) is influenced by its genotypic context, manifested in the present case by the configuration of 2-9 and 7-178.

A further result is noteworthy: marked intraindividual variability across the testing period poses limitations on predictions in advanced age from values measured in youth. Within strains, the only significant correlations were between IGF1-150 and IGF1-450 within Strain 1 (rho $= .42$, $p < .03$) and between IGF1-150 and IGF1-750 within Strain 3 (rho $= .72$, $p < .013$). In the total population, the only significant correlation was between IGF1-150 and IGF1-450 (rho $= .26$, $p < .015$).

CONCLUSION

The broad expectation of the study was that there would be manifestations of complex causation. This expectation was well realized. An initial nomination of an interactive QTL relationship was affirmed in an amended form (early death incidence rather than population median difference), but only in one of the four test strains. Neither of the other two nominated singleton QTLs exhibited significant correlation with age at death in any strain. A specific rearing environment was influential in one strain only. And so on.

Observations of causal theorists on hierarchical control systems (e.g., Salthe, 1985; Simon, 1996) constitute a particularly appropriate vantage point for the striving to find "the" mechanism of a particular gerontological phenotype. A given level of such a hierarchical system may be responsive only to the relevant output signals from adjacent levels. The recipient level may be utterly indifferent to the details about how that output was generated. These considerations indicate that there may be an optimal explanatory level for any particular stratum of phenomena, and that the more particularized or reductive searches may result in less generalizable explanatory gain.

The broad conclusion that emerges from this study is the ubiquity of interaction. This strongly indicates that there is no single best group or strain of animals, no single optimal controlled environment, no optimal level(s) of a manipulated variable for investigation of the complex processes of aging. This complexity may be encountered as a major nuisance in the search for the dynamics of aging. The argument can be made, however, that specific examples of interaction "hot-spots" are research targets whose study may be particularly fruitful. The operational starting point is that, to a question about the effectiveness of any given variable in a gerontological scenario, the initial answer should be—"it depends"—perhaps on a very large number of factors.

The foregoing discussion underlines the complexities of designing research whose goal is to uncover mechanisms of aging and, in particular, the significant caution that should be exercised before extrapolating results obtained to more general populations. Even given the overwhelming body of evidence that genetic inheritance plays a major role in aging processes, the identification of specific genes or genetic loci affecting longevity is impacted by factors that are often ignored in current and previous studies. The present work suggests lifetime experiences (or absence of experiences), birth order, and environmental conditions, among others, may play a role in determining length of life. In addition, outcome measures such as the average longevity of a population may not reveal potentially deleterious effects on early- or late-life mortality associated with particular genetic configurations. Phenotypes such as BMD, plasma level of insulin-like growth hormone, body fat, and so forth were shown to be of very low predictability for length of life, and then only for particular genetic/age configurations. The inability to reproduce our earlier results, despite similarity of population genetics and environmental conditions, indicates additional as yet unknown variables. We conclude that the generalizability of data obtained in particular genetic and environmental configurations, in both laboratory animal populations and in human populations should be viewed with caution. Similarly, extrapolation of experimental data to expectations of outcome in free-living populations should be done with great care.

ACKNOWLEDGMENTS

This work was supported by The Ellison Medical Foundation, grant AG-SS-1727-06.

REFERENCES

Barzilai, N., Guarente, L., Kirkwood, T. B., Partridge, L., Rando, T. A., & Slagboom, P. E. (2012). The place of genetics in ageing research. *Nature Reviews Genetics, 13*, 589–594.

Foreman, J. E., Lionikas, A., Lang, D. H., Gyekis, J. P., Krishnan, M., Sharkey, N. A., . . . Blizard, D. A. (2009). Genetic architecture for hole-board behaviors across substantial time intervals in young, middle-aged and old mice. *Genes, Brain and Behavior*, *8*(7), 714–727.

Gelman, R., Watson, A., Bronson, R., & Yunis, E. (1988). Murine chromosomal regions correlated with longevity. *Genetics*, *118*, 693–704.

Heller, D. A., Ahern, F. M., Stout, J. T., & McClearn, G. E. (1998). Mortality and biomarkers of aging in heterogeneous stock (HS) mice. *The Journals of Gerontology Series A: Biological Sciences and Medical Sciences*, *53*(3), B217–B230.

Jiang, J. C., Kirchman, P. A., Zagulski, M., Hunt, J., & Jazwinski, S. M. (1998). Homologs of the yeast longevity gene LAG1 in Caenorhabditis elegans and human. *Genome Research*, *8*, 1259–1272.

Lang, D. H., Gerhard, G. S., Griffith, J. W., Vogler, G. P., Vandenbergh, D. J., Blizard, D. A., . . . McClearn, G. E. (2010). Quantitative trait loci (QTL) analysis of longevity in C57BL/6 by DBA/2 (BXD) recombinant inbred mice. *Aging Clinical and Experimental Research*, *22*(1), 8–19.

McClearn, G. E., Johansson, B., Berg, S., Pedersen, N. L., Ahern, F., Petrill, S. A., & Plomin, R. (1997). Substantial genetic influence on cognitive abilities in twins 80 or more years old. *Science*, *276*, 1560–1563.

Neafsey, P. J. (1990). Longevity hormesis. *Mechanisms of Ageing and Development*, *51*, 1–31.

Olshansky, S. J., Perry, D., Miller, R. A., & Butler, R. N. (2006). In pursuit of the longevity dividend. *The Scientist*, *20*, 28–36.

Salmon, A. B., Murakami, S., Bartke, A., Kopchick, J., Yasumura, K., & Miller, R. A. (2005). Fibroblast cell lines from young adult mice of long-lived mutant strains are resistant to multiple forms of stress. *American Journal of Physiology: Endocrinology and Metabolism*, *289*, E23–E29.

Salthe, S. N. (1985). *Evolving hierarchical systems: Their structure and representation*. New York, NY: Columbia University Press.

Simon, H. A. (1996). *The sciences of the artificial* (3rd ed.). Cambridge, MA: The MIT Press.

Sonntag, W., Csiszar, A., deCabo, R., Ferrucci, L., & Ungvari, Z. (2012). Diverse roles of growth hormone and Insulin-like Growth Factor-1 in mammalian aging: Progress and controversies. *The Journals of Gerontology Series A: Biological Sciences and Medical Sciences*, *67*(6), 587–598.

CHAPTER 9

Networks in the Biology of Aging

Powerful Tools for a Complex Process

Mark A. McCormick and Daniel E. L. Promislow

ABSTRACT

Aging is a fundamental biological process of great interest. However, despite a tremendous research effort, there are still many unknowns when it comes to understanding even the basic mechanisms that underlie this trait. On the one hand, as this book illustrates, there is much hope—several signaling pathways have now been shown to greatly influence aging and lifespan in diverse organisms, including mammals. These findings suggest that at least some aging pathways have been conserved over deep evolutionary time and that lessons learned from yeast, worms, flies, and mice could well apply to humans. On the other hand, perhaps more than any other widely studied biological phenomenon, both the causes and consequences of aging are exceedingly complex.

The complex nature of aging means that a single genetic or environmental perturbation will not guarantee an increase in healthy days (for yeast or worms) or years (for humans). Rather, the underlying mechanisms of aging are likely to include many pathways, and the interactions among those pathways are likely to take place within and across many different levels of organization, from DNA and RNA to proteins, to metabolites, and ultimately to the physiological processes—and the failure of these processes—that determine whether an organism lives or dies.

http://dx.doi.org/10.1891/0198-8794.34.243

In this chapter, we argue that a focus on molecular networks has the potential to help us understand the proximate mechanisms of aging and age-related diseases and to explain at least some of the enormous variation in patterns of aging that we see in genetically variable populations. Moreover, we suggest that by examining the way in which network structure or function both shapes and is shaped by aging, we can refine theoretical models, and so better explain the proximate and evolutionary determinants of aging.

INTRODUCTION

Organisms alive today represent the end product of an extraordinary lineage; a lineage that has experienced over 3 billion years of continued natural selection for growth and development, reproduction, and survival. This same selection pressure has given rise to exquisite mechanisms to maintain and repair organisms in the face of a constant onslaught of biotic and abiotic damaging agents. Why, then, can a genome able to replicate throughout the millennia not avoid the inexorable decline in physiological function that happens as organisms age?

Why Aging Exists

Biologists have offered two kinds of answer to this question. The first answer, an evolutionary one, was put forward by Sir Peter Medawar (1952) in his "mutation accumulation" theory. Inspired by Haldane's (1942) work on Huntington's disease, Medawar started with the assumption that germ-line mutations could have age-specific effects. Consider a mutation in humans that decreases survival rate by some fraction, but only after the age of 60 years. Carriers of this mutation will have passed the novel allele on to their children and grandchildren long before they experience its deleterious effects. Because of this, natural selection would have little power to remove the mutation from the population. In general, as Medawar's thought experiment illustrates and as subsequent mathematical modeling proves (W. D. Hamilton, 1966), the strength of selection declines with age. And because of this decline, as we age we expect an ever-increasing number of deleterious mutations, passed down from our ancestors, to be expressed. A derivative of Medawar's theory—George Williams' (1957) "antagonistic pleiotropy" theory—posits that selection could actually *favor* some of these late-acting deleterious alleles if they had early-acting beneficial effects (de Keizer, Laberge, & Campisi, 2010).

The Complexity of Aging

These evolutionary models, developed in the 1940s and the 1950s, offer fundamental explanations for why aging occurs but are agnostic about the proximate mechanisms that explain how aging occurs. In fact, until molecular biologists showed otherwise, most evolutionary biologists concluded that evolutionary theory implied that aging would be a highly polygenic trait, caused by a large number of loci each of small effect, and that we would be unlikely to identify single genes with large effects on aging. Of course, as we have already noted, recent decades have shown that single-gene mutations, and the pathways in which these genes participate, can greatly affect the lifespan, health span, and rate of aging in multiple, evolutionarily distant organisms (Gems & Partridge, 2001; Jia, Chen, & Riddle, 2004; Kaeberlein et al., 2005; Kapahi et al., 2004; Kenyon, 2005; Piper, Selman, McElwee, & Partridge, 2008; Tatar, Bartke, & Antebi, 2003). In addition, single compounds acting on these regulatory pathways have also been shown to have remarkable effects on aging (Harrison et al., 2009). However, closer inspection points to a more complex story.

Although aging can be greatly modified by single-gene mutations that in many cases affect individual signaling pathways, developing a complete picture of these signaling pathways, from initial source to all final targets, has proven remarkably difficult. Much excellent work has been done in identifying downstream targets, but often this has left us still far from a real understanding of the mechanisms that lead to the decline of function with age, or that postpone this decline in long-lived mutant or drug-treated organisms. A representative example is the *daf-2* or *age-1* insulin signaling pathway in *Caenorhabditis elegans* (Dorman, Albinder, Shroyer, & Kenyon, 1995; Friedman & Johnson, 1988; Kenyon, Chang, Gensch, Rudner, & Tabtiang, 1993), which was one of the earliest pathways shown genetically to have a dramatic effect on aging in a model organism and which has received more attention than any other aging pathway. Early in the study of this pathway, it was realized that the FOXO family transcription factor *daf-16* was a relevant and necessary downstream effector (Kenyon et al., 1993; K. Lin, Dorman, Rodan, & Kenyon, 1997; Ogg et al., 1997). As a result of these findings, multiple groups have studied the likely transcriptional targets of DAF-16, specifically in the context of lifespan-extending *daf-2* or *age-1* mutations, in the hopes of revealing more about the proximal mechanisms involved (Halaschek-Wiener et al., 2005; McElwee, Bubb, & Thomas, 2003; McElwee, Schuster, Blanc, Thomas, & Gems, 2004; Murphy, 2006; Murphy et al., 2003; Oh et al., 2006; Schuster et al., 2010; H. Yu & Larsen, 2001). These studies have been carried out using diverse methods and platforms for assaying transcript level as well as chromosomal locus occupation. In each case much has been added to what we know about the targets of this pathway, and in each case interesting downstream genes have been identified that have statistically significant effects on aging and lifespan. Overall, however, these data sets are more discordant than overlapping. Furthermore, no subset of the identified targets in this pathway has been identified whose perturbation can come close to the magnitude of effect on lifespan of *age-1* or *daf-2* mutations themselves. One possibility that these results leave open is that, although modifying regulatory genes that modulate multiple downstream effectors might allow large changes in lifespan and health span, the downstream targets themselves might have to act in large ensembles to produce these same dramatic effects, with no single target or small combination of targets sufficient.

The studies described earlier suggest that even within a fairly small module of genes, epistatic interactions might be a critical part of the overall function of the pathway. There are other factors that further complicate the situation. First, epistatic interactions might be important not only between genes within the same pathway but also more broadly speaking. For example, although overexpression of a human superoxide dismutase (hSOD) gene in flies can extend lifespan in *Drosophila* (Parkes et al., 1998), when placed in different natural genetic backgrounds, this same gene can lose its effect on lifespan (Spencer, Howell, Wright, & Promislow, 2003). Other lifespan studies have found that genetic background influences the effects not only of genetic manipulations but also of diet restriction in both mice (Liao et al., 2011) and yeast (Schleit et al., 2013). Second, screens for worm aging genes routinely turn up a large number of genes in different pathways. However, when carried out in different labs, these studies show little overlap, even when studying the same mutants in the same genetic background (Yanos, Bennett, & Kaeberlein, 2012). Third, Greer et al. (2011) have shown that epigenetically encoded changes in lifespan because of deficiencies in the H3K4me3 methylation complex can be passed down through multiple generations. Finally, and perhaps most importantly, the large-effect genes that we discover in the lab might have little effect on variation in longevity in natural populations. Genome-wide association studies (GWAS) examine the effects on some trait of interest of allelic variation at all segregating loci in a population. These studies, made possible by whole-genome sequencing, have had great success in identifying loci that explain variation in complex traits (such as aging). However, although longevity is highly heritable (genome-wide variation explains 20%–50% of the total variance in longevity), GWAS identify loci that typically explain just 1%–2% of the total variation at best (Walter et al., 2011). This pattern from GWAS has led us to wonder whether complex interactions among these many genes might account, at least in part, for the unexplained or "missing" heritability.

So we are left with a challenging situation. A large body of evolutionary theory tells us that aging should happen but tells us little about its underlying mechanisms. And mechanistic studies suggest that variation in rates of aging in natural populations could be extremely complex genetically, leaving open the question of whether what we learn about the genetics of aging from lab studies applies to natural populations. How, then, are we to determine what the many complex genetic factors are that shape aging, and to explain why they do so?

Aging Research in a World of High-Throughput Biology

All of these complications point to the need to be able to look at a large number of genes (or other factors) and their interactions simultaneously. Recent advances in high-throughput biology make all this possible. First, large-scale screens have now been undertaken for genes that influence aging in yeast (*Saccharomyces cerevisiae*; Kaeberlein et al., 2005; Matecic et al., 2010; Powers, Kaeberlein, Caldwell, Kennedy, & Fields, 2006), worms (*C. elegans*; Dillin et al., 2002; B. Hamilton et al., 2005; Hansen, Hsu, Dillin, & Kenyon, 2005; S. S. Lee et al., 2003), and fruit flies (*Drosophila melanogaster*; Funakoshi et al., 2011; Y. L. Lin, Seroude, & Benzer, 1998; Liu et al., 2009; Paik et al., 2012; H. D. Wang, Kazemi-Esfarjani, & Benzer, 2004), among others. Second, we can now easily collect whole-transcriptome data to compare organisms at different ages (Budovskaya et al., 2008; Lund et al., 2002; McCarroll et al., 2004; Vinuela, Snoek, Riksen, & Kammenga, 2010; Zahn et al., 2007), short-lived versus long-lived genotypes (Fisher & Lithgow, 2006; Slack et al., 2010), and individuals treated with lifespan-extending treatments such as caloric restriction (Estep, Warner, & Bulyk, 2009; Oita, Mazzatti, Lim, Powell, & Merry, 2009; Swindell, 2009). Third, we now have easy access to published repositories of large data sets such as genomes, interactomes, functional annotations, and ontologies. And finally, freely available computational tools allow us to analyze these data with relative ease.

Networks and Aging

We can think of an organism as a set of interacting elements, from the simplest molecules that make up the metabolome, to the physiological interactions within and between organ systems, to the higher level interactions that occur between individuals and between an individual and the environment in which it lives. To understand these complex interactions, we can take advantage of the tools that have been developed over the years, initially by physicists and social scientists, and more recently by bioinformaticians.

Network-based analysis has been able to greatly aid in the dissection of diverse complex phenomena, such as expression patterns of gap genes (Kozlov, Surkova, Myasnikova, Reinitz, & Samsonova, 2012) and pair-rule genes (von Dassow, Meir, Munro, & Odell, 2000) in the developing *Drosophila* embryo, as well as the development and evolution of mammalian teeth (Salazar-Ciudad & Jernvall, 2002), among many others.

Increasingly, these powerful methods are being applied to questions about aging. In what follows, we will introduce several questions that have benefited from a network approach. These include the following: (a) Do so-called "aging genes" have a different network architecture than other genes?; (b) Can we use network analysis to predict whether or not a gene will impact aging?; and (c) How does network structure change with age?

Before we tackle these various questions, we will start with an introduction of some of the basic concepts in network science.

NETWORKS IN AGING

Networks are Powerful Tools for Dissecting Complex Phenomena

A biological network is made up a series of *nodes* (also known as *vertices*), each of which is connected by a set of *edges* to *k* other nodes. For example, a specific node might be a metabolite and its edges might be biochemical interactions that link that metabolite to other metabolites. Links can be defined in different ways. For example, we might consider two metabolites as linked if we know that one is the immediate downstream product of another in a metabolic pathway. Alternatively, we can define metabolites or other molecules as linked if they correlate with one another across different environmental conditions, different tissues, or different genotypes. This latter is of particular interest because it ties together the study of networks with the study of genetically variable (i.e., "natural") populations.

We can further distinguish networks based on the type of edges they contain. For some types of networks, edges can have directionality. For example, in signaling pathways, we can define an upstream protein and a downstream one. For other networks, only the existence of the edge is informative and there is no directionality, as in physical protein–protein interactions. These two types of graphs are referred to, respectively, as directed and undirected graphs or networks. Starting with Euler's famous mathematical work on the bridges of Königsberg (Euler, 1758), the tools of *graph theory* have been used to understand all kinds of networks (including biological ones). Although we will not delve into the mathematics here, we will provide a few definitions that will be useful later on.

The structure of a network can be summarized as a short text table listing all node–node pairs individually. The graphical and tabular representations of the same simple undirected graph are shown next in Figure 9.1 and Table 9.1, respectively, to illustrate this concordance.

Note that here, it is irrelevant which of the two connected nodes is listed under the header "NODE 1," and which is under "NODE 2." If this were a directed

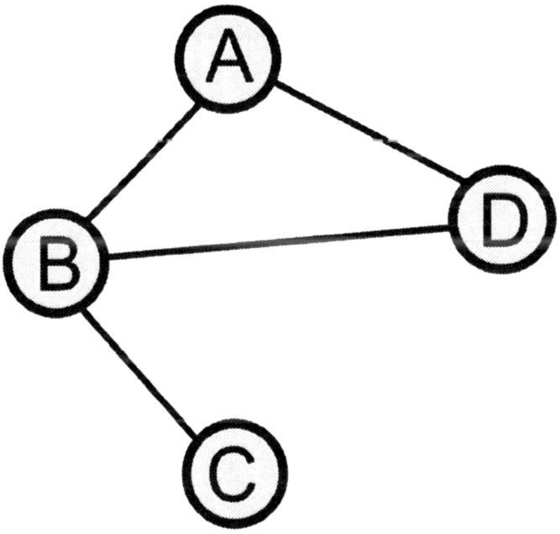

FIGURE 9.1 A simple, undirected graph.

TABLE 9.1
A Simple, Undirected Graph in Tabular Form

NODE 1	NODE 2
A	B
A	D
B	D
B	C

graph, we could add this information simply by insisting that the "from" column and "to" column be made clear, as shown in Figure 9.2 and Table 9.2 next.

Because of this, it is easy to portably save even very complex networks as reasonably sized tables, and to move these simple tables between network analysis software platforms. If the node names, rather than "A" or "B," are sufficiently unique identifiers of the gene, protein, metabolite, and so forth of interest, then the same software that is used to display the table as a visual graph can append additional data such as functional category, pathway, and so forth often by directly polling online repositories.

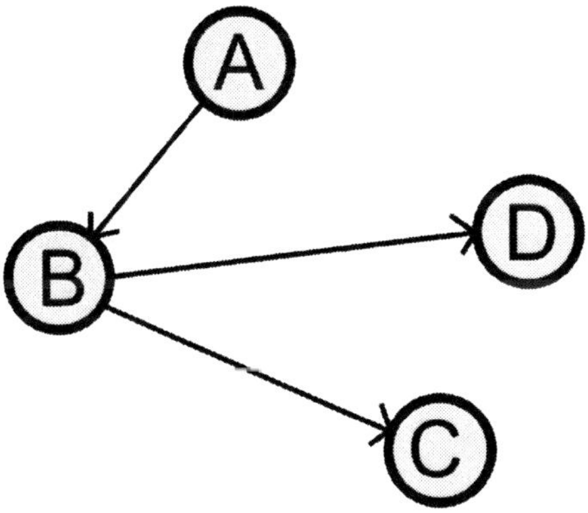

FIGURE 9.2 A simple, directed graph.

TABLE 9.2
A Simple, Directed Graph in Tabular Form

From	To
A	B
B	C
B	C

Structural Properties of Networks

In addition to defining a network in terms of which nodes are connected to which other nodes, we can also define numerous structural properties of the network. Here we describe a few that have been used to better understand the function of biological networks.

Connectivity

We define the number of edges that connect to a given node as its connectivity, denoted by the letter k. In a directed network, we can distinguish between k_{in} and k_{out}.

Degree Distribution

The degree distribution refers to the frequency distribution of values of k among all nodes in the network. For example, imagine that we have a network with 100 nodes, and we randomly assign 100 edges between randomly chosen pairs of nodes. Some nodes might be chosen multiple times just by chance, whereas others might be chosen just once or not at all. The frequency distribution of k for this random network will be Poisson (see Figure 9.3).

Interestingly, many different kinds of networks, including biological networks, depart dramatically from this random graph. Most "real-world" networks come much closer to a Power law distribution, defined as $f(k) = k^{-\gamma}/\zeta(k)$ (Albert & Barabási, 2002; see Figure 9.4; $\zeta(k)$ is the *zeta* function, which simply normalizes the function so all the frequencies sum to 1).

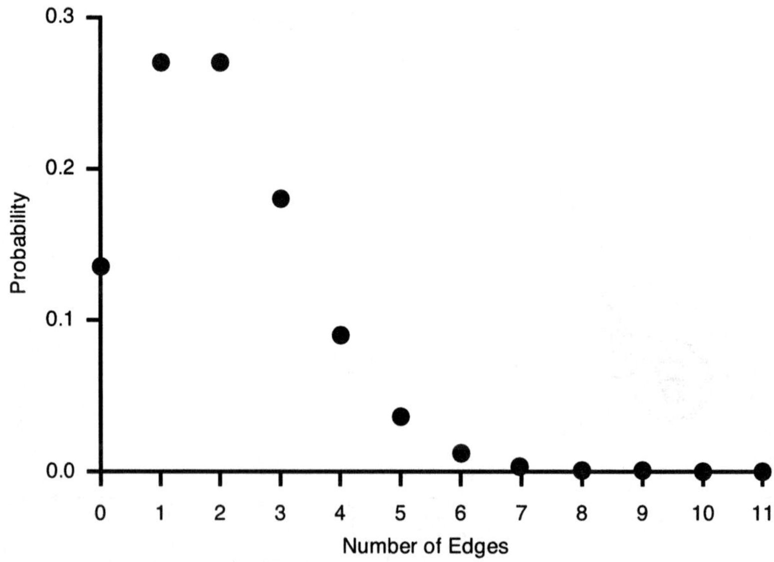

FIGURE 9.3 Distribution of edges in a graph with 100 nodes and 100 randomly assigned edges.

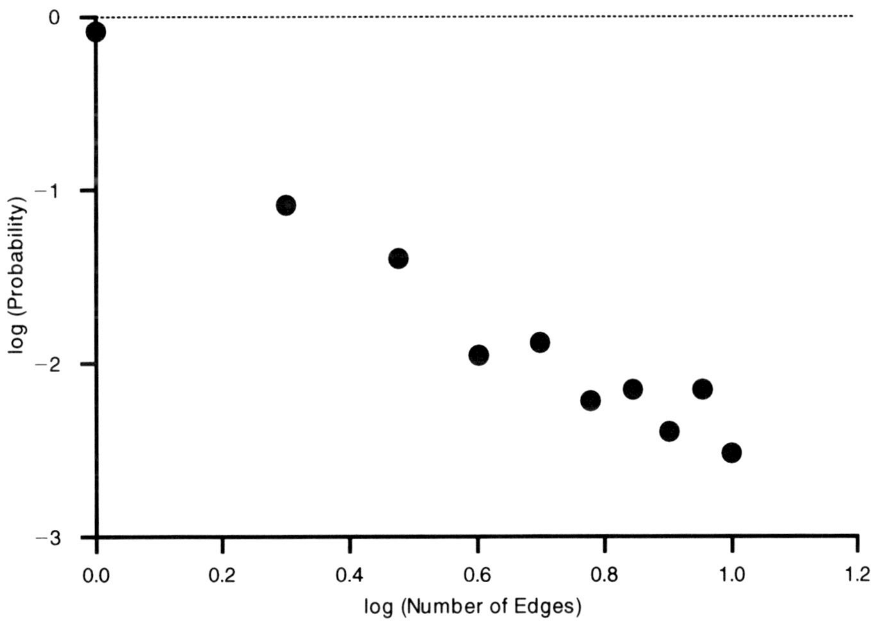

FIGURE 9.4 Distribution of edges in a simulated scale-free (power-law described) network, for connectivity up to 11. Note that the power law distribution is a straight line on a log-log scale.

Centrality

In addition to determining how connected a particular node is, we can also define various attributes that describe its location in relation to other nodes in the network. These include such factors as *closeness*, the average distance between a specific node and all other nodes, and *betweenness*, the relative frequency with which a particular node must be traversed to go from each node to each other node.

Modularity

Biological networks often can be described in terms of groups of "subnetworks" that form the overall network. Within a large network, we can define subnetworks, or *modules*, as groups of nodes whose connectivity between one another is greater, on average, than the connectivity to other nodes within the same network but outside of the module.

Motif

In directed networks, we can identify specific *motifs* that arise between small groups of nodes. For example, a feedback motif is defined as A→B, B→C, and C→A, whereas a feedforward motif is defined as A→B, B→C, and A→C

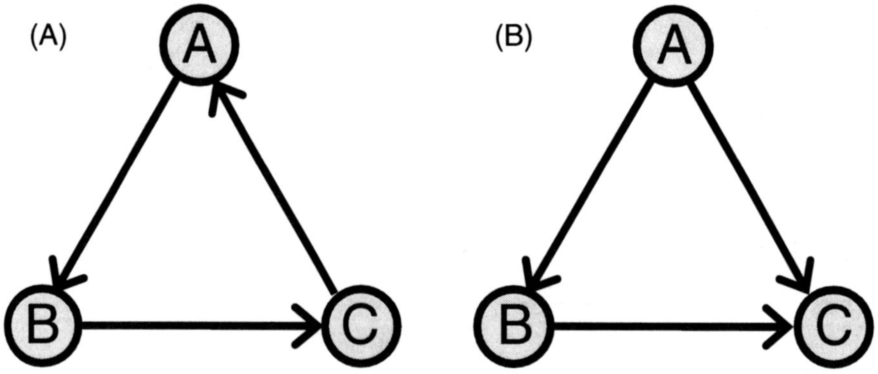

FIGURE 9.5 Two examples of three-node motifs in a directed network, including (A) a feedback loop and (B) a feedforward loop.

(see Figure 9.5). The frequency of different motifs can vary among networks with different functions (Shen-Orr, Milo, Mangan, & Alon, 2002; Yeger-Lotem et al., 2004).

Using Networks to Ask Biological Questions in Aging

Recent advances in the identification of genes that affect aging and lifespan, and even more recent advances in tools for network analysis of biological data, have allowed researchers to ask a range of interesting and insightful questions about aging. For example, Tacutu et al. (2012) constructed a protein–protein interaction network for known worm and human longevity genes, and found that these networks have a high power to predict novel genes that influence longevity in *C. elegans*. J. Wang, Zhang, Wang, Chen, and Zhang (2009) constructed a network containing both aging-related genes and human disease genes and were able to show that disease genes are significantly closer to aging genes in the network than would be expected by chance, and also to show that disease-related genes can be clustered into two broad groups, with one of these groups containing those disease genes that are especially connected to genes involved in aging. Finally, Xue et al. (2007) constructed a protein–protein interaction network of genes involved in aging in *Drosophila* and in the human brain. Inspection of these networks revealed that genes highly involved in connections between modules in their networks were more likely to be involved in aging, and that aging might decrease network stability by acting at key regulatory nodes in the network. In all of these examples, the key advance comes from recognizing that we can learn about the basic biology of aging if we examine not only the age-related changes that occur in the level of particular genes, proteins, or metabolites but also if we examine age-related changes in the strength and direction of the *connections* between these molecules. Next we discuss a few examples of this in greater detail.

Aging-Related Genes and Connectivity

One of the earliest studies on genetic networks and aging appeared in 2004 (Promislow, 2004). Promislow (2004) was interested in using a network approach to test the antagonistic pleiotropy (AP) theory of aging. Promislow argued that if aging genes come about because they are selected for early-life advantages despite late-life disadvantages, they must exhibit multiple disparate phenotypes, which would suggest that they should exhibit higher connectivity. A network analysis using 13,231 pairwise interactions in the budding yeast, *S. cerevisiae*, found that genes reported to affect senescence (replicative lifespan) had higher average connectivity than would be expected by chance. Moreover, genes that had more functions based on the gene ontology database also had higher connectivity. Although not proof of the AP model, this result was at least consistent with it. One caveat is that our search for genes that affect aging is far from saturated, as has been commented on elsewhere (McCormick & Kennedy, 2012), and thus should be expected to be biased toward more severe and easily detectable phenotypes. Because genes or proteins with a higher connectivity should be more likely to exhibit a more severe phenotype, it is also possible that they may be overrepresented in the findings to date for this reason, and these possibilities are not mutually exclusive. Interestingly, Promislow's findings have now been replicated in other species, including flies (Ferrarini, Bertelli, Feala, McCulloch, & Paternostro, 2005) and humans (Bell et al., 2009; Budovsky et al., 2009).

In a separate work, a model based on simulated evolution of protein–protein interaction networks indicates that evolutionarily old proteins should have higher connectivities and be more centrally embedded in their networks (Peterson, Presse, Peterson, & Dill, 2012). This finding, combined with the finding earlier, suggests the possibility that proteins that greatly influence lifespan and aging are likely to be ancient and conserved, and this is further supported by the fact that not only is aging found in species as evolutionarily distant as yeast and humans, but in many cases the same proteins have been also shown to dramatically affect aging across this vast evolutionary distance.

Using Networks to Predict Gene Function

Our standard approach for identifying novel genes associated with aging has been to carry out a forward genetic (e.g., mutagenesis) screen, a reverse genetic (e.g., RNAi) screen, or with the advent of whole-genome sequencing, GWAS.

But a series of network studies points to a more computational approach. If we assume that biomolecules (e.g., genes, proteins, metabolites) tend to interact with other biomolecules of similar function, then molecules that are closely linked to a gene known to affect aging should have a higher than random probability of also being associated with aging. Using this logic, several labs have successfully predicted genes and proteins associated with aging and longevity (Witten & Bonchev, 2007).

Other studies using a network approach have yielded important insights into aging. In one case (Lorenz, Cantor, & Collins, 2009), a transcriptional perturbation model (Gardner, di Bernardo, Lorenz, & Collins, 2003) of the yeast Snf1-signaling pathway, using a system of first-order ordinary differential equations, was able to identify new modulators of Snf1 and assign them roles in altering yeast chronological lifespan. Other work has shown that a network model can be constructed to attempt to reconcile some of the disparate theoretical predictions and existing experimental results in aging (Kirkwood & Kowald, 1997; Kowald & Kirkwood, 1996).

How Does Network Structure Change With Age

We have all observed the physical manifestations of aging in our own species, either in ourselves or our older friends and relations—grey hair and wrinkles, compromised physiological function, cognitive decline, and more. Moreover, some around us seem to age much more slowly than others, presumably because of some combination of environmental and genetic factors that vary among us. We know there is a genetic basis to the rate at which we age, but drawing the causal link from genotype to phenotype is far from straightforward. One way to do this might be to focus on aging not at the most downstream phenotypes but much closer to the genes themselves. For instance, we could consider how aging affects the network of interacting genes and metabolites which, in turn, lead to the physiological changes that we observe.

With this in mind, Southworth, Owen, and Kim (2009) looked at transcriptional data from 16- and 24-month old mice. Here, a "weighted co-expression network" was constructed for each of the two time points. In a *co-expression* network, edges are drawn between any pair of genes whose expression levels are significantly correlated (in this case, across different cell types). The weight of the edge (from 0 to 1) is proportional to the absolute value of the correlation coefficient and can be visualized by a thickness or color scale encoding of the edge, for example. In Southworth et al.'s study, a *difference* network was constructed in which a new weighting of each edge was representative of an increase or decrease in correlation between the two nodes, from 16 to 24 months. A simple example of an undirected difference network is given in Figure 9.6.

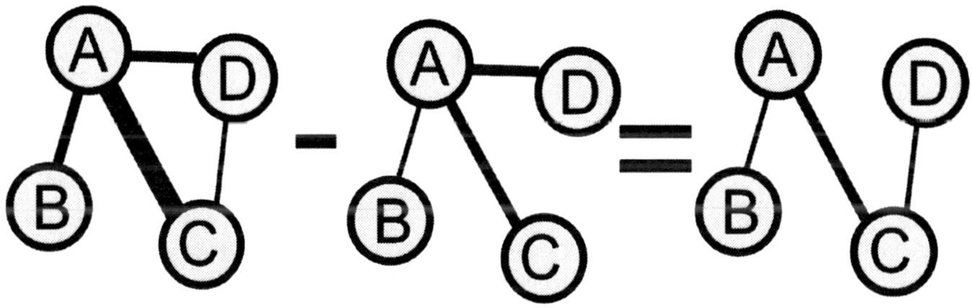

FIGURE 9.6 A simple, undirected difference network. Note that as the edge weights are encoded by thickness only, this simple example cannot accommodate negative differences, which would call for a more complex encoding (e.g., color). From "Aging mice show a decreasing correlation of gene expression within genetic modules," by L. K. Southworth, A. B. Owen, and S. K. Kim, 2009, *PLoS Genetics*, 5, p. e1000776.

This analysis of gene expression in different tissues in mice revealed that within modules of genes whose expression levels were correlated across tissues, the strength of these correlations declined with age. This phenotype would not easily have been uncovered without a network-level approach. Thus, it is as though the integrity of the genetic network declines with age. Their result also points to the specific possibility that targets of the NF-κB transcription factor might be particularly affected by this loss of correlation in expression. Given that previous work has shown an increase in the variability of expression with age (Bahar et al., 2006; Somel, Khaitovich, Bahn, Paabo, & Lachmann, 2006), these results suggest that an important overall phenotype of aging might be a global disruption of connectedness in regulation. In a more recent review, Soltow, Jones, and Promislow (2010) suggest that just as moving from a gene-by-gene approach to the global perspective of networks can shed new light on a complex process such as aging, so moving from a focus on the proximal genes to a focus on age-related changes in metabolomic networks might further improve our ability to uncover patterns in the changes of aging between long and short-lived organisms, and between different-aged individuals within natural populations, including humans (Z. Yu et al., 2012).

THE JUGGERNAUT OF DATA ACCUMULATION

The earlier review of examples illustrating the use of networks to study aging is necessarily brief and incomplete—we are still in the early stages. But the appearance of such studies will surely accelerate, just as the appearance of data used in such studies has accelerated. In the following section, we introduce the reader to a few resources for obtaining and analyzing data.

The rapidly increasing availability of very large interaction data sets will synergistically improve the power of all network analyses, including those of aging. For any established multigene, multiprotein, multimetabolite, and so forth network analysis pipeline, ongoing increases in cumulative published data set sizes will be a rising tide that lifts all boats. As an illustrative example, Figure 9.7 considers the cumulative total number of physical, co-expression, and genetic interactions curated in GeneMANIA (Warde-Farley et al., 2010) for *S. cerevisiae*. Large jumps in available data in 2007 and 2009 are noticeable in the years of publication of landmark studies in the physical interaction (I. Lee, Li, & Marcotte, 2007) and genetic interaction (Costanzo et al., 2010) totals, respectively. It is worth noting that very little usable data on this scale was available in any category before 1998. A table of the raw data used in Figure 9.7 with PMIDs for all interaction sources is available at https://sites.google.com/site/networksinaging2014/.

At first glance, this might suggest a windfall that any biologist would be hard-pressed not to collect, but it is possible, even tempting, to paint oneself into a corner in several ways only to end up cut off from the full benefit of these trends. Interestingly, as we begin thinking about the analysis of biological networks, we also need to consider the social networks in which we work.

Avoiding Culs-de-Sac: The Value of Data Portability in Accessing Big Data

Open, well documented file formats are crucial to effective interoperability of large data sets; their value cannot be overstated (Stallman, 2005). In many projects in network biology and other large-scale analyses of biological data, painstakingly reentering and reformatting published and existing data can take up the lion's share of a scientist's time. A few precautions early on in a foray into network analysis can pay large dividends later in time saved. Firstly, the use of proprietary, restricted, or incompletely documented file formats introduces insidious obstacles to large-scale comparison of various data sets. Often, a network analysis might start with a small network, or much more commonly as a project with no intended network analysis at all, and at this time the value of portable and open data formats may pale in comparison to other perceived considerations. Later, if the project becomes larger in scope, or grows to attempt comparison to broader sources of published data, problems with orphan file formats will be greatly magnified and much harder to correct retroactively.

Another obstacle to data portability is the use of nonunique gene identifiers. The most commonly human-readable gene names for most organisms are both nonunique (some unrelated genes will have been given synonymous common names) and nonexhaustive (many predicted open reading frames [ORFs]

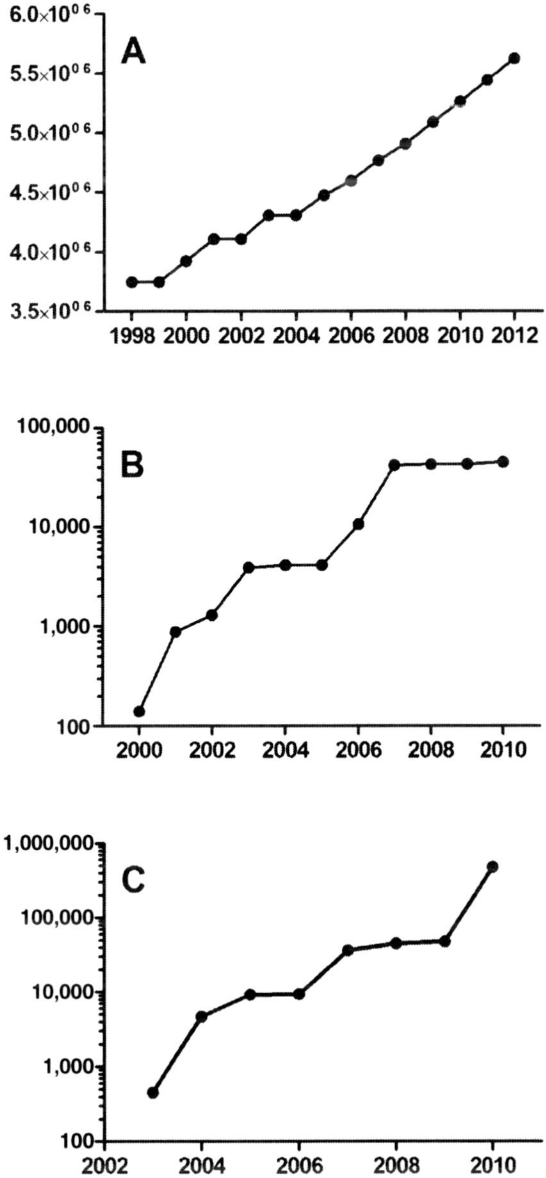

FIGURE 9.7 A windfall. Shown in this figure are the cumulative total gene–gene interactions for dated sources in the online network analysis tool GeneMANIA, in three categories of interaction for the budding yeast *S. cerevisiae*. A: Gene co-expression; B: Physical protein–protein interaction; and C: Gene interaction (as assayed, e.g., by synthetic phenotype).

do not have assigned common names). Including a comprehensive unique gene identifier (ID) for your organism as one field (e.g., one column in your table or spreadsheet) from the outset will pay disproportionate dividends to you or a collaborator or successor as a project expands in size or scope. Similar considerations exist for protein and metabolite identifiers. Tools for facilitating comprehensive ID use and other useful resources for network analysis are described in the following text.

A BRIEF INTRODUCTION TO NETWORK TOOLS FOR THE AGING BIOLOGIST

We have argued here that we have reached a time when high-throughput data are common, and these data are beginning to be used to construct networks with the aim of better understanding the mechanistic and evolutionary causes and consequences of aging. Fortunately, we are also seeing very rapid progression and development of the tools and resources required for biological network analysis. Although this makes it possible for readers with a wide range of abilities to carry out such studies, it also means that any snapshot of the current state of the art will both age rapidly and be nonexhaustive when new. Nevertheless, we hope that an introduction to some powerful and easy-to-use tools will speed their adoption and use by those readers who are aging biologists and not necessarily network specialists (yet), and that this warrants the inclusion here of this overview. A more in-depth treatment can be found in Berger, Peng, and Singh's (2013) study.

Gene Repositories and Concordances

In the past, one source of frustration in organizing large data sets for network analyses has been conversion between competing sets of unique and comprehensive gene, protein, or metabolite identifiers. Many online databases have now added bulk-query tools that largely automate this process. For *S. cerevisiae*, for example, the Saccharomyces Genome Database (Cherry et al., 2012) now hosts YeastMine (Balakrishnan et al., 2012), a data warehousing and mining interface. Among the many, more powerful, network analysis related capabilities that are described in detail in its online video tutorials, YeastMine allows users to easily append multiple sets of unique *S. cerevisiae* gene identifiers to any list of genes while allowing easy user control over interpretation of any synonymous genes found, allowing for quick and easy conversion between competing gene identifiers. Similarly, the *C. elegans* online genome repository, WormBase (Yook et al., 2012), hosts the WormMart iteration of the BioMart data mining tool (Baker, 2012), which also facilitates easy data set annotation and gene ID conversion in this organism. More generally, for data sets involving other or multiple organisms, there are organism-agnostic tools specifically designed to convert gene names, including the DAVID Gene ID Conversion tool (Huang da et al., 2008). Careful planning at the outset regarding file formats and unique node identifiers can slash overhead time for investigators entering the world of network analysis.

Published Data Set Repositories

A very large global transcriptional profiling data compendium is accessible at the NCBI Gene Expression Omnibus (Edgar, Domrachev, & Lash, 2002), and excellent tutorials on using and querying this database have been written (Barrett & Edgar, 2006a, 2006b).

Easy Visualization and Analysis: GeneMANIA and Cytoscape

The GeneMANIA web-based network graphing tool is an excellent low-barrier-to-entry introduction to network tools for simply graphing interactions, in this case between genes and/or their encoded proteins (Warde-Farley et al., 2010). It allows user-selectable auto import of large sets already formatted and annotated interaction data for seven common model organisms to leverage against your own pathways or targets of interest, and easy import of additional interaction data. It also allows export of networks in tabular form as well as export of network edge-node graphs. For offline usage, GeneMANIA is also available as an App Store plugin for Cytoscape (Montojo et al., 2010).

Cytoscape (Smoot, Ono, Ruscheinski, Wang, & Ideker, 2011) is perhaps the most widely used software for dealing with biological networks. It is relatively easy to begin to use, and its default capabilities extend to sophisticated network analysis. In addition, there are more than 150 specialized plugins (Saito et al., 2012) available to extend its basic capabilities.

Going Further

Although the capabilities of the tools described earlier increase with each release, investigators who intend analyses more complex than those afforded by these tools might be faced with learning simple programming, using the R statistical computing environment or a scripting language such as Perl or Python. There are many published and online guides and tutorials for these tools. An excellent more extensive overview is provided in Dudley and Butte (2009). For the R statistical computing environment (http://cran.r-project.org), in addition to the online tutorials and vignettes, we find Dalgaard (2008) an especially useful resource for those also in need of a statistical refresher course. For Perl, Schwartz, Foy, and Phoenix (2011), and for Python, Lutz (2009) and Shaw (2010) provide excellent introductions.

CONCLUSION

Although much more is known about genes and compounds that can modulate lifespan and aging with each passing year, it is still very early in the development of our understanding of the modulation and perhaps regulation of aging. Although individual genes and in some cases pathways have been shown to greatly affect lifespan and health span, and downstream targets have been identified, no single proximal effector has emerged as singularly important, and we do not have a clear mechanistic picture in most of these cases despite the dramatically altered phenotypes under study. Work to date using a global network-based approach has shown that genes involved in senescence are more connected than would be expected at random, and that modular correlation of gene transcription decreases with age, among other findings. Moving forward, the rapid accumulation of experimental data on all fronts will increase the power of network approaches in analyzing complex phenomena such as aging. This effect, combined with rapid improvements in ease of use and interface design of network analysis tools, point to greatly increased use of network methods in studying aging in the near future, perhaps with exciting results. It is hoped that the final brief introduction to some of the tools used in this type of analysis may contribute to this trend.

ACKNOWLEDGMENTS

This work was supported by NIH Training Grant T32 AG000266 to Mark A. McCormick and NIH AG038746 to Daniel E. L. Promislow.

REFERENCES

Albert, R., & Barabási, A.-L. (2002). Statistical mechanics of complex networks. *Reviews of Modern Physics*, *74*, 47–97.

Bahar, R., Hartmann, C. H., Rodriguez, K. A., Denny, A. D., Busuttil, R. A., Dolle, M. E., . . . Vijg, J. (2006). Increased cell-to-cell variation in gene expression in ageing mouse heart. *Nature*, *441*, 1011–1014.

Baker, M. (2012). Quantitative data: Learning to share. *Nature Methods*, *9*, 39–41.

Balakrishnan, R., Park, J., Karra, K., Hitz, B. C., Binkley, G., Hong, E. L., . . . Cherry, J. M. (2012). YeastMine—An integrated data warehouse for *Saccharomyces cerevisiae* data as a multipurpose tool-kit. *Database: The Journal of Biological Databases and Curation*, *2012*, bar062.

Barrett, T., & Edgar, R. (2006a). Gene expression omnibus: Microarray data storage, submission, retrieval, and analysis. *Methods in* Enzymology, *411*, 352–369.

Barrett, T., & Edgar, R. (2006b). Mining microarray data at NCBI's Gene Expression Omnibus (GEO)*. *Methods in Molecular Biology*, *338*, 175–190.

Bell, R., Hubbard, A., Chettier, R., Chen, D., Miller, J. P., Kapahi, P., . . . Hughes, R. E. (2009). A human protein interaction network shows conservation of aging processes between human and invertebrate species. *PLoS Genetics*, *5*, e1000414.

Berger, B., Peng, J., & Singh, M. (2013). Computational solutions for omics data. *Nature Reviews. Genetics*, *14*, 333–346.

Budovskaya, Y. V., Wu, K., Southworth, L. K., Jiang, M., Tedesco, P., Johnson, T. E., & Kim, S. K. (2008). An *elt-3/elt-5/elt-6* GATA transcription circuit guides aging in *C. elegans*. *Cell*, *134*, 291–303.

Budovsky, A., Tacutu, R., Yanai, H., Abramovich, A., Wolfson, M., & Fraifeld, V. (2009). Common gene signature of cancer and longevity. *Mechanisms of Ageing and Development*, *130*, 33–39.

Cherry, J. M., Hong, E. L., Amundsen, C., Balakrishnan, R., Binkley, G., Chan, E. T., . . . Wong, E. D. (2012). Saccharomyces Genome Database: The genomics resource of budding yeast. *Nucleic Acids Research*, *40*, D700–D705.

Costanzo, M., Baryshnikova, A., Bellay, J., Kim, Y., Spear, E. D., Sevier, C. S., . . . Boone, C. (2010). The genetic landscape of a cell. *Science*, *327*, 425–431.

Dalgaard, P. (2008). *Introductory Statistics with R* (2nd ed.). New York, NY: Springer Publishing.

de Keizer, P. L., Laberge, R. M., & Campisi, J. (2010). p53: Pro-aging or pro-longevity? *Aging*, *2*, 377–379.

Dillin, A., Hsu, A. L., Arantes-Oliveira, N., Lehrer-Graiwer, J., Hsin, H., Fraser, A. G., . . . Kenyon, C. (2002). Rates of behavior and aging specified by mitochondrial function during development. *Science*, *298*, 2398–2401.

Dorman, J. B., Albinder, B., Shroyer, T., & Kenyon, C. (1995). The *age-1* and *daf-2* genes function in a common pathway to control the lifespan of *Caenorhabditis elegans*. *Genetics*, *141*, 1399–1406.

Dudley, J. T., & Butte, A. J. (2009). A quick guide for developing effective bioinformatics programming skills. *PLoS Computational Biology*, *5*, e1000589.

Edgar, R., Domrachev, M., & Lash, A. E. (2002). Gene Expression Omnibus: NCBI gene expression and hybridization array data repository. *Nucleic Acids Research*, *30*, 207–210.

Estep, P. W., III, Warner, J. B., & Bulyk, M. L. (2009). Short-term calorie restriction in male mice feminizes gene expression and alters key regulators of conserved aging regulatory pathways. *PLoS One*, *4*, e5242.

Euler, L. (1758). Solutio problematis ad geometriam situs pertinentis. *Novi Commentarii Academiae Scientarium Imperialis Petropolitanque*, *7*, 9–28.

Ferrarini, L., Bertelli, L., Feala, J., McCulloch, A. D., & Paternostro, G. (2005). A more efficient search strategy for aging genes based on connectivity. *Bioinformatics*, *21*, 338–348.

Fisher, A. L., & Lithgow, G. J. (2006). The nuclear hormone receptor DAF-12 has opposing effects on *Caenorhabditis elegans* lifespan and regulates genes repressed in multiple long-lived worms. *Aging Cell*, *5*, 127–138.

Friedman, D. B., & Johnson, T. E. (1988). A mutation in the *age-1* gene in *Caenorhabditis elegans* lengthens life and reduces hermaphrodite fertility. *Genetics*, *118*, 75–86.

Funakoshi, M., Tsuda, M., Muramatsu, K., Hatsuda, H., Morishita, S., & Aigaki, T. (2011). A gain-of-function screen identifies *wdb* and *lkb1* as lifespan-extending genes in *Drosophila. Biochemical and Biophysical Research Communications*, *405*, 667–672.

Gardner, T. S., di Bernardo, D., Lorenz, D., & Collins, J. J. (2003). Inferring genetic networks and identifying compound mode of action via expression profiling. *Science*, *301*, 102–105.

Gems, D., & Partridge, L. (2001). Insulin/IGF signalling and ageing: Seeing the bigger picture. *Current Opinion in Genetics and Development*, *11*, 287–292.

Greer, E. L., Maures, T. J., Ucar, D., Hauswirth, A. G., Mancini, E., Lim, J. P., . . . Brunet, A. (2011). Transgenerational epigenetic inheritance of longevity in *Caenorhabditis elegans. Nature*, *479*, 365–371.

Halaschek-Wiener, J., Khattra, J. S., McKay, S., Pouzyrev, A., Stott, J. M., Yang, G. S., . . . Riddle, D. L. (2005). Analysis of long-lived *C. elegans daf-2* mutants using serial analysis of gene expression. *Genome Research*, *15*, 603–615.

Haldane, J. B. S. (1942). *New paths in genetics* (1st ed.). London, United Kingdom: Harper.

Hamilton, B., Dong, Y., Shindo, M., Liu, W., Odell, I., Ruvkun, G., & Lee, S. S. (2005). A systematic RNAi screen for longevity genes in *C. elegans. Genes & Development*, *19*, 1544–1555.

Hamilton, W. D. (1966). The moulding of senescence by natural selection. *Journal of Theoretical Biology*, *12*, 12–45.

Hansen, M., Hsu, A. L., Dillin, A., & Kenyon, C. (2005). New genes tied to endocrine, metabolic, and dietary regulation of lifespan from a *Caenorhabditis elegans* genomic RNAi screen. *PLoS Genetics*, *1*, 119–128.

Harrison, D. E., Strong, R., Sharp, Z. D., Nelson, J. F., Astle, C. M., Flurkey, K., . . . Miller, R. A. (2009). Rapamycin fed late in life extends lifespan in genetically heterogeneous mice. Nature, *460*, 392–395.

Huang da, W., Sherman, B. T., Stephens, R., Baseler, M. W., Lane, H. C., & Lempicki, R. A. (2008). DAVID gene ID conversion tool. *Bioinformation*, *2*, 428–430.

Jia, K., Chen, D., & Riddle, D. L. (2004). The TOR pathway interacts with the insulin signaling pathway to regulate *C. elegans* larval development, metabolism and life span. *Development*, *131*, 3897–3906.

Kaeberlein, M., Powers, R. W., III, Steffen, K. K., Westman, E. A., Hu, D., Dang, N., . . . Kennedy, B. K. (2005). Regulation of yeast replicative life span by TOR and Sch9 in response to nutrients. *Science*, *310*, 1193–1196.

Kapahi, P., Zid, B. M., Harper, T., Koslover, D., Sapin, V., & Benzer, S. (2004). Regulation of lifespan in *Drosophila* by modulation of genes in the TOR signaling pathway. *Current Biology*, *14*, 885–890.

Kenyon, C. (2005). The plasticity of aging: Insights from long-lived mutants. *Cell*, *120*, 449–460.

Kenyon, C., Chang, J., Gensch, E., Rudner, A., & Tabtiang, R. (1993). A *C. elegans* mutant that lives twice as long as wild type. *Nature*, *366*, 461–464.

Kirkwood, T. B., & Kowald, A. (1997). Network theory of aging. *Experimental Gerontology*, *32*, 395–399.

Kowald, A., & Kirkwood, T. B. (1996). A network theory of ageing: The interactions of defective mitochondria, aberrant proteins, free radicals and scavengers in the ageing process. *Mutation Research*, *316*, 209–236.

Kozlov, K., Surkova, S., Myasnikova, E., Reinitz, J., & Samsonova, M. (2012). Modeling of gap gene expression in *Drosophila* Kruppel mutants. *PLoS Computational Biology*, *8*, e1002635.

Lee, I., Li, Z., & Marcotte, E. M. (2007). An improved, bias-reduced probabilistic functional gene network of baker's yeast, *Saccharomyces cerevisiae*. *PLoS One*, *2*, e988.

Lee, S. S., Lee, R. Y., Fraser, A. G., Kamath, R. S., Ahringer, J., & Ruvkun, G. (2003). A systematic RNAi screen identifies a critical role for mitochondria in *C. elegans* longevity. *Nature Genetics*, *33*, 40–48.

Liao, C. Y., Rikke, B. A., Johnson, T. E., Gelfond, J. A., Diaz, V., & Nelson, J. F. (2011). Fat maintenance is a predictor of the murine lifespan response to dietary restriction. *Aging Cell*, *10*, 629–639.

Lin, K., Dorman, J. B., Rodan, A., & Kenyon, C. (1997). *daf-16*: An HNF-3/forkhead family member that can function to double the life-span of *Caenorhabditis elegans*. *Science*, *278*, 1319–1322.

Lin, Y. J., Seroude, L., & Benzer, S. (1998). Extended life-span and stress resistance in the *Drosophila* mutant *methuselah*. *Science*, *282*, 943–946.

Liu, Y. L., Lu, W. C., Brummel, T. J., Yuh, C. H., Lin, P. T., Kao, T. Y., . . . Wang, H. D. (2009). Reduced expression of alpha-1,2-mannosidase I extends lifespan in *Drosophila melanogaster* and *Caenorhabditis elegans*. *Aging Cell*, *8*, 370–379.

Lorenz, D. R., Cantor, C. R., & Collins, J. J. (2009). A network biology approach to aging in yeast. *Proceedings of the National Academy of Science of the United States of America*, *106*, 1145–1150.

Lund, J., Tedesco, P., Duke, K., Wang, J., Kim, S. K., & Johnson, T. E. (2002). Transcriptional profile of aging in *C. elegans*. *Current Biology*, *12*, 1566–1573.

Lutz, M. (2009). *Learning python* (4th ed.). Sebastopol, CA: O'Reilly Media.

Matecic, M., Smith, D. L., Pan, X., Maqani, N., Bekiranov, S., Boeke, J. D., & Smith, J. S. (2010). A microarray-based genetic screen for yeast chronological aging factors. *PLoS Genetics*, 6, e1000921.

McCarroll, S. A., Murphy, C. T., Zou, S., Pletcher, S. D., Chin, C. S., Jan, Y. N., . . . Li, H. (2004). Comparing genomic expression patterns across species identifies shared transcriptional profile in aging. *Nature Genetics*, 36, 197–204.

McCormick, M. A., & Kennedy, B. K. (2012). Genome-scale studies of aging: Challenges and opportunities. *Current Genomics*, *13*, 500–507.

McElwee, J., Bubb, K., & Thomas, J. H. (2003). Transcriptional outputs of the *Caenorhabditis elegans* forkhead protein DAF-16. *Aging Cell*, 2, 111–121.

McElwee, J. J., Schuster, E., Blanc, E., Thomas, J. H., & Gems, D. (2004). Shared transcriptional signature in *Caenorhabditis elegans* Dauer larvae and long-lived *daf-2* mutants implicates detoxification system in longevity assurance. *Journal of Biological Chemistry*, *279*, 44533–44543.

Medawar, P. B. (1952). *An unsolved problem of biology* (1st ed.). London, United Kingdom: H.K. Lewis.

Montojo, J., Zuberi, K., Rodriguez, H., Kazi, F., Wright, G., Donaldson, S. L., . . . Bader, G. D. (2010). GeneMANIA Cytoscape plugin: Fast gene function predictions on the desktop. *Bioinformatics*, *26*, 2927–2928.

Murphy, C. T. (2006). The search for DAF-16/FOXO transcriptional targets: Approaches and discoveries. *Experimental Gerontology*, *41*, 910–921.

Murphy, C. T., McCarroll, S. A., Bargmann, C. I., Fraser, A., Kamath, R. S., Ahringer, J., . . . Kenyon, C. (2003). Genes that act downstream of DAF-16 to influence the lifespan of *Caenorhabditis elegans*. *Nature*, *424*, 277–283.

Ogg, S., Paradis, S., Gottlieb, S., Patterson, G. I., Lee, L., Tissenbaum, H. A., & Ruvkun, G. (1997). The Fork head transcription factor DAF-16 transduces insulin-like metabolic and longevity signals in *C. elegans*. *Nature*, *389*, 994–999.

Oh, S. W., Mukhopadhyay, A., Dixit, B. L., Raha, T., Green, M. R., & Tissenbaum, H. A. (2006). Identification of direct DAF-16 targets controlling longevity, metabolism and diapause by chromatin immunoprecipitation. *Nature Genetics*, *38*, 251–257.

Oita, R. C., Mazzatti, D. J., Lim, F. L., Powell, J. R., & Merry, B. J. (2009). Whole-genome microarray analysis identifies up-regulation of Nr4a nuclear receptors in muscle and liver from diet-restricted rats. *Mechanisms of Ageing and Development*, *130*, 240–247.

Paik, D., Jang, Y. G., Lee, Y. E., Lee, Y. N., Yamamoto, R., Gee, H. Y., . . . Park, J. J. (2012). Misexpression screen delineates novel genes controlling *Drosophila* lifespan. *Mechanisms of Ageing and Development*, *133*(5), 234–245.

Parkes, T. L., Elia, A. J., Dickinson, D., Hilliker, A. J., Phillips, J. P., & Boulianne, G. L. (1998). Extension of *Drosophila* lifespan by overexpression of human SOD1 in motorneurons. *Nature Genetics*, *19*, 171–174.

Peterson, G. J., Presse, S., Peterson, K. S., & Dill, K. A. (2012). Simulated evolution of protein-protein interaction networks with realistic topology. *PLoS One*, *7*, e39052.

Piper, M. D., Selman, C., McElwee, J. J., & Partridge, L. (2008). Separating cause from effect: How does insulin/IGF signalling control lifespan in worms, flies and mice? *Journal of Internal Medicine*, *263*, 179–191.

Powers, R. W., III, Kaeberlein, M., Caldwell, S. D., Kennedy, B. K., & Fields, S. (2006). Extension of chronological life span in yeast by decreased TOR pathway signaling. *Genes & Development*, *20*, 174–184.

Promislow, D. E. L. (2004). Protein networks, pleiotropy and the evolution of senescence. *Proceedings. Biological Sciences/The Royal Society*, *271*, 1225–1234.

Saito, R., Smoot, M. E., Ono, K., Ruscheinski, J., Wang, P. L., Lotia, S., . . . Ideker, T. (2012). A travel guide to Cytoscape plugins. *Nature Methods*, *9*, 1069–1076.

Salazar-Ciudad, I., & Jernvall, J. (2002). A gene network model accounting for development and evolution of mammalian teeth. *Proceedings of the National Academy of Sciences of the United States of America*, *99*, 8116–8120.

Schleit, J., Johnson, S. C., Bennett, C. F., Simko, M., Trongtham, N., Castanza, A., . . . Kaeberlein, M. (2013). Molecular mechanisms underlying genotype-dependent responses to dietary restriction. *Aging Cell*, *12*, 1050–1061.

Schuster, E., McElwee, J. J., Tullet, J. M., Doonan, R., Matthijssens, F., Reece-Hoyes, J. S., . . . Gems, D. (2010). DamID in *C. elegans* reveals longevity-associated targets of DAF-16/FOXO. *Molecular Systems Biology*, *6*, 399.

Schwartz, R. L., Foy, B. D., & Phoenix, T. (2011). *Learning perl* (6th ed.). Sebastopol, CA: O'Reilly Media.

Shaw, Z. A. (2010). *Learn python the hard way*. Retrieved from http://learnpythonthehardway.org/book/

Shen-Orr, S. S., Milo, R., Mangan, S., & Alon, U. (2002). Network motifs in the transcriptional regulation network of *Escherichia coli*. *Nature Genetics*, *31*, 64–68.

Slack, C., Werz, C., Wieser, D., Alic, N., Foley, A., Stocker, H., . . . Partridge, L. (2010). Regulation of lifespan, metabolism, and stress responses by the *Drosophila* SH2B protein, Lnk. *PLoS Genetics*, *6*, e1000881.

Smoot, M. E., Ono, K., Ruscheinski, J., Wang, P. L., & Ideker, T. (2011). Cytoscape 2.8: New features for data integration and network visualization. *Bioinformatics*, *27*, 431–432.

Soltow, Q. A., Jones, D. P., & Promislow, D. E. L. (2010). A network perspective on metabolism and aging. *Integrative and Comparative Biology*, *50*, 844–854.

Somel, M., Khaitovich, P., Bahn, S., Paabo, S., & Lachmann, M. (2006). Gene expression becomes heterogeneous with age. *Current Biology*, *16*, R359–R360.

Southworth, L. K., Owen, A. B., & Kim, S. K. (2009). Aging mice show a decreasing correlation of gene expression within genetic modules. *PLoS Genetics*, *5*, e1000776.

Spencer, C. C., Howell, C. E., Wright, A. R., & Promislow, D. E. L. (2003). Testing an 'aging gene' in long-lived *Drosophila* strains: Increased longevity depends on sex and genetic background. *Aging Cell*, *2*, 123–130.

Stallman, R. (2005). Free community science and the free development of science. *PLoS Medicine*, *2*, e47.

Swindell, W. R. (2009). Genes and gene expression modules associated with caloric restriction and aging in the laboratory mouse. *BMC Genomics*, *10*, 585.

Tacutu, R., Shore, D. E., Budovsky, A., de Magalhaes, J. P., Ruvkun, G., Fraifeld, V. E., & Curran, S. P. (2012). Prediction of *C. elegans* longevity genes by human and worm longevity networks. *PLoS One*, *7*, e48282.

Tatar, M., Bartke, A., & Antebi, A. (2003). The endocrine regulation of aging by insulin-like signals. *Science*, *299*, 1346–1351.

Vinuela, A., Snoek, L. B., Riksen, J. A., & Kammenga, J. E. (2010). Genome-wide gene expression regulation as a function of genotype and age in *C. elegans*. *Genome Research*, *20*, 929–937.

von Dassow, G., Meir, E., Munro, E. M., & Odell, G. M. (2000). The segment polarity network is a robust developmental module. *Nature*, *406*, 188–192.

Walter, S., Atzmon, G., Demerath, E. W., Garcia, M. E., Kaplan, R. C., Kumari, M., . . . Franceschini, N. (2011). A genome-wide association study of aging. *Neurobiology of Aging*, *32*, 2109, e2115–e2128.

Wang, H. D., Kazemi-Esfarjani, P., & Benzer, S. (2004). Multiple-stress analysis for isolation of *Drosophila* longevity genes. *Proceedings of the National Academy of Sciences of the United States of America, 101*, 12610–12615.

Wang, J., Zhang, S., Wang, Y., Chen, L., & Zhang, X. S. (2009). Disease-aging network reveals significant roles of aging genes in connecting genetic diseases. *PLoS Computational Biology, 5*, e1000521.

Warde-Farley, D., Donaldson, S. L., Comes, O., Zuberi, K., Badrawi, R., Chao, P., . . . Morris, Q. (2010). The GeneMANIA prediction server: Biological network integration for gene prioritization and predicting gene function. *Nucleic Acids Research, 38*, W214–W220.

Williams, G. C. (1957). Pleiotropy, natural selection, and the evolution of senescence. *Evolution, 11*, 398–411.

Witten, T. M., & Bonchev, D. (2007). Predicting aging/longevity-related genes in the nematode *Caenorhabditis elegans. Chemical Biodiversity, 4*, 2639–2655.

Xue, H., Xian, B., Dong, D., Xia, K., Zhu, S., Zhang, Z., . . . Han, J. D. (2007). A modular network model of aging. *Molecular Systems Biology, 3*, 147.

Yanos, M. E., Bennett, C. F., & Kaeberlein, M. (2012). Genome-wide RNAi longevity screens in *Caenorhabditis elegans. Current Genomics, 13*, 508–518.

Yeger-Lotem, E., Sattath, S., Kashtan, N., Itzkovitz, S., Milo, R., Pinter, R. Y., . . . Margalit, H. (2004). Network motifs in integrated cellular networks of transcription-regulation and protein-protein interaction. *Proceedings of the National Academy of Sciences of the United States of America, 101*, 5934–5939.

Yook, K., Harris, T. W., Bieri, T., Cabunoc, A., Chan, J., Chen, W. J., . . . Sternberg, P. W. (2012). WormBase 2012: More genomes, more data, new website. *Nucleic Acids Research, 40*, D735–D741.

Yu, H., & Larsen, P. L. (2001). DAF-16-dependent and independent expression targets of DAF-2 insulin receptor-like pathway in *Caenorhabditis elegans* include FKBPs. *Journal of Molecular Biology, 314*, 1017–1028.

Yu, Z., Zhai, G., Singmann, P., He, Y., Xu, T., Prehn, C., . . . Wang-Sattler, R. (2012). Human serum metabolic profiles are age dependent. *Aging Cell, 11*, 960–967.

Zahn, J. M., Poosala, S., Owen, A. B., Ingram, D. K., Lustig, A., Carter, A., . . . Becker, K. G. (2007). AGEMAP: A gene expression database for aging in mice. *PLoS Genetics, 3*, e201.

CHAPTER 10

Nature, Nurture, and Chance

Their Roles in Interspecific and Intraspecific Modulations of Aging

George M. Martin

ABSTRACT

The constitutional genome, its environment, and a range of stochastic events all interact to produce virtually unique patterns of lifespan and health span. This is certainly the case for genetically heterogeneous organisms living in the wild, but there is growing evidence of considerable variations even among inbred organisms maintained in the laboratory. When one compares different species, it is clear that the dominant variable is the constitutional genome. I shall argue, however, that stochastic events are the dominant variables among members of the same species. Somatic mutations clearly play important roles. Leslie Orgel's protein synthesis error catastrophe remains a potential mechanism because it has been insufficiently tested in vivo. The recent discovery of widespread random clonal monoallelic expression in the laboratory of Andrew Chess provides yet another layer of complexity. Perhaps the most cogent explanation of the growing phenotypic variations among aging cohorts, however, are increasing drifts in gene expression with age, presumably epigenetic in origin, but conceivably also driven by posttranscriptional mechanisms. I shall argue that such drifts evolved because they proved adaptive to groups of organisms in unpredictable environments, but that age-related expansions of such variegated gene expressions will have escaped the force of natural selection and are responsible for a wide range of quasi-geriatric pathologies, both proliferative and degenerative.

http://dx.doi.org/10.1891/0198-8794.34.267

INTRODUCTION

All biologists and most laymen are aware that how they age is a composite of both one's inherited set of gene (Nature) and one's complex set of environmental experiences (Nurture). Much less attention is given, however, to the potentially important roles of various stochastic events (Chance). The goal of this chapter is to provide overviews of how Nature, Nurture, and Chance can differentially modulate lifespan and the wide range of phenotypes that, collectively, can be defined as health span (i.e., how long one can live in the absence of significant disease and disability). We shall approach this subject from the point of view of the relative contributions of Nature, Nurture, and Chance to differences *between* species (interspecific variation) versus differences among individuals *within* a species (intraspecific variation). With respect to the former (interspecific variation), we conclude that by far the greatest contribution to variations in lifespan (and presumably, health span) is the constitutional genotype. With respect to the latter (intraspecific variation), we review the current state of the evidence supporting major roles of various classes of stochastic events.

Research on the genomic basis of intraspecific differences in lifespan ("comparative biogerontology" or "comparative geroscience") is of enormous relevance to the human condition and is ripe for exploitation, given the current revolution in genome sciences. Interspecific differences in noncoding RNA sequences and their relevance for the regulation of gene expression represents a particularly cogent opportunity for researchers interested in the biological basis of lifespan plasticity. The major emphasis of this chapter, however, will be on stochastic contributions to differential trajectories of aging within a species, particularly within our species. The goal will be to encourage more research on this comparatively neglected topic, especially as regards the role of epigenetic drifts in gene expression. Particularly important will be efforts to falsify or support a hypothesis that may explain the quasi-stochastic distributions of a wide range of proliferative and degenerative pathologies observed in aging human subjects (Martin, 2012). That hypothesis proposes that drifts in gene expression (whether epigenetic or posttranscriptional) evolved as an adaptive response to environmental challenges early in the life course, but with deleterious effects postreproductively (i.e., an antagonistic pleiotropic mechanism of aging; Martin, 2009).

INTERSPECIFIC VARIATIONS IN LIFESPAN

The Role of the Constitutional Genome

Why does a typical laboratory mouse live for a maximum of around 3–4 years while humans often survive into the 10th decade? It should be obvious that this is not attributable to such environmental variables as diet or exposure to ionizing

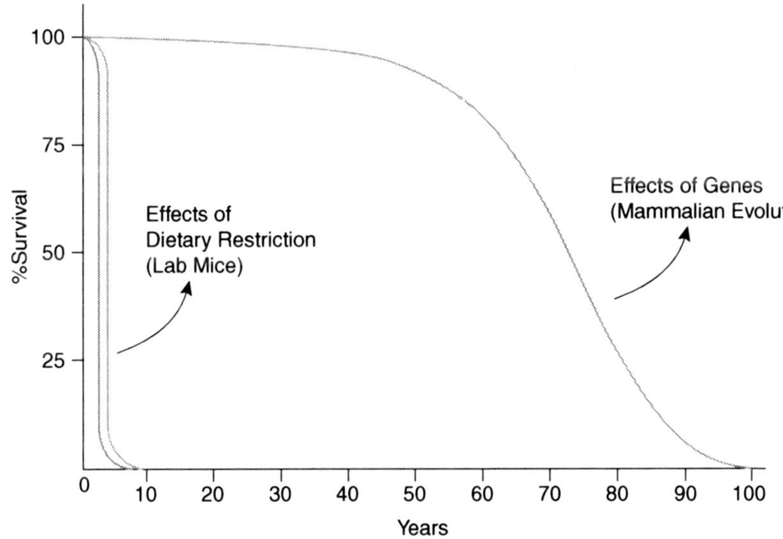

FIGURE 10.1 Constitutional genetic events dominate interspecific variations in lifespan. The figure illustrates survival curves for typical strains of laboratory mice compared to that of humans. A 40% restriction of calories, a widely documented environmental intervention for enhancing the lifespans of many (but not all) strains of mice by about 50% is barely discernible with the scaling of this X axis. By contrast, evolution has managed an enormous increase in lifespan in the lineage leading to our species. This was achieved via changes in the constitutional genome.

radiation. The biggest variable is how evolution has tinkered with the genomes of these two species (see Figure 10.1).

As regards stochastic events, there is neither compelling evidence that the rates of somatic mutation in mice are sufficiently different from those of humans to account for this difference nor is there any evidence that key genetic loci like tumor suppressor genes or oncogenes are more likely to sustain mutations than other loci. Even if that were the case for both of these scenarios, however, the ultimate cause in such differences should be found in the constitutional genomes. The same argument could be made for differential degrees of age-related epigenetic drifts of gene expression. This is not to say, of course, that environmental factors and chance events are not playing some roles in the different trajectories of aging between different mammalian species. As emphasized in Figure 10.2, however, the "the dominant circle" in this Venn diagram is the genome. (The precise relative contributions of Nature, Nurture, and Chance illustrated in Figures 10.2 and 10.4 are, of course, mere "guesstimates.")

Speaking of nonhuman primates, it is important to point out the great opportunities for research in comparative geroscience. A classical 1975 paper by

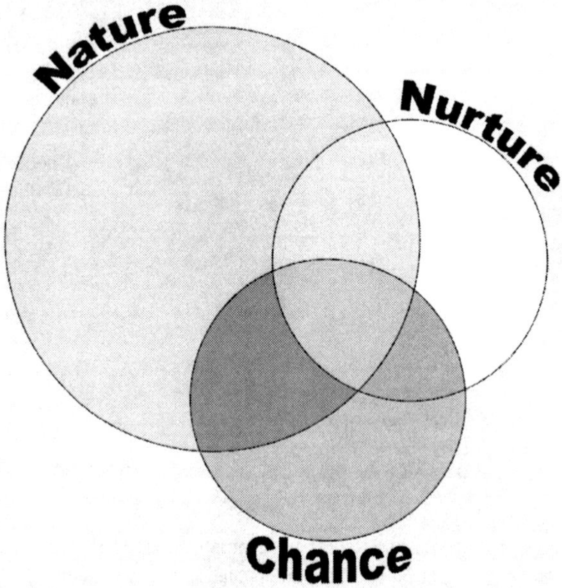

FIGURE 10.2 *Interspecific* variations in health span and lifespan. The Venn diagram follows the logic of Figure 10.1. Although environmental factors (Nurture) and stochastic events (Chance) likely play some roles in explaining interspecific differences in the health spans and lifespans, the major contribution comes from the constitutional genome (Nature). The suggested proportions of these various contributions are imprecise, given the lack of reliable data and this gross generalization of many interspecific comparisons.

my University of Washington colleague, Mary Claire King, and her mentor, the late Alan Wilson, concluded that the marked phenotypic differences between a chimpanzee and a human are very unlikely to be explained by differences in the amino acid sequences of their respective proteins because those investigated were virtually identical (King & Wilson, 1975). Almost certainly, the differential features of development, aging, and associated disease susceptibilities are attributable, in large part, to differences in the way genes are regulated by the so-called "dark matter" of DNA. We have lots of noncoding RNA candidates to explore (Gomes, Nolasco, & Soares, 2013) in the context of the plasticity of the lifespan that, in chimpanzees and humans, exhibit approximately twofold differences. Research on exploring the genetic basis for the differential phenotypes of these two primate species have already demonstrated the value of this approach for our understanding of the evolution of both coding and noncoding sequences (Berglund, Pollard, & Webster, 2009).

INTRASPECIFIC VARIATIONS IN LIFESPAN

The Role of the Constitutional Genome

The use of genome-wide association studies (GWAS) as a means of discovering differential genetic susceptibilities to age-related diseases has reached "industrial strength," with studies that include more than 100,000 human subjects (Sabater-Lleal et al., 2013). Typical findings reveal large numbers of loci, each with small effects, as well as interesting differences among ethnically distinct populations. For the case of dementias of the Alzheimer type, three dominant loci have been widely documented for the early onset familial types; the vastly more common late onset cases (older than the age of ~60 years) is greatly influenced by a polymorphism at the *APOE* locus, but increasing numbers of loci with small effect are now being discovered via GWAS, exome sequencing, and full genome sequencing studies. A recent review suggests that up to 50% of the heritability of that group of disorders can be explained by variants at four loci, however—three loci defined by autosomal dominant mutations for early onset disease (*APP*, *PS1*, *PS2*) and the *APOE* polymorphism (Tanzi, 2012).

Heritability of adult lifespan in humans is approximately 25% (Brooks-Wilson, 2013). Robust replications have been documented for associations of exceptional longevity with two genetic loci—*APOE* and *FOXO3A* (Brooks-Wilson, 2013). There have been several suggestions for why the allele of *APOE* survives in modern populations (Kulminski et al., 2013; Rusted et al., 2013). My favorite hypothesis, of course, is my own! The tradeoff I have suggested is resistance of the E4 allele, among our early African ancestors, against lipophilic pathogens, because the E4 allele is deficient in delivering lipids to pathogens whose effective replications are dependent on the host for lipids (Martin, 1999). The late Joshua Lederberg suggested an excellent candidate for such a pathogen—*Trypanosoma brucei brucei*—which may still be endemic in many parts of Africa.

FOXO3A is a member of a family of forkhead transcription factors. Remarkably, it is homologous to the key downstream transcription factors in the IGF1 signaling pathways in both *Caenorhabditis elegans* and *Drosaphila melanogaster*. Leaky mutations in those pathways established the first "public" mechanism of aging. Mutations in that pathway that substantially enhance lifespans have also been demonstrated in laboratory mice (Brown-Borg & Bartke, 2012). The precise mechanisms by which polymorphic variants of *FOXO3A* contribute to enhanced longevity of humans require more research. Suggested functions of this transcription factor have included the triggering of apoptosis (Ekoff et al., 2007), the response to hyperglycemic stress (Raju, Kannan, & Abraham, 2013), the neuronal response to oxidative stress (Uranga, Katz, & Salvador, 2013), an antagonistic interaction with the *MYC* oncogene, and their roles in cellular bioenergetics, reactive oxygen metabolism, and adaptation to hypoxia (Peck, Ferber, & Schulze, 2013) and the implementation of a protective pro-autophagy gene program in old hematopoietic stem cells (Warr et al., 2013).

The search for genetic mutations responsible for human segmental progeroid syndromes (Martin, 1978) has revealed at least one underlying common pathogenetic mechanism—the failure to maintain genomic stability (Martin, 2005). Not surprisingly, however, there is evidence of pathogenetic heterogeneity (Tivey, Brook, Rokicki, Kipling, & Davis, 2013).

The Role of the Environment

My impression from having attended numerous meetings on the biology of aging for the past 50 years or so is that far more attention has been given to genetic factors than to environmental factors. Some objective evidence to support this impression comes from a PubMed search (at the time of this writing) for "aging AND genetics" versus "aging AND environment." The former yielded more than twice as many publications (42,093/17,206 = 2.45). Perhaps research on "gerontogens" (Martin, 1987) is more difficult than research on "gerontogenes" (T. E. Johnson & Lithgow, 1992). What we really need more research on is the interaction between these two domains (T. E. Johnson et al., 2000). This is the correct pathway toward the realization of our dream of "personalized" or "precision" medicine. It is exemplified by the field of pharmacogenetics—the "low hanging fruit" of precision medicine. A cogent example is the role of Nrf2 in the modulation of xenobiotic-metabolizing enzymes and their importance in the chemoprevention of cancer (Wu et al., 2013).

Just as I have done for the case of progeroid syndromes (Martin, 1982), I find it useful to classify gerontogens into two broad groups: segmental gerontogens, which involve multiple aspects of the senescent phenotype, and unimodal gerontogens, in which predominantly one aspect of the senescent phenotype is impacted.

Cigarette smoke was perhaps the most important segmental gerontogen of the 20th century and continues to have major impacts on health span and lifespan in this century. For an illuminating history of tobacco smoking, readers would enjoy the following informative website, thanks to the Boston University Medical Center: http://academic.udayton.edu/health/syllabi/tobacco/history.htm#health. Most of us now are fully aware of the fact that there are numerous carcinogens in cigarette smoke and that it is a major cause of the most common form of lung cancer, bronchogenic squamous cell carcinoma. (It is not of major significance for the pathogenesis of adenocarcinoma of the lung, however.) Surprisingly, few of us are fully aware of the severe deleterious effects of cigarette smoke and their relevance for aging. Some, but not all of these myriad effects appear in the following reviews: Martin, 1987; Bernhard, Moser, Backovic, and Wick, 2007; Wainer, 2001. The latter French meta-analysis of the effects of cigarette smoking on female fertility is particularly impressive because it deals with a classical aging-associated phenotype. The overall impact of smoking on mortality from any cause has been well documented (Gellert, Schottker, & Brenner, 2012). Detailed pathophysiological mechanistic investigations of the impact of various components of cigarette smoking on its numerous targets remains comparatively neglected, with the exception of the many studies documenting carcinogenic and mutagenic effects.

Two compelling examples of unimodal gerontogens can be cited. One is exposure of the skin to ultraviolet (UV) rays (Chung et al., 2001). The DNA damaging and carcinogenic effects of UV have been well documented (Nakanishi, Niida, Murakami, & Shimada, 2009). A second example is the rapid induction of Parkinson's disease via the administration of 1-Methyl-4-phenyl-1,2,3,6-tetrahydropyridine, a chemical agent that, when metabolized by glial monoamine oxidase B, is neurotoxic for dopaminergic neurons (Bove & Perier, 2012). The rapid induction of Parkinson's disease was first detected among young adults who had been exposed to contaminants in illicit narcotics (Kopin, 1987).

The Role of Chance

There is a surprisingly long history of scholarship on the role of chance events in the modulation of a range of phenotypes in a wide range of organisms in which genetic and environmental factors have been substantially controlled. I am grateful to an epidemiologist, George Davey Smith, for bringing to my attention several pioneering studies; these are discussed in a fascinating review based on his 2011 John Snow Lecture (Smith, 2011). One such recently reviewed study on phenotypic variability among inbred mice and rats lasted some thirty years and came to the conclusion that there is "a third component causing random variability beside environment and genotype" (title from Gartner, 2012). More recent studies with model organisms include an impressively wide range of phenotypes among inbred marbled crayfish within a well-controlled laboratory environment (Vogt, 2010). By far, the most compelling model system for such investigations is the N2 strain of *C. elegans*. These hermaphroditic organisms are identical twins as regards their constitutional genetics. Although they are usually grown on petri dishes with *E. coli* as a food source, they can be grown as suspension cultures with well-defined media under apparently identical conditions, yet exhibit striking variability in individual lifespans (Vanfleteren, De Vreese, & Braeckman, 1998). There are in fact overlaps in the distributions of lifespans between wild type and an exceptionally long-lived mutant organism (*age-1*; Kirkwood et al., 2005); these authors also provide a thoughtful list of various potential sources of stochastic variations, both during development and within adult organisms. Two of the authors (Finch and Kirkwood), both leading gerontologists, had previously published a valuable book on the subject of chance events in aging in which the emphasis was on developmental events (Finch & Kirkwood, 2000).

An important *C. elegans* paper from the laboratory of Tom Johnson was consistent with a key role of nonheritable stochastic events in the differential modulations of lifespans, as revealed by a small heat shock promoter driving a green fluorescent promoter (Rea, Wu, Cypser, Vaupel, & Johnson, 2005); long-lived "bright" and short-lived "dull" fluorescent living worms could be sorted and their progeny could be re-analyzed for those phenotypes, which once again exhibited marked variability. Subsequent studies, however, were more consistent with substantial heritability of these phenotypes (Cypser et al., 2013). We await more detailed information on subsequent generations of single copy transgenic worms with exceptionally strong or exceptionally weak expression (Mendenhall et al., 2012).

The mechanism that most clearly couples a stochastic event to a specific senescent phenotype in mammals (cancer) is somatic mutation. Two individuals, including identical twins, may have the same flux of somatic mutations, but one unlucky twin may suffer mutations in oncogenes and tumor suppressor genes while the other may have mutations in nonfunctional pseudogenes. The dominant type of malignant neoplasm in humans involves epithelial cell types (carcinoma). There is strong evidence that the frequencies of somatic mutation in normal diploid human epithelial cells increase as a function of donor age (Martin et al., 1996). A wide range of chromosomal mutations also increase dramatically in epithelial cells with aging, at least in mice (Martin, Smith, Ketterer, Ogburn, & Disteche, 1985).

Although the frequencies of some carcinomas—for example, ductal infiltrative carcinoma of the breast—do not continue to exhibit age-specific increases in frequencies during the last decades of the usual lifespan, this could be explained by the fact that the target organ undergoes atrophy, with adipose tissue replacing the vulnerable epithelial target cells for the case of aging breast tissue. Carcinogenesis is a multi-hit process probably eventually requiring the emergence of mutator strains—cells with substantial increases in their intrinsic rates of mutation (Loeb, 1998); the target cells have to have lifespans long enough to reach that critical stage of oncogenesis.

A second potentially important stochastic mechanism of aging could involve transcriptional and/or translational errors in protein synthesis. One such formal theory was developed by the late Leslie Orgel, who shortly pointed out a flaw in his "protein synthesis error catastrophe theory," however (Orgel, 1970). Although several experiments do not support that theory (see, e.g., Edelmann

& Gallant, 1977; Pendergrass, Martin, & Bornstein, 1976), my own view is that these ideas still require more investigation, particularly those employing in vivo mammalian experiments (Martin & Bressler, 2000).

A third and much more recent candidate for connecting senescent phenotypes to random events is the evidence that there is random silencing of chromosomal alleles leading to somatic mosaicism in which patches of tissues are either monoallelic for the paternal or maternal chromosome (i.e., haploinsufficient) or normal diploid (Gimelbrant, Hutchinson, Thompson, & Chess, 2007). This had been well established for the case of the X chromosome, but the fact that hundreds of autosomal genes could be involved was quite unexpected. Of special interest is the involvement of the beta amyloid precursor gene (*APP*) on Chromosome 21. It had been well-known that patients with the Down syndrome (trisomy 21) invariably exhibit the neuropathological features of Alzheimer's disease (AD)—early evidence that the APP protein played a key role in the pathogenesis of that disease. It will now be important to discover if individuals who have only one copy of that gene in critical regions of the medial temporal cortex are resistant to AD.

A fourth stochastic mechanism is of special interest to this author and is the basis of an antagonistic pleiotropic theory of aging (Martin, 2009). There is now strong evidence of a gradual drift in gene expression throughout the life course of human identical twins (Fraga et al., 2005; Talens et al., 2012). The term "epigenetic drift" is now well embedded in the literature to describe these variations in gene expression and does indeed describe the most likely mechanism of variegated gene expression. Polymerase chain reaction (PCR) assays of a wide range of genes expressed in individual myocardial cells isolated from the hearts of young and old mice have consistently revealed increased cell-to-cell variegation of gene expression in the old mice (Bahar et al., 2006). It will be important, however, to continue to explore stochastic variations in the several posttranscriptional steps of protein synthesis.

One can imagine that different degrees of variegated gene expression evolved in the context of particular ecologies during speciation. In environments with unpredictable types and concentrations of cytotoxic agents, it would be risky to have each cell type within a vulnerable tissue display identical patterns of gene expression. Consider, for example, exposure to cadmium, a highly toxic metal. Some degree of "bet hedging" or "epigenetic gambling" of gene expression might ensure exceptionally high levels of protective proteins such as metallothioneins within critical cells of some individuals and thus ensure their survival and subsequent reproduction. Given the evidence cited earlier that aging is associated with increasing degrees of variegated gene expression, one can also imagine that it could lead to the loss of physiological homeostasis and the emergence of age-related disease and dysfunction. Thus, variegated gene expression may be adaptive during the early phases of the life course, but deleterious postreproductively—an antagonistic pleiotropic theory of aging.

As a pathologist, the author has been puzzled by what one could call the "quasi-stochastic" distributions of a wide range of geriatric pathologies, particularly for proliferative and degenerative lesions (Martin, 2012). Although specific types of tissue are impacted by specific types of lesions, the distributions within those tissues are typically stochastic. Epigenetic drifts leading to altered patterns of gene expression for loci involved in proliferative homeostasis could result in a wide range of pathologies (Martin, 1979). One such pathology is hyperplasia. I suggest that clonal expansions of hyperplastic lesions are the first steps in oncogenesis. Increased rates of DNA synthesis in such tissues would then be expected to lead to increased probabilities of somatic mutations in driver mutations for neoplastic transformation. Evidence that there are in fact such nonneoplastic clonal expansions surrounding adenocarcinomas of the colon has been published (Salk et al., 2009).

Classical examples of quasi-stochastic distributions are seen in the two most prevalent age-related neurodegenerative disorders, AD and Parkinson's disease (Martin, 2012). Figure 10.3 illustrates a speculative and simplified

FIGURE 10.3 Postdevelopmental bumps in the Waddington landscape. The diagram in the upper left hand corner is a reproduction of the famous "canalization" drawing by the late Conrad Waddington (http://en.wikipedia.org/wiki/Conrad_Waddington), who imagined that the amazing feats of differentiation of a fertilized ovum into diverse cell types was like a marble rolling down different tracks of gene expression. He imagined that these different trajectories are determined by epigenetic events, as the underlying DNA sequences remain unchanged. The figure suggests that there can be "bumps" (perturbations) in these various tracks of differentiation as a result of epigenetic drifts in patterns of gene expression. The figure provides a hypothetical scenario whereby such epigenetic drifts can result in the multifocal neuritic plaques that are characteristic of dementias of the Alzheimer type. The columns represent genetic loci whose expressions are either involved in modulating the synthesis or the degradation of the beta amyloid protein, the putative proximal neurotoxic moiety (currently thought to act via oligomers). On the synthetic side are three loci involved in the processing of the beta amyloid precursor protein. High expression of an alpha secretase diminishes the synthesis of Abeta while high expression of beta and gamma secretases enhance its synthesis. Upward-pointing arrows indicate different degrees of high expression, whereas downward-pointing arrows indicate different degrees of diminished expression. On the degradation side are shown two major pathways for the clearance of Abeta peptides—the insulin degrading enzyme (IDE) and neprilysin. Examples of stochastic drifts in gene expression are shown in three cells in young, middle aged, and old brains. The rectangular box at the bottom of the figure (Cell 3) indicates a pattern of gene expression representing "a perfect storm" of altered gene expression, one that is sufficient to create a sufficient amount of Abeta peptide to initiate the creation of a neuritic plaque and presumably create damage to neighboring synapses. As pointed out in the text, there are several additional genetic loci differential expression at which could contribute to or prevent the creation of "a perfect storm."

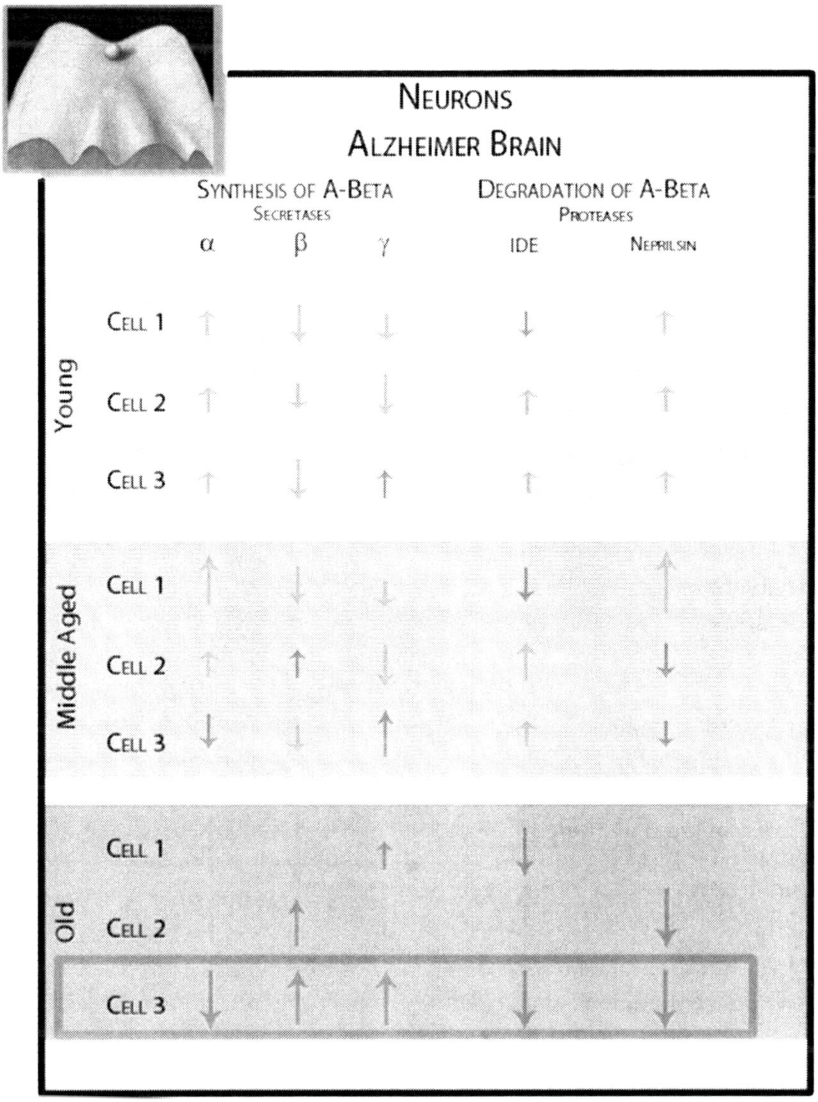
Neurons
Alzheimer Brain
Synthesis of A-Beta
Secretases
α
β
γ
Degradation of A-Beta
Proteases
IDE
Neprilsin
Young
Cell 1
Cell 2
Cell 3
Middle Aged
Cell 1
Cell 2
Cell 3
Old
Cell 1
Cell 2
Cell 3

scenario for how stochastic drifts in gene expression during aging could lead to a "perfect storm" for the creation of neuritic plaques as a result of critical levels of enhanced rates of synthesis of amyloid beta (Abeta) peptides together with critical levels of diminished gene expressions for gene products involved in the clearance of Abeta peptides. Several loci not shown on the graph are quite likely to be also involved, certainly including *APOE* (Holtzman, Herz, & Bu, 2012). There may therefore be various patterns of gene expression that could lead to such "perfect storms." The diagram in the upper left hand corner of Figure 10.3 is the famous "canalization" figure of Conrad Waddington (Goldberg, Allis, & Bernstein, 2007).

CONCLUSIONS

We have seen how Nature, Nurture, and Chance work together to modulate health span and lifespan, both as they apply to differences among species (see Figure 10.1) and differences among individuals within species (see Figure 10.4). This author will "stick his neck out" (see Figure 10.4) and make the case that the most important variables underlying the striking differences in human patterns of aging involve stochastic events, particularly age-related drifts in gene expression. Epigenetic alterations appear to be the most likely explanation for these drifts in gene expression. Such drifts are likely to exhibit both qualitative and quantitative differences among families of genetic loci and among individuals within a given population. The evolutionary theory of their origins make several predictions, the most important of them being the evolution of different alleles at key loci responsible for modulating the rates and extents of epigenetic drift. Our laboratory is currently involved in somatic cell genetic experiments attempting to support or falsify that hypothesis. If such a locus or loci were identified, it is not inconceivable that targeted drugs could be developed to decrease the degree of drift in gene expression during aging and thus ensure longer health spans and lifespans for outpatients, if the underlying theory is in fact correct.

The aforementioned conclusions do not minimize the importance of rare constitutional mutations that result in dramatic accelerations in patterns of aging—for example, autosomal recessive null mutations in the RecQ helicase/endonuclease mutation responsible for the Werner syndrome (Yu et al., 1996) or the dominant autosomal mutations responsible for Huntington's disease. "Lady Luck" also plays a big role in the kinds of de novo germ line mutations we might be born with, of course. Moreover, the inherited trinucleotide repeats responsible for Huntington's disease can undergo stochastic differential expansions

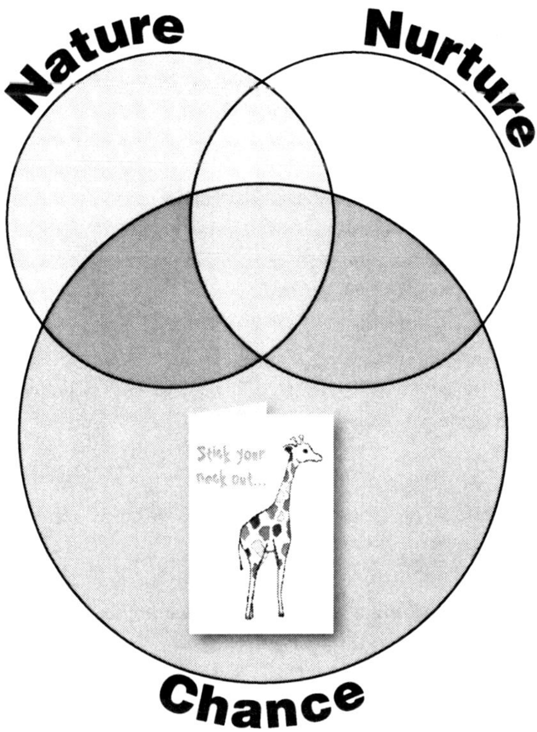

FIGURE 10.4 *Intraspecific* variation in health span and lifespan. In contrast to what is shown in Figure 10.2, the author "sticks his neck out" to propose the hypothesis that stochastic events (Chance) are the major contributors to variations in health span and lifespan among individuals within species.

during meiosis (Yoon, Dubeau, de Young, Wexler, & Arnheim, 2003); this could also happen in somatic cells.

The emphasis on stochastic events in this chapter also does not trivialize the enormous importance of nature–nurture interactions in the modulations of various patterns of aging, including the variability of the response to putative interventions. It is astonishing, for example, that it took some 81 years since the seminal 1929 experiment of Clive McKay before the scientific community demonstrated that a standard methodology of dietary restriction in mice (40% restriction of calories) produced a remarkable range of both positive and negative impacts on the lifespans of recombinant inbred strains (Liao, Rikke, Johnson, Diaz, & Nelson, 2010). In going forward toward the development of new interventions that retard various processes of aging and the emergence of age-related disorders (the use of rapamycin analogues, for example; S. C. Johnson, Rabinovitch, & Kaeberlein, 2013), we must never lose sight of the importance of considering dose–response and nature–nurture interactions in the determination of the outcomes of such interventions.

REFERENCES

Bahar, R., Hartmann, C. H., Rodriguez, K. A., Denny, A. D., Busuttil R. A., Dollé, M. E., . . . Vijg, J. (2006). Increased cell-to-cell variation in gene expression in ageing mouse heart. *Nature*, *441*, 1011–1014.

Berglund, J., Pollard, K. S., & Webster, M. T. (2009). Hotspots of biased nucleotide substitutions in human genes. *PLoS Biology*, *7*, e26.

Bernhard, D., Moser, C., Backovic, A., & Wick, G. (2007). Cigarette smoke—An aging accelerator? *Experimental Gerontology*, *42*, 160–165.

Bove, J., & Perier, C. (2012). Neurotoxin-based models of Parkinson's disease. *Neuroscience*, *211*, 51–76.

Brooks-Wilson, A. R. (2013). Genetics of healthy aging and longevity. *Human Genetics*, *132*(12), 1323–1338.

Brown-Borg, H. M., & Bartke, A. (2012). GH and IGF1: Roles in energy metabolism of long-living GH mutant mice. *The Journals of Gerontology. Series A, Biological Sciences and Medical Sciences*, *67*, 652–660.

Chung, J. H., Lee, S. H., Youn, C. S., Park, B. J., Kim, K. H., Park, K. C., . . . Eun, H. C. (2001). Cutaneous photodamage in Koreans: Influence of sex, sun exposure, smoking, and skin color. *Archives of Dermatology*, *137*, 1043–1051.

Cypser, J. R., Wu, D., Park, S. K., Ishii, T., Tedesco, P. M., Mendenhall, A. R., & Johnson, T. E. (2013). Predicting longevity in C. elegans: Fertility, mobility and gene expression. *Mechanisms of Ageing and Development*, *134*, 291–297.

Edelmann, P., & Gallant, J. (1977). On the translational error theory of aging. *Proceedings of the National Academy of Sciences of the United States of America*, *74*, 3396–3398.

Ekoff, M., Kaufmann, T., Engstrom, M., Motoyama, N., Villunger, A., Jönsson, J. I., . . . Nilsson, G. (2007). The BH3-only protein Puma plays an essential role in cytokine deprivation induced apoptosis of mast cells. *Blood*, *110*, 3209–3217.

Finch, C. E., & Kirkwood, T. B. L. (2000). *Chance, development, and aging*. New York, NY: Oxford University Press.

Fraga, M. F., Ballestar, E., Paz, M. F., Ropero, S., Setien, F., Ballestar, M. L., . . . Esteller, M. (2005). Epigenetic differences arise during the lifetime of monozygotic twins. *Proceedings of the National Academy of Sciences of the United States of America*, *102*, 10604–10609.

Gartner, K. (2012). A third component causing random variability beside environment and genotype. A reason for the limited success of a 30-year long effort to standardize laboratory animals? *International Journal of Epidemiology*, *41*, 335–341.

Gellert, C., Schottker, B., & Brenner, H. (2012). Smoking and all-cause mortality in older people: Systematic review and meta-analysis. *Archives of Internal Medicine*, *172*, 837–844.

Gimelbrant, A., Hutchinson, J. N., Thompson, B. R., & Chess, A. (2007). Widespread monoallelic expression on human autosomes. *Science, 318*, 1136–1140.

Goldberg, A. D., Allis C. D., & Bernstein, E. (2007). Epigenetics: A landscape takes shape. *Cell, 128*, 635–638.

Gomes, A. Q., Nolasco, S., & Soares, H. (2013). Non-coding RNAs: Multi-tasking molecules in the cell. *International Journal of Molecular Sciences, 14*, 16010–16039.

Holtzman, D. M., Herz, J., & Bu, G. (2012). Apolipoprotein E and apolipoprotein E receptors: Normal biology and roles in Alzheimer disease. *Cold Spring Harbor Perspectives in Medicine, 2*, a006312.

Johnson, S. C., Rabinovitch, P. S., & Kaeberlein, M. (2013). mTOR is a key modulator of ageing and age-related disease. *Nature, 493*, 338–345.

Johnson, T. E., Cypser, J., de Castro, E., de Castro, S., Henderson, S., Murakami, S., . . . Link, C. (2000). Gerontogenes mediate health and longevity in nematodes through increasing resistance to environmental toxins and stressors. *Experimental Gerontology, 35*, 687–694.

Johnson, T. E., & Lithgow, G. J. (1992). The search for the genetic basis of aging: The identification of gerontogenes in the nematode Caenorhabditis elegans. *Journal of the American Geriatrics Society, 40*, 936–945.

King, M. C., & Wilson, A. C. (1975). Evolution at two levels in humans and chimpanzees. *Science, 188*, 107–116.

Kirkwood, T. B., Feder, M., Finch, C. E., Franceschi, C., Globerson, A., Klingenberg, C. P., . . . Westendorp, R. G. (2005). What accounts for the wide variation in life span of genetically identical organisms reared in a constant environment? *Mechanisms of Ageing and Development, 126*, 439–443.

Kopin, I. J. (1987). MPTP: An industrial chemical and contaminant of illicit narcotics stimulates a new era in research on Parkinson's disease. *Environmental Health Perspectives, 75*, 45–51.

Kulminski, A. M., Culminskaya, I., Arbeev, K. G., Ukraintseva, S. V., Arbeeva, L., & Yashin, A. I. (2013). Trade-off in the effect of the APOE gene on the ages at onset of cardiocascular disease and cancer across ages, gender, and human generations. *Rejuvenation Research, 16*, 28–34.

Liao, C. Y., Rikke, B. A., Johnson, T. E., Diaz, V., & Nelson, J. F. (2010). Genetic variation in the murine lifespan response to dietary restriction: From life extension to life shortening. *Aging Cell, 9*, 92–95.

Loeb, L. A. (1998). Cancer cells exhibit a mutator phenotype. *Advances in Cancer Research, 72*, 25–56.

Martin, G. M. (1978). Genetic syndromes in man with potential relevance to the pathobiology of aging. *Birth Defects Original Article Series, 14*, 5–39.

Martin, G. M. (1979). Proliferative homeostasis and its age-related aberrations. *Mechanisms of Ageing and Development, 9*, 385–391.

Martin, G. M. (1982). Syndromes of accelerated aging. *National Cancer Institute Monograph, 60*, 241–247.

Martin, G. M. (1987). Interactions of aging and environmental agents: The gerontological perspective. *Progress in Clinical and Biological Research, 228*, 25–80.

Martin, G. M. (1999). APOE alleles and lipophylic pathogens. *Neurobiology of Aging 20*, 441–443.

Martin, G. M. (2005). Genetic modulation of senescent phenotypes in Homo sapiens. *Cell, 120*, 523–532.

Martin, G. M. (2009). Epigenetic gambling and epigenetic drift as an antagonistic pleiotropic mechanism of aging. *Aging Cell*, *8*, 761–764.

Martin, G. M. (2012). Stochastic modulations of the pace and patterns of ageing: Impacts on quasi-stochastic distributions of multiple geriatric pathologies. *Mechanisms of Ageing and Development*, *133*, 107–111.

Martin, G. M., & Bressler, S. L. (2000). Transcriptional infidelity in aging cells and its relevance for the Orgel hypothesis. *Neurobiology of Aging*, *21*, 897–900; discussion 3–4.

Martin, G. M., Ogburn, C. E., Colgin, L. M., Gown, A. M., Edland, S. D., & Monnat, R. J., Jr. (1996). Somatic mutations are frequent and increase with age in human kidney epithelial cells. *Human Molecular Genetics*, *5*, 215–221.

Martin, G. M., Smith, A. C., Ketterer, D. J., Ogburn, C. E., & Disteche, C. M. (1985). Increased chromosomal aberrations in first metaphases of cells isolated from the kidneys of aged mice. *Israel Journal of Medical Sciences*, *21*, 296–301.

Mendenhall, A. R., Tedesco, P. M., Taylor, L. D., Lowe, A., Cypser, J. R., & Johnson, T. E. (2012). Expression of a single-copy hsp-16.2 reporter predicts life span. *The Journals of Gerontology. Series A, Biological Sciences and Medical Sciences*, *67*, 726–733.

Nakanishi, M., Niida, H., Murakami, H., & Shimada, M. (2009). DNA damage responses in skin biology—Implications in tumor prevention and aging acceleration. *Journal of Dermatological Science*, *56*, 76–81.

Orgel, L. E. (1970). The maintenance of the accuracy of protein synthesis and its relevance to ageing: A correction. *Proceedings of the National Academy of Sciences of the United States of America*, *67*, 1476.

Peck, B., Ferber, E. C., & Schulze, A. (2013). Antagonism between FOXO and MYC Regulates Cellular Powerhouse. *Frontiers in Oncology*, *3*, 96.

Pendergrass, W. R., Martin, G. M., & Bornstein, P. (1976). Evidence contrary to the protein error hypothesis for in vitro senescence. *Journal of Cellular Physiology*, *87*, 3–13.

Raju, I., Kannan, K., & Abraham, E. C. (2013). FOXO3a serves as a biomarker of oxidative stress in human lens epithelial cells under conditions of hyperglycemia. *PloS One*, *8*, e67126.

Rea, S. L., Wu, D., Cypser, J. R., Vaupel, J. W., & Johnson, T. E. (2005). A stress-sensitive reporter predicts longevity in isogenic populations of Caenorhabditis elegans. *Nature Genetics*, *37*, 894–898.

Rusted, J. M., Evans, S. L., King, S. L., Dowell, N., Tabet, N., & Tofts, P. S. (2013). APOE e4 polymorphism in young adults is associated with improved attention and indexed by distinct neural signatures. *NeuroImage*, *65*, 364–373.

Sabater-Lleal, M., Huang, J., Chasman, D. I., Naitza, S., Dehghan, A., Johnson, A. D., . . . O'Donnell C. J. (2013). A multi-ethnic meta-analysis of genome-wide association studies in over 100,000 subjects identifies 23 fibrinogen-associated loci but no strong evidence of a causal association between circulating fibrinogen and cardiovascular disease. *Circulation, 128*(12), 1310–1324.

Salk, J. J., Salipante, S. J., Risques, R. A., Crispin, D. A., Li, L., Bronner, M. P., . . . Loeb, L. A. (2009). Clonal expansions in ulcerative colitis identify patients with neoplasia. *Proceedings of the National Academy of Sciences of the United States of America, 106*, 20871–20876.

Smith, G. D. (2011). Epidemiology, epigenetics and the "Gloomy Prospect": Embracing randomness in population health research and practice. *International Journal of Epidemiology, 40*, 537–562.

Talens, R. P., Christensen, K., Putter, H., Willemsen, G., Christiansen, L., Kremer D, . . . Heijmans, B. T. (2012). Epigenetic variation during the adult lifespan: Cross-sectional and longitudinal data on monozygotic twin pairs. *Aging Cell, 11*, 694–703.

Tanzi, R. E. (2012). The genetics of Alzheimer disease. *Cold Spring Harbor Perspectives in Medicine*, 2(10).

Tivey, H. S., Brook, A. J., Rokicki, M. J., Kipling, D., & Davis, T. (2013). p38 (MAPK) stress signalling in replicative senescence in fibroblasts from progeroid and genomic instability syndromes. *Biogerontology, 14*, 47–62.

Uranga, R. M., Katz, S., & Salvador, G. A. (2013). Enhanced phosphatidylinositol 3-kinase (PI3K)/Akt signaling has pleiotropic targets in hippocampal neurons exposed to iron-induced oxidative stress. *The Journal of Biological Chemistry, 288*, 19773–19784.

Vanfleteren, J. R., De Vreese, A., & Braeckman, B. P. (1998). Two-parameter logistic and Weibull equations provide better fits to survival data from isogenic populations of Caenorhabditis elegans in axenic culture than does the Gompertz model. *The Journals of Gerontology. Series A, Biological Sciences and Medical Sciences, 53*, B393–B403; discussion B404–B408.

Vogt, G. (2010). Suitability of the clonal marbled crayfish for biogerontological research: A review and perspective, with remarks on some further crustaceans. *Biogerontology, 11*, 643–669.

Wainer, R. (2001). Smoking and ovarian fertility. *Gynecologie, Obstetrique & Fertilite, 29*, 881–887.

Warr, M. R., Binnewies, M., Flach, J., Reynaud, D., Garg, T., Malhotra, R., . . . Passegué, E. (2013). FOXO3A directs a protective autophagy program in haematopoietic stem cells. *Nature, 494*, 323–327.

Wu, T. Y., Khor, T. O., Lee, J. H., Cheung, K. L., Shu, L., Chen, C., & Kong, A. N. (2013). Pharmacogenetics, pharmacogenomics and epigenetics of Nrf2-regulated xenobiotic-metabolizing enzymes and transporters by dietary phytochemical and cancer chemoprevention. *Current Drug Metabolism, 14*, 688–694.

Yoon, S. R., Dubeau, L., de Young, M., Wexler, N. S., & Arnheim, N. (2003). Huntington disease expansion mutations in humans can occur before meiosis is completed. *Proceedings of the National Academy of Sciences of the United States of America, 100*, 8834–8838.

Yu, C. E., Oshima, J., Fu, Y. H., Wijsman, E. M., Hisama, F., Alisch, R., . . . Schellenberg, G. D. (1996). Positional cloning of the Werner's syndrome gene. *Science*, *272*, 258–262.

Index

Note: Page references followed by "*f*" and "*t*" denote figures and tables